BASIC NUTRITION AND
DIET THERAPY

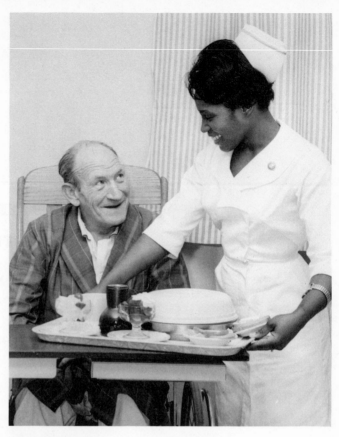

SECOND EDITION

THE MACMILLAN COMPANY

BASIC NUTRITION
AND
DIET THERAPY

CORINNE H. ROBINSON

Consultant in Nutrition Education · Professor
of Nutrition, Emeritus, and Formerly Head,
Department of Nutrition and Food, DREXEL
UNIVERSITY, PHILADELPHIA
Formerly Instructor, Nutrition and Diet Therapy
JEFFERSON MEDICAL COLLEGE HOSPITAL SCHOOL OF
NURSING, PHILADELPHIA

COLLIER-MACMILLAN LIMITED, LONDON

Fourth Printing, 1971

Earlier edition © copyright 1965 by Corinne H. Robinson

Figures 5–1, 7–3, 8–1, 9–2, 9–3, 10–1, 11–2, 11–3, 11–4, and 11–5 herein are reproduced from the third printing (1969) of C. H. Robinson, *Proudfit-Robinson's Normal and Therapeutic Nutrition*, 13th ed. (New York: The Macmillan Company, 1967). Also reproduced from this source are the flavorings for meat, poultry, fish, eggs, and vegetables. Frontispiece courtesy of Thomas Jefferson University Hospital.

Library of Congress catalog card number: 70–92084

THE MACMILLAN COMPANY
866 THIRD AVENUE, NEW YORK, NEW YORK 10022
COLLIER-MACMILLAN CANADA, LTD., TORONTO, ONTARIO

Printed in the United States of America

PREFACE TO THE SECOND EDITION

Nutritional well-being is a national and international concern of the health professions, social organizations, governments, and the lay public. Today's nurse has an important role to fulfill in helping people to maintain health through good nutrition, as well as in giving nutritional care to the ill person. The nurse may be employed within the hospital or extended care facility, in the community agency, or in the home. In recognition of the varied responsibilities of the nurse for nutritional care, this text places substantial emphasis upon the principles of normal nutrition and includes practical applications for the nurse in her own daily life as well as in the maintenance of the health of people with whom she works. Modified diets for ill persons are viewed as a point of departure from the normal diet rather than an orientation to specific diseases. The individualization of dietary planning in terms of nutritional requirements, economic practicality, psychologic needs, and cultural and individual preferences is continuously stressed.

The second edition of this textbook, like the first, is directed primarily to students of practical and vocational nursing, and to those in associate-degree programs of nursing. It is intended for use in a basic course that will prepare students for applying the principles of nutrition in relatively simple situations. Some of the more complex problems of nutrition that require considerable professional planning and supervision are described briefly to give the technical nurse sufficient background information to assist in nursing care.

Prerequisite courses in chemistry and physiology are not essential to the use of this book. The organization within each chapter permits the instructor to omit selected sections when the time allotment is very limited or when the high-school preparation of the students has included no science courses whatsoever. Moreover, the text is so written that considerable flexibility is possible in choosing the topical sequence for a course. Review questions at the end of each chapter, supplementary references, and several new summary tables will be helpful as study guides.

As in the first edition, the book is organized in four units. Each chapter has been revised to conform to the 1968 Recommended Daily Dietary Allowances and to include new developments in the field of nutrition. Several chapters have been reorganized and substantially rewritten. Many new illustrations, revised charts and tables, and current references have been included.

Unit I, "Introduction to Food and Nutrition—Individual and Community Goals," is intended to give the student an overview of the many meanings of nutrition, the problems of nutrition in the community, the nutritive processes of the body, and the practical guides for the correlation of nutritional requirements and dietary planning. Through the study of this unit, the student is helped to develop her own personal and professional goals in the study of nutrition. The discussion of digestive processes, formerly appearing in the several chapters pertaining to the nutrients, has now been brought together in one chapter (Chap. 3).

Unit II, "The Nutrients," includes information on the functions, utilization, food sources, recommended allowances, and effects of deficiency for the essential nutrients. The chapters on minerals and vitamins have been rewritten, with the fat-soluble and water-soluble vitamins being presented in two chapters. Following a discussion of the interrelated ways in which the minerals and vitamins function, each of these nutrients is discussed with respect to its specific functions, daily allowances, food sources, and problems of deficiency. Pertinent information on several mineral elements and vitamins has been added to provide the background essential for the 1968 Recommended Daily Dietary Allowances and for some of the newer developments in diet therapy. Summary tables for the important minerals and vitamins appear at the end of the chapters.

A new feature of this unit is a section on food fallacies and facts in each of the chapters. With this arrangement the reader is able to refute the fallacies with the principles pertaining to the specific nutrient being studied.

"Practical Planning for Good Nutrition," Unit III, places greater emphasis upon dietary planning for various age groups and includes a section on the emergency food supply (Chap. 16). "Basic Principles and Procedures for Food Preparation" (Chap. 17) has been rewritten to emphasize the nurse's role in giving practical guidance to patients concerning the maintenance of nutritive quality and food palatability of the Four Food Groups.

"Diet Therapy," Unit IV, provides additional guidelines for the most widely used modified diets with respect to daily food allowances, food lists from which to choose, sample menus, and controls to be exercised in food preparation. Two new tables at the end of Chapter 18 summarize the nutritional considerations for some common symptoms and laboratory findings and for specific diseases. Among the important additions and revisions to this unit are "Dietary Calculations with Food Exchange Lists" as a separate chapter (Chap. 20), a discussion of the prevention of obesity and the hazards of fad diets in weight control, a reorganization of the chapter on fat-restricted and fat-controlled diets, the inclusion of diet lists for fat-controlled diets from the booklets of the American Heart Association, and a regimen for the potassium-restricted diet.

Appendix A includes a table of the nutritive composition of over 500 food items, a table of the food exchange lists, and a height-weight table for men and women. Appendix B, a list of reference materials, cites books that are useful to the student as well as professional, government, and commercial sources of reliable teaching aids. An expanded glossary is provided in Appendix C.

Instructors in nursing programs throughout the United States have provided many valuable suggestions in their replies to a questionnaire. The ideas submitted were sincerely appreciated, and most of them have been incorporated into this edition of the text. Useful commentary on nutrition education in nursing programs by Miss Elizabeth J. Sweeney, director of the Program of Practical Nursing, Thomas Jefferson University Hospital, is also acknowledged. Photographs of clinical situations were supplied by the Thomas Jefferson University Hospital. Special thanks are due Miss Margaret C. McClean, instructor of nutrition, who made the arrangements for the photographs; Miss Doris E. Bowman, director of the School of Nursing; Mrs. Marie C. Bookhammer, director of public relations; Mr. Ed Brinker, photographer; Miss Elizabeth Lippincott, director, Dietary Department; and to nurses and patients appearing in the photographs. Appreciation is also expressed for a number of photographs provided by governmental agencies, trade organizations, and companies.

The author has again had the privilege of working with Miss Joan C. Zulch, medical editor of The Macmillan Company, who has provided many creative ideas for the new edition and who can invariably be counted upon to set the highest standards for converting manuscript to book. Most especially, my husband, Howard West Robinson, through his helpful criticism and genuine understanding has contributed immeasurably to the completion of this book.

C. H. R.

CONTENTS

ix

Unit III
Practical Planning for Good Nutrition

Unit IV
Diet Therapy

Appendixes

INTRODUCTION TO FOOD AND NUTRITION— INDIVIDUAL AND COMMUNITY GOALS

FOOD, NUTRITION, AND HEALTH

BREAD—THE STAFF OF LIFE

From birth to death food is a dominant factor in our lives. In a single year, on a three-meal-a-day basis, we eat well over 1000 meals. We know that the food we eat is necessary for our very being—we know it provides the energy for the quiet breathing at night and the full activity of the day—we know too that it builds, maintains, and regulates muscles and bones, nerves and brain, eyes, hair, and all our physical body.

But food does much more than nourish, for most of us enjoy eating. Food makes us feel secure and happy; we use food as a link in our friendships, as an expression of pleasure during our holidays, and as a symbol of our religious life.

Food is the world's biggest business. A large part of the world's work is concerned with the growing, processing, and preparation of food. In the United States one farm worker produces enough food for 25 persons, but think of all the people who work in the factories that process the food, in the markets that sell the food, or in restaurants, institutions, and homes that serve the food. We spend an important amount of our income for food. We have food in abundance and in variety. Our surpluses sometimes become political issues, but we also share these surpluses with the less fortunate.

Most of the world's people spend the greater part of their working days and most of their income for food. In some countries of the world three fourths or more of the working population is directly concerned with

3

growing food; yet it seldom manages to grow quite enough. Tonight millions of the world's people will go to bed more or less hungry. Is it any surprise that these people are discontented, diseased, and die an early death?

From this brief introduction you can see that good nutrition depends upon the understanding, knowledge, and cooperation of many people. Good nutrition alone cannot guarantee good health, but without good nutrition health cannot be at its best.

SOME DEFINITIONS

Before we can begin the study of nutrition, some definitions need to be made.

Food is that which nourishes the body. No two foods are alike in their ability to nourish, because no two foods contain identical amounts of nutrients.

Nutrients are those chemical substances in food that are needed by the body. More than 50 nutrients are known to be required. They are divided into these six classes: proteins and amino acids; fats and fatty acids; carbohydrates; mineral elements; vitamins; and water.

Nutrition refers to the processes in the body for making use of food. It includes eating the correct foods for the body's needs; digestion of foods so that the body can use the nutrients; absorption of the nutrients into the blood stream; use of the individual nutrients by the cells in the body; and elimination of waste.

Dietetics is the practical application of the science of nutrition to the feeding of people. It deals with the planning of meals according to individual physiologic and psychologic needs and the selection, care, preparation, and service of food. Its practice requires understanding of the sciences of nutrition and of foods, management for the use of money and materials, and art in planning, preparation, and service.

GOOD AND POOR NUTRITION

Nutritional status is the condition of health as it is related to the use of food by the body. Nutritional status is evident in some very obvious ways we can all see, such as changes in weight. However, an accurate measure of nutritional status can be made only by the expert examination that a physician can give and through a variety of blood and urine tests that can be done only in a laboratory. Some contrasts in good and poor nutrition are listed in Table 1–1. You should remember that other reasons for poor health might be lack of sleep, poor sanitation, poor housing, and so on.

TABLE 1–1   SOME CONTRASTS IN NUTRITION

Good Nutrition	Poor Nutrition
Normal weight for height, body frame, and age	Overweight; underweight; failure to grow; sudden loss of weight
Erect posture; arms and legs straight; abdomen in; chest up; chin in	Poor posture: chest forward; rounded shoulders; protruding abdomen
Firm, strong muscles; moderate padding of fat	Thin, flabby muscles; lack of padding of fat, or excessive fat
Firm, clear skin with good color; healthy, pink mucous membranes	Dry, scaly, pale skin; pale mucous membranes
Well-formed jaw and even teeth	Poorly formed jaw with teeth poorly aligned
Soft, glossy hair	Dull, dry hair
Clear, bright eyes, not unduly sensitive to light	Dull eyes, sensitive to light; burning, itching; circles and puffiness under eyes
Good appetitite and digestion	Poor appetite; complaints of indigestion
Abundance of energy and endurance	Listlessness, fatigue, and lack of endurance
Resistance to disease	Many infections; longer convalescence from disease
Ability to concentrate	Short attention span
Cooperative, interested, agreeable, cheerful	Irritable, apathetic, worried, depressed

NUTRITION AS A SCIENCE

Throughout all of history man has written about food and its effects on the body. Ancient Egyptian writings on tablets of stone record the use of food for the treatment of numerous diseases. In the Old Testament of the Bible we can learn much about the foods available to the Jewish people, the religious symbolism of food, and the laws governing the use of food. Hippocrates, the famous Greek physician who lived several hundred years before Christ, wrote of the proper foods for treating disease. He observed, "Persons who are naturally very fat are apt to die earlier than those who are slender." [1] The thinking of Hippocrates, Galen, and other philosophers governed the whole practice of medicine down through the Middle Ages.

[1] G. Lusk, *Nutrition* (New York: Paul B. Hoeber, Inc., 1933), p. 8.

People have learned throughout the ages that some foods were more nourishing than others, and that some plants were, in fact, poisonous and could not be eaten. Along with this experience a great deal of superstition about foods also arose. Some of these false notions are believed even today by many people. The science of nutrition developed only after the groundwork had been laid for the sciences of chemistry and physiology, and had its beginning in the late eighteenth century—just about the time of the American Revolution.

Antoine Lavoisier (1743–1794) is sometimes called the "Father of the Science of Nutrition." Through experiments on animals and on one of his associates he noticed that more air was breathed in when food was eaten than when it was not, and that more air was breathed in as the activity increased. He showed that the more a man worked, the more food he needed. He showed that the amount of oxygen necessary was related to the amount of food used by the body for the production of energy.

During the nineteenth century scientists in Europe and in the United States furthered the study of energy metabolism, discovered the nature of proteins and amino acids, established that the body needed certain mineral salts, analyzed foods, and began to question whether certain other substances were also necessary. The discovery of vitamins is a story of the last 70 years. Most of our understanding of the functioning of nutrients in the body, the nutritive values of foods, the body's requirements for nutrients, and the role of nutrition in health and disease also belongs to the last 60 or 70 years. Thus it must be emphasized that nutrition is indeed one of the youngest sciences.

Scientists learn about nutrition through laboratory studies on experimental animals and on human beings. Many animals are used for such studies, including rats, mice, guinea pigs, hamsters, chickens, dogs, cattle, monkeys, and even microorganisms. In fact, many of the early nutrition studies were conducted so that farmers might know how to obtain the best quality of beef, or the most production of milk, or the most rapid growth of chickens, and so on.

Rats have been most widely used for nutrition studies because they can be studied over an entire life-span to see the effects of various diets on growth, reproduction, and length of life. They are easy to care for, they can be fed synthetic diets that are carefully controlled, and they are relatively inexpensive.

Not all of the results obtained on animals can be applied directly to humans. Many human volunteers have participated in studies to determine the amounts of nutrients required for good health.

Studies conducted on animals and on humans usually measure certain physical changes; for example, growth in height and weight, skin condition, and many other conditions that a physican can note. The amount of nutrients in the food intake and the amount of specific substances excreted

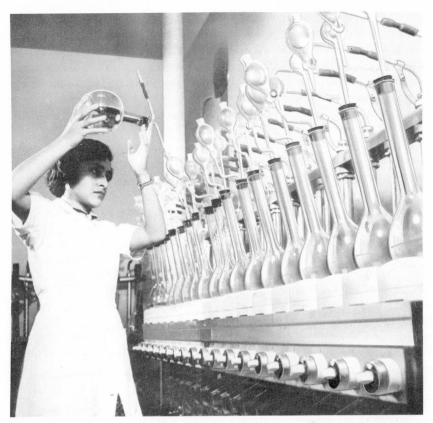

FIGURE 1-1 Research in many laboratories leads to increased understanding of the science of nutrition. In this instance a laboratory technician at the Institute of Nutrition of Central America and Panama determines the protein value of a vegetable-protein mixture. (*Courtesy, UNICEF.*)

in the urine and feces may be measured in balance experiments. Thus, if the intake and excretions are equal, the subject is said to be in *balance* or *equilibrium*. Many constituents may also be measured in the blood and tissues, for changes in diet will, sooner or later, bring about changes in the level of certain substances in the blood. The techniques of the physician, biologist, physiologist, chemist, and nutritionist are required in nutrition research. (See Fig. 1-1.)

You can see that the researcher in nutrition must have many years of professional education in the sciences. The dietitian who is responsible for feeding groups of people in a hospital, school, or any institution must have a thorough college preparation in the study of nutrition and practical experience in its application. The college teacher of nutrition is a person who has specialized in the study of nutrition at the graduate level.

To summarize, when you study nutrition, you become aware that this is a well-organized science with a tremendous body of knowledge and with a continuing need for research. The understanding of the intricacies of nutrition requires professional education. There is no room for the food faddist or the quack who tries to substitute oratory, unrealistic promises, and emotional appeal for sound knowledge and wise applications to the healthful feeding of people.

TEAMWORK IN NUTRITION

As a nurse you are part of the professional team that cares for the sick. The physician is the captain of this team, and many people with varying skills work under his direction: nurses, dietitians, social workers, physical therapists, occupational therapists, laboratory technicians, and others. You are also a member of the nursing team that includes professional nurses, practical or vocational nurses, nurse's aides, and orderlies. (See Fig. 1–2.)

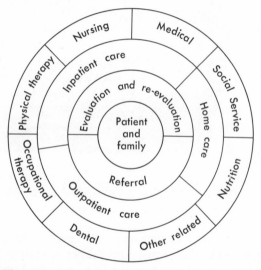

FIGURE 1–2 The concentric circles of comprehensive care radiate out from the patient and his family. (*Courtesy, Miss Geraldine Piper, and the* Journal of the American Dietetic Association.)

Nutrition teamwork means that the physician prescribes the diet; the dietitian supervises the planning of menus and the purchase and preparation of food for all patients and personnel; the nurse helps the patient at mealtime and records the acceptance of the meal. The nurse and dietitian may consult with the physician concerning any nutritional problems presented by the patient. The dietitian and nurse may work together in planning the modified diet for the patient and in the various stages of education of the patient.

YOUR RESPONSIBILITY IN NUTRITION

First of all, you have a responsibility to *yourself*. You will personally benefit from good nutrition, for you will look and feel better; you will be better able to meet the demands of your profession; and you will set an example for others.

You have a responsibility to your *family*. Perhaps this lies in planning and preparing better meals for the family, in helping a child to develop good food habits, or in guiding an elderly person in making adjustments in his diet according to a doctor's prescription. Perhaps this is a responsibility you will assume more fully at some later time.

You have a responsibility as a *nurse*. Nutrition is an essential part of the total care of a patient. You will need an appreciation of what food means to the patient, how illness changes his feelings about food, and how to help him with his day-to-day meals. See Chapter 18 for specific details on the nutritional care of patients.

You have a responsibility as a *citizen*. Because you are a nurse, many people look to you for an example and for advice. You will need to know how to answer simple questions. But you will also need to know when to refer people to physicians if questions concerning diagnosis and treatment are asked. You can give your support to the school lunch program and other activities that improve the nutrition of people. You can take a positive stand for any action by the community government aimed toward better nutrition.

GOALS FOR NUTRITION STUDY

If you accept seriously the responsibilities outlined, you will find the following goals to be helpful in the study of nutrition:

Understanding and appreciation of:
    the relation of food and nutrition to health, happiness, efficiency, and
        long life for yourself as well as for others
    the meanings of food to people—religious, cultural, social, psychologic,
        and economic; respect for individual differences
    the importance of having the right attitude toward food
    the opportunities to help people in the selection of a good diet
    the difficulties involved in changing food habits
    the importance of nutrition to the recovery of the patient
    the need for teamwork in the improvement of nutrition of people
    your responsibility for the nutritional care of patients
Knowledge concerning:
    basic principles of nutrition
        functions of the nutrients
        requirements for nutrients by various age groups

foods as sources of nutrients
principles of meal planning and preparation
    cost of food
    retention of nutrients
    palatable food
    attractive service
principles for modifying the diet for disease conditions
reliable sources of information on nutrition
Ability to:
select your own diet for good nutrition
interpret labeling and advertising of food products
make adjustments in meal plans for low-cost diets
plan, prepare, and serve simple attractive meals
follow directions for planning a modified diet
help patients at mealtime
observe food intake of patients and report to nursing supervisor or dietitian
answer simple questions posed by patients
work with the supervising nurse, dietitian, and physician in caring for the patient
make use of community resources in helping the patient to care for himself

REVIEW QUESTIONS AND PROBLEMS

1. Define nutrient, nutrition, nutritional status.

2. List some signs of good nutrition.

3. In addition to poor diet what factors might be responsible for poor health?

4. Look for advertisements on food in magazines and newspapers. Discuss the good features of these advertisements. What are some of the bad features?

5. Start a file for articles on food and nutrition from current newspapers and magazines. From time to time compare the content of these articles with what you learn in your study of nutrition.

6. Examine the list of goals for nutrition. As you proceed in the study of nutrition, evaluate yourself against these goals. Are there other aims you should include?

REFERENCES

Rasmussen, S. *Foundations of Practical and Vocational Nursing.* New York: The Macmillan Company, 1967, pp. 1–11.
Robinson, C. H. *Proudfit-Robinson's Normal and Therapeutic Nutrition,* 13th ed. New York: The Macmillan Company, 1967, Chaps. 1 and 2.

NUTRITION IN THE COMMUNITY

Nutrition in the United States

The patterns of American diet have resulted from a bountiful and varied food supply and from the cultural impact of many nationality backgrounds. The creativity of the food technologist, the skill of the food engineer, and the speed of transportation from east to west and from north to south have all contributed to the variety of readily available foods.

CHANGING PATTERNS OF LIVING

Americans today have more money, more education, more leisure, and more opportunity to travel both here and abroad. More women work than ever before and they depend more upon their families for the purchase and preparation of the food. The market has a greater wealth of food choices, more snack items, and more convenience foods. Children eat more well-balanced lunches at school, and adults eat more meals in cafeterias at their places of work. They eat in restaurants more often and enjoy many unusual foods from all parts of the world. As a family, Americans eat together less often. They are subject to fashions in foods just as they are to fashions in clothing; for example, tossed green salads with blue-cheese dressing, baked potato with sour cream, and meats cooked at an open hearth.

11

NUTRITIONAL PROBLEMS

The quality of health is affected when there is too much food, too little food, or the wrong kind of food. Obesity is widely recognized as a public health problem because it is associated with diabetes, gallbladder disease, and heart disease. Moreover, diets high in saturated fat, high in cholesterol, or too high in calories are among the factors leading to coronary disease as the principal cause of death in the United States.

Dental decay is almost universally present, even in young children, and leads in early life to considerable loss of teeth as well as expensive dental repair work. Somewhat later in life many people lose their teeth because of faulty gum structures. Those who lose their teeth often are unable to chew satisfactorily, and they may not eat the foods necessary for good health.

The extent of malnutrition in the United States is not known. Nevertheless, according to a preliminary report of a nutrition status study conducted in four states by the United States Public Health Service, it is more widely prevalent than had been generally believed. Dr. Arnold E. Schaefer reported to the Senate Committee on Nutrition and Human Needs that 17 per cent of the 12,000 people studied were undernourished to the point of being "real medical risks."[1] In this study one of three children under six years was anemic, and growth was stunted in 3.5 per cent. Mental retardation sometimes accompanies growth failure in young children. Several nutritional deficiency diseases are increasing although their prevention is both easy and inexpensive. These are goiter resulting from iodine deficiency, rickets caused by lack of vitamin D, and night blindness brought about by inadequate vitamin A. Total blindness was a potential threat for a significant number of children.

FAULTY FOOD HABITS

A survey of family food consumption was conducted by the United States Department of Agriculture in 1965. Surprisingly, only 50 per cent of all families had diets classified as "good," as compared with 60 per cent in 1955. A good diet was one that provided the Recommended Dietary Allowances for seven nutrients. About three diets in ten failed to furnish the full allowances for calcium, ascorbic acid, and vitamin A. (See Fig. 2-1.)

The quality of the American diet is directly related to income. People at the lowest income level had poor diets four times as often as those at the highest income level. (See Fig. 2-2.) But the fact that some people at higher income levels also had poor diets indicates that adequate nutrition education has not reached as many people as it should.

[1] "Nutrition," *Time*, January 31, 1969, p. 74.

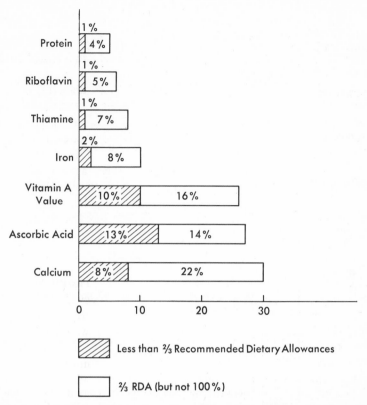

Less than ⅔ Recommended Dietary Allowances

⅔ RDA (but not 100%)

FIGURE 2–1 Calcium, vitamin A, and ascorbic acid are the nutrients most frequently supplied at levels below the Recommended Dietary Allowances according to data from the family dietary survey of 1965. *(Courtesy, Agricultural Research Service, U.S. Department of Agriculture.)*

Insufficient money, ignorance of the essential foods for an adequate diet, poor facilities for preparing food, and lack of skills must share the blame for the malnutrition seen in this country. The following points need to be recognized in setting up programs for improved nutrition.

1. Infants, preschool children, adolescent girls, and pregnant women are the most vulnerable to the effects of poor food habits.

2. Milk, deep-green and yellow vegetables, and citrus fruits require greater emphasis in dietary planning. The trend among Americans today seems to be away from milk as a beverage, substituting coffee, tea, soft drinks, and fruit-ades.

3. The use of convenience foods has greatly increased and no doubt will continue to do so. Homemakers need much more assistance in making the best choices for the money they can spend because the products are so numerous.

4. Snacks are too often made up of foods high in starches, sugars, and fats but providing little by way of other nutrients. These snacks may lead to

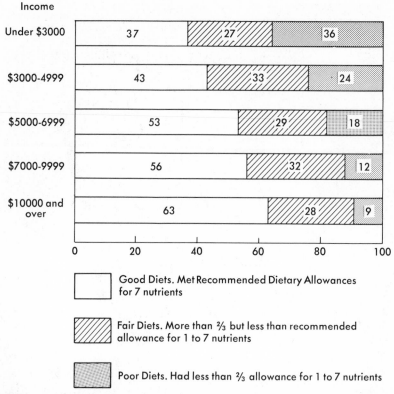

Income

FIGURE 2–2 As income goes down the percentage of people having a good diet also goes down. Lack of income is not the sole reason for inadequate diets, however. Note that only 63 per cent of people at the highest income level had good diets. (*Data from family dietary survey, 1965, Courtesy Agricultural Research Service, U.S. Department of Agriculture.*)

excessive weight gain, they may replace nutritionally essential foods, or they may destroy the appetite for meals. Teen-agers especially need to learn to control the quality and the amounts of snack foods that they consume.

5. Breakfast is often skipped. Lack of time, uninteresting foods, and poor appetite are usually given as reasons. It is hard to make up in the rest of the day for the nutrients that a good breakfast can provide.

6. Lunch is likely to be skimpy, or may consist of high-calorie foods low in nutrients.

7. Too many meals are eaten in a hurry with little enjoyment of them.

Nutritional improvement means public concern for the poor. It means much greater emphasis on nutrition education for people of all ages. Elementary and secondary schools must strengthen their classroom programs in nutrition; school feeding programs need to be expanded; and all segments of the population must be reached through wider use of mass

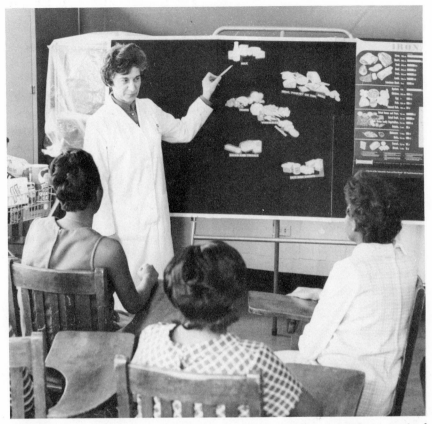

FIGURE 2–3 Education: Mothers-to-be are very receptive to guidance in food selection given by a nutritionist. (*Courtesy, Thomas Jefferson University Hospital.*)

media such as television, radio, and newspapers and magazines. (See Fig. 2–3.)

FOOD FADDISM AND QUACKERY

People of ancient times believed that foods possessed many remarkable qualities. They believed, for example, that to eat flesh foods would make one fierce and warlike; to eat the heart of an animal would give courage; to eat fish would develop the brain; and so on. These superstitions seem downright silly to us. Yet you could surely list many beliefs that are not based on sound information that you, your family, and your friends subscribe to about food.

People today are more interested in health, food, and nutrition than at any previous time. They read more about food and nutrition in magazines and books and hear much on radio and television. Because many of them are not educated in the science of nutrition they find it difficult to decide what is true and what is exaggerated or false. This situation provides a real opportunity for quacks to make some money. Today millions of people are being misled into believing that a particular food possesses some miracle properties and that it can cure such specific diseases as diabetes, cancer, arthritis, and many others. When people believe such false claims about food they may neglect going to a physician for advice. When finally they do go because they are not improving, it may be too late for treatment.

Some people may eat an inadequate diet because the quack has claimed that certain foods should be omitted from the diet. Other people have spent so much for the fad item that they don't have enough money left to buy nutritious foods. This is often true of elderly persons who have been misled into thinking their health problems would be solved by eating some "wonder" food.

A number of widely prevalent fallacies pertaining to food will be more specifically identified in the chapters that follow.

IDENTIFYING THE FOOD QUACK

It is not always easy to determine who is a food quack. Often he is handsome, a good speaker, very clever, and sounds convincing. But you should become suspicious if he talks about specific foods or supplements as "wonder foods," "miracle foods," "health foods," "organically grown foods," "nature's own foods," "food cures," or a "secret formula." The faddist and quack claim special virtues for foods such as yogurt, blackstrap molasses, raw sugar, honey, sea salt, stone-ground flour, vegetable juices, wheat germ oil, and foods grown without chemical fertilizers.

No single food possesses unique qualities for health. Rather, good nutrition is served by any combination of foods that will provide the necessary nutrients. The Food and Drug Administration considers a food to be misbranded if it is called a "health" food. (See also Chap. 15.)

The food quack appeals to the emotions and makes extravagant claims for his product: youth, beauty, glamour, long life, cure of disease. He is out to sell something, whether it be a book, appliance, or food product. Many of his products are sold from door to door, often with "money back" guarantees to cure some disease in a matter of weeks or months. The product is usually more expensive than similar products sold in food markets.

The food quack may tell you that the food in grocery stores is robbed of its nutritional values because it has been grown on depleted soil or because processes such as canning or dehydration have removed most of the nutrients. He accuses the medical profession of not giving the full facts to the public, and he claims that he is being persecuted by scientists and the government. He quotes frequently from the scientific literature and sounds very learned. A careful search of his sources will often show that he has lifted sentences out of books and journals and is placing his own interpretation upon them.

RELIABLE SOURCES OF INFORMATION

The best defense against food misinformation and faddism is through sound nutrition education at all levels—in the elementary and high school, in industry, through health agencies in the community. A number of individuals who work in a community may be especially helpful in providing sound information:

Nutritionists from city, county, and state offices of health
Dietitians who are members of the American Dietetic Association
Nutritionists in county and state extension offices
Professors of nutrition in colleges and universities
Physicians

Much sound nutrition information is published by professional organizations, government agencies, and industry groups. A partial list of groups that distribute inexpensive or free materials will be found in Appendix B.

Nutrition, a World Concern

INTERNATIONAL NUTRITION PROBLEMS

The central problem in nutrition today is that millions of people in underdeveloped countries of the world do not have enough to eat. Yet, each day approximately 100,000 persons are added to the world's population, and they, too, must somehow be fed. Asia contains one third of the earth's land surface, but it must feed two thirds of the world's people. Thus, supplying more food to keep up with the increase in population as well as trying to improve the state of nutrition is truly a staggering problem.

Infants and young children suffer most from the lack of food. The death rate among infants in many countries is appallingly high. Of infants who survive the first year, many will die before the age of five. The infants and children fail to grow, they are quite susceptible to infection, and many of them die of protein malnutrition known as *kwashiorkor*. Even though these severely malnourished children live, their mental development may have been permanently retarded.

Other deficiency diseases are still quite prevalent in many parts of the world. Anemias caused by lack of iron and of the B-complex vitamins are frequent. Goiter is widespread in areas where there is a lack of iodine. Beriberi occurs because of lack of thiamine; pellagra from lack of niacin; xerophthalmia and blindness from lack of vitamin A; and rickets from lack of vitamin D. As you study nutrition, the characteristics of some of these diseases will become more familiar.

INTERNATIONAL ORGANIZATIONS

Much is being done to improve the lot of people in the underdeveloped countries. Various agencies of our government and numerous charitable organizations are pledged to providing aid in many ways: direct food supplies from our surplus; technical assistance in the development of agriculture and industry; education of youth; education of homemakers in food preparation, child care, and sanitation; and many other ways. Several organizations of the United Nations illustrate the peaceful efforts of that great international body.

The *Food and Agriculture Organization* (FAO) aims especially to improve the growth, distribution, and storage of food. To carry out its aims it might be involved in such widely different activities as irrigation for crops; development of varieties of grain that will grow in a given climate; sponsoring home economics programs to show people how to prepare their foods and to better feed their families; and setting up a canning factory.

The *World Health Organization* (WHO) aims to eliminate diseases of all kinds, including those that relate to nutrition. It works closely with FAO. Diseases such as malaria and others keep millions from working. When people are treated for these diseases they are able to work and produce food for themselves and their families. WHO works closely with communities to improve the sanitation through insect control, water supplies, housing, and waste disposal.

The *United Nations Children's Fund* (UNICEF) is concerned with all aspects of the health and welfare of children everywhere. We are probably most familiar with the work of this group through the distribution of nonfat dry milk to prevent and treat the protein deficiency disease kwashiorkor.

The *United Nations Education, Scientific, and Cultural Organization* (UNESCO) aims to eliminate illiteracy and thus to help people through education to use science and to understand cultural forces for the improvement of their lives.

REVIEW QUESTIONS AND PROBLEMS

1. Prepare a list of false ideas about foods that you have heard. What is your basis for saying that each is false?

2. What are some ways by which you can identify a quack?

3. What nutritional problems do you know of in your community?

4. List some food habits of people you know that could be improved. What are some ways you would use to try to help them?

5. Find five examples of materials prepared by food manufacturers that are useful in obtaining a better diet.

6. What organizations in your community include nutrition as part of their work?

7. Prepare a report for your class on a state, national, or international organization that has the major goal of promoting good nutrition.

REFERENCES

Adelson, S. F. "Changes in Diets of Households, 1955 to 1965," *J. Home Econ.*, **60**:448, 1968.

Beeuwkes, A. M. "Characteristics of the Self-Styled Scientist," *J. Amer. Diet. Ass.*, **32**:627, 1956.

Food Facts Talk Back. Chicago: The American Dietetic Association, 1957.

Maddox, G. "The Superstitious Side of Eating," *Today's Health*, **41**:48, December 1963.

Schultz, G. "Food Taboos," *Today's Health*, **42**:28, February 1964.

Smith, R. L. "The Bunk About Health Foods," *Today's Health*, **43**:24, October 1965.

White, P. L. *Let's Talk About Food*. Chicago: The American Medical Association, 1967.

THE NUTRIENTS AND THEIR UTILIZATION

NUTRIENTS AND BODY COMPOSITION

Whatever you eat turns into you. It is quite reasonable to suppose that there is a relationship between the substances present in the body and the kinds of nutrients present in food. Also it is quite reasonable to suppose that the body can be properly built and maintained only if the correct materials are available.

The cell is the unit of body structure. Cells in different body tissues carry out specific kinds of functions; thus liver, bone, muscle, and blood cells differ from each other. Likewise, the kinds and amounts of nutrients that make up cells vary from one type of cell to another. At least 50 nutrients are required by the cells of the body.

Four chemical elements account for 96 per cent of the body weight. They are carbon, hydrogen, oxygen, and nitrogen. Water is by far the most abundant compound in the body; it accounts for about two thirds of the body weight. Protein represents roughly one fifth of the body weight, and fat constitutes one fifth, more or less, of the body weight. The proportions of these major body constituents will vary widely from individual to individual. Obviously, a lean person will have a much lower proportion of fat than an overweight person. A baby has a higher proportion of body water than an adult.

Carbohydrate, so important in the diet for its energy value, actually is present only in limited amounts in body tissues. Somewhat less than a pound occurs in the adult body in the forms of liver and muscle glycogen and the blood sugar.

Mineral matter accounts for about 4 per cent of the body weight, but a wide variety of mineral elements is needed for the structure of the tissues. The total store of vitamins in the body would not add up to a single ounce.

FUNCTIONS OF FOOD

Some nutrients function in three categories, whereas others are restricted to one or two classes of functions.

Nutrients that furnish energy: carbohydrates, fats, proteins
Nutrients that build and maintain body tissues: water, proteins, fats, carbohydrates, mineral elements
Nutrients that regulate body functions: water, mineral elements, vitamins, proteins, fats, carbohydrates

DIGESTION

Digestion includes the mechanical and chemical processes by which foods are broken down to their nutrients so that they may be absorbed into the circulation. Mechanical and chemical changes take place simultaneously on the carbohydrates, fats, and proteins in foods. (See Fig. 3–1.)

The mechanical processes include the chewing of food, the churning actions in the stomach, and the muscular contractions of the intestinal tract. The rhythmic contractions, known as peristalsis, break up food into smaller and smaller particles, mix them intimately with the digestive juices, and continually move the food mass along the intestinal tract.

The chemical reactions in digestion involve the addition of water to the protein, fat, and carbohydrate molecules and their splitting up into nutrients that the tissues can use. This process is known as *hydrolysis.* The final end products of digestion are:

Carbohydrates to the simple sugars—glucose, fructose, galactose
Fats to fatty acids and glycerol
Proteins to amino acids

Enzymes. The chemical reactions require helpers called *enzymes.* Sometimes enzymes are called living catalysts. A catalyst is any substance that hastens a chemical reaction but does not itself become a part of the compounds that are formed.

Enzymes are composed of specific proteins. They are named for the substance upon which they act; for example, *protease* is an enzyme that

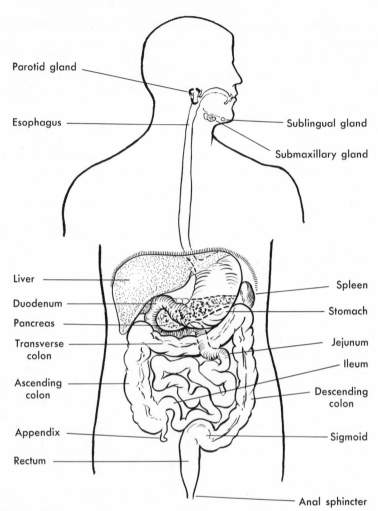

FIGURE 3-1 The digestive tract. (*Adapted from Youmans, W. B.,* Human Physiology, *2nd ed. New York: The Macmillan Company, 1962.*)

digests protein, and *oxidase* is involved in the addition of oxygen. Each enzyme is highly individual in its action. An enzyme that digests fat will not digest starch. Some enzymes act only in an acid medium, such as the stomach, whereas others act only in an alkaline medium, as in the small intestine. See Table 3-1 for a summary of enzyme activity.

Digestion in the mouth. The digestion of food begins in the mouth with the chewing of food and its mixing with saliva. Chewing is important because it increases the surface area of the food particles for later digestive action. Saliva contains *amylase*, a starch-splitting enzyme, but food remains in the mouth for such a short time that only a small amount of starch can be broken down to dextrins and maltose.

TABLE 3–1 SUMMARY OF CHEMICAL REACTIONS IN DIGESTION

Site of Activity	Enzyme	Substrate	Products of Enzyme Activity
Mouth	Salivary amylase (ptyalin)	Cooked starch	Dextrins, maltose
Stomach	Protease (pepsin)	Proteins	Proteoses, peptones, polypeptides
	Rennin	Milk casein	Calcium caseinate
	Lipase	Emulsified fats	Fatty acids, glycerol
Small intestine	Pancreatic juice		
	Protease (trypsin)	Proteins	Proteoses, peptones, polypeptides, some amino acids
	Lipase (steapsin)	Fats	Di- and monoglycerides, fatty acids, glycerol
	Amylase (amylopsin)	Starch	Maltose
	Intestinal juice		
	Peptidases (erepsin)	Peptones, poly-peptides	Amino acids
	Sucrase	Sucrose	Glucose, fructose
	Maltase	Maltose	Glucose (2 molecules)
	Lactase	Lactose	Glucose, galactose

Digestion in the stomach. The stomach serves as a temporary store-house for food, brings about partial digestion of protein, and prepares food for further digestion in the small intestine. The food is con-tinually churned and mixed with gastric juice until it reaches a liquid consistency known as *chyme.* Rhythmic contractions move the chyme toward the pylorus where small portions are gradually released through the pyloric sphincter into the duodenum.

Gastric juice contains hydrochloric acid, pepsin, rennin, mucin, and other substances. Hydrochloric acid has several important functions: (1) it swells the proteins so as to make them more easily attacked by the enzymes; (2) it provides the acid medium necessary for the action of pepsin; (3) it increases the solubility of calcium and iron salts so that they are more readily absorbed; and (4) it reduces the activity of harmful bacteria that may have been present in the food.

The protease pepsin splits proteins to smaller molecules called pro-teoses and polypeptides. Very little digestion of carbohydrates and fats occurs in the stomach. In the upper (cardiac) portion of the stomach the salivary amylase continues to act upon starch to change it to dextrins and maltose. As soon as the food mass is mixed with hydrochloric acid this action ceases. Lipase in the stomach has some effect on emulsified fats as in milk, cream, butter, and egg yolk, but most of the hydrolysis of fats takes place in the small intestine.

Digestion in the small intestine.   Most of the digestive activity takes place in the small intestine, which includes the duodenum, the jejunum, and the ileum. Bile, manufactured by the liver and stored in the gall-bladder, is essential for fat digestion. As soon as fats enter the duodenum the secretion of a hormone, *cholecystokinin,* is stimulated. Cholecystokinin causes the gallbladder to contract and to release bile into the duodenum. Bile emulsifies the fats, that is, breaks them down into tiny globules so that the fat-splitting enzymes have greater contact with the fat molecules.

As soon as acid chyme enters the duodenum another hormone, *secretin,* is produced. This is carried by the blood stream to the pancreas where it stimulates the secretion of pancreatic juice. The pancreas also pours its secretion into the duodenum. Pancreatic amylase splits starch to maltose; a protease, *trypsin,* breaks down proteins and polypeptides to much smaller molecules; and lipase, *steapsin,* completes the digestion of fats to fatty acids and glycerol.

Intestinal juice produced by the walls of the intestines contains protein- and sugar-splitting enzymes. Lactase splits lactose to the simple sugars glucose and galactose; maltase acts on the maltose molecule to yield glucose; and sucrase brings about the hydrolysis of sucrose to glucose and fructose. A group of enzymes known as *peptidases* completes the break-down of proteins and polypeptides to amino acids.

Function of the large intestine.   The large intestine includes the cecum, colon, rectum, and anal canal. Digestion and the absorption of nutrients have been essentially completed by the time the food mass reaches the large intestine, but much water and digestive juices are re-absorbed so that the intestinal contents gradually take on a solid consistency. The feces contain the fibers of food, small amounts of undigested food, mucus, bacteria, and broken-down cellular wastes.

DIGESTIBILITY OF FOOD

By digestibility is meant the completeness of digestion and also the ease or speed of digestion. The efficiency of digestion is remarkably high. On the average 98 per cent of the carbohydrate, 95 per cent of the fat, and 92 per cent of the protein in the food eaten is digested and absorbed.

Fibers and seeds are not digested. Therefore, a diet made up of many fruits, vegetables, and whole-grain products could have a digestibility of carbohydrate of only 85 per cent. The completeness of digestion is greatly reduced in some disorders of the gastrointestinal tract such as severe diarrhea. In some hereditary diseases such as celiac disease, cystic fibrosis of the pancreas, and lactose intolerance, the enzymes for the digestion of fats and carbohydrates may be missing so that much fat or starch is eliminated in the feces.

The speed of digestion varies widely according to the size of the meal and the composition of the diet and also depends upon certain psychologic factors. As little as nine hours or as much as 48 hours may elapse from the time food is eaten until the wastes are eliminated. Small meals will remain in the stomach for a far shorter time than will large meals. Foods that are poorly chewed are likely to require a longer time for digestion.

Foods are sometimes said to "stick to the ribs." In other words, they stay in the stomach longer so that they delay hunger contractions and are therefore more satisfying. They are said to have high *satiety* value. A breakfast of juice and dry toast, being chiefly carbohydrate, has little satiety value. But a breakfast of juice, toast, eggs, and bacon also contains proteins and fats. Because the digestion takes somewhat longer in the stomach, this meal would be more satisfying. An excessive amount of fat, especially in the form of fried foods, slows up digestion so much that some discomfort results.

Extractives in meat increase the flow of digestive juices. A cup of broth or bouillon is sometimes used at the beginning of a meal to stimulate the appetite and to increase the digestive action. The secretion of digestive juices is also increased by the pleasant sight, smell, and taste of food. On the other hand, the secretion is likely to be decreased when foods are unattractively served or when the surroundings are unpleasant. An individual who is excessively tired or who is under emotional stress such as fear, grief, or anger often experiences digestive upsets or may be unable to take food.

ABSORPTION

The intestinal wall is lined with 4 to 5 million tiny fingerlike projections called *villi*. The villi increase the surface area of the intestines tremendously so that the nutrients may be rapidly absorbed into the circulation. Each villus is supplied with small capillaries that take up the simple sugars, amino acids, glycerol, some fatty acids, water-soluble vitamins, and minerals. Lacteals, which are part of the lymph circulation, are also present in each villus. Most of the fatty acids, various fat molecules, and fat-soluble vitamins are taken up by the lacteals and enter the lymph circulation.

METABOLISM

Metabolism is an inclusive term that describes all the changes that take place in the body. *Anabolism* is a more specific term that is used to indicate the building up of complex substances from simpler substances.

Building new bone, or hemoglobin, or muscle tissue would be examples of anabolism. *Catabolism,* by contrast, refers to the breaking down of complex substances into simpler substances. The breakdown of glucose or fatty acids to yield energy is an example of catabolism.

The term "dynamic equilibrium" is sometimes used to indicate that the processes of anabolism and of catabolism are continuously taking place and that the one is equal to the other. In growing children, during pregnancy, and during recovery from illness the processes of anabolism are greater than those of catabolism. On the other hand, excessive catabolism takes place with high fever, during acute illness, following surgery, fractures, and burns, or when certain hormones are produced in excessive amounts by the body.

The innumerable reactions in metabolism also require the activity of enzymes. Many of these enzymes require another substance called a *coenzyme* in addition to the protein. One of the important functions of vitamins and certain mineral elements is to act as coenzymes.

Hormones are substances produced by glands of the body. They maintain a system of checks and balances on metabolism. To name just a few: thyroxine, produced by the thyroid gland, regulates energy metabolism; insulin, produced in the pancreas, controls the level of the blood sugar; an adrenal hormone controls the amount of sodium retained or excreted.

In addition to (1) ingestion, (2) digestion, and (3) absorption, metabolism includes these categories.

4. Transportation of the nutrients to the cells where they are needed and of the wastes to the organs of excretion is the function of the blood circulation.

5. Respiration. In the lungs oxygen is taken into the blood so that the nutrients may be combined with oxygen (oxidized). Through the lungs carbon dioxide is given off as a waste.

6. Utilization. Within every cell are found hundreds of enzymes that bring about the appropriate functions in terms of energy, building or maintenance, and regulation. In a complex series of steps glucose combines with oxygen to release the energy for the body's work. Fats, likewise, are oxidized for energy. Carbohydrates and fats may be stored as potential energy in the form of adipose tissue. Amino acids may be used to build new cells, to form hormones or enzymes, or as a source of energy. Mineral elements too may enter into the structure of the cell or into any one of many activities. An important aspect of the study in the chapters to follow will be concerned with more detail of the functions of the nutrients.

7. Excretion of wastes is accomplished by the kidney, which removes nitrogenous wastes, water, mineral salts, and excess water-soluble vitamins; by the bowel, which eliminates indigestible fiber, bile pigments, cholesterol and other products of metabolism, and bacterial wastes; by the skin,

through which water, mineral salts, and some nitrogenous wastes are removed; and by the lungs, which remove carbon dioxide and water.

REVIEW QUESTIONS AND PROBLEMS

1. Name the three functions of food in the body. What functions are performed by fats, by carbohydrates, by mineral elements, by proteins, by vitamins?

2. Define metabolism, anabolism, catabolism, enzyme, hormone.

3. Name three enzymes in the digestion of foods, and tell what they do.

4. What percentage of food eaten is digested under normal circumstances?

5. What products result from the complete digestion of proteins, fats, carbohydrates?

6. List five factors that may determine the speed with which a meal is digested.

7. What relation exists between the oxygen you breathe in and the food you eat?

8. How could you explain the fact that your output of urine may be less on a very warm day when you are exercising vigorously?

9. What kinds of waste products are excreted in the urine? Refer to a table of constituents in the urine.

REFERENCES

Rasmussen, S. *Foundations of Practical and Vocational Nursing.* New York: The Macmillan Company, 1967, Chap. 34.

Robinson, C. H. *Proudfit-Robinson's Normal and Therapeutic Nutrition*, 13th ed. New York: The Macmillan Company, 1967, Chap. 3.

4

GUIDES FOR NUTRITIONAL PLANNING

Do you weigh what you should? Are you getting enough protein? Is a small glass of tomato juice a good substitute for a small glass of orange juice? How much milk should you drink each day?

Almost everything we do is according to some design. We use recipes for cooking, patterns for sewing, and rules for behavior. Likewise, we have certain guides to answer questions such as the above and to help us in the maintenance of good nutrition and health. Let us examine more closely some of the guides that can be especially useful.

STANDARDS OF BODY WEIGHT

Probably no aspect of one's health is more often discussed than one's weight. Some people are trying to take off pounds, others are trying to put on pounds, and still others are fortunate in weighing just what they should. How do you measure up according to the standards of height and weight?

During the teen years boys and girls reach their full height, but in the early twenties they continue to mature somewhat in their body frame and muscle development. The adult is at the peak of his physical development between 20 and 30 years of age. Many people, however, continue to gain somewhat throughout life, so that the average weights for men and women at 35, 45, and 55 years are steadily increased.

Medical and insurance authorities have shown that it is not desirable for men and women to continue to gain throughout their lives. Height

28

and weight tables are, therefore, set up on the basis of weight at age 25 to 30 years. See Table A–3. One should aim to keep the desirable weight for one's height and body frame at age 25 years for the rest of one's life.

In using this table, some differences are allowed for body frame. Some people with small bones—small wrists, narrow shoulders, and narrow hips—would be classified as "low." Other people of a generally stocky build—large wrists, broad shoulders, wide hips—would have a desirable weight range between "median" and "high." You should note that the heights indicated in this table are without shoes and that the weights are without clothing.

At best, height-weight tables are only an approximate guide to body fatness. Many athletes could be considered overweight by these standards but the excess weight results from well-developed muscles and not fat. On the other hand, some inactive people may be of normal weight but have little muscular development and much body fat. Many physicians use the thickness of fat layers under the skin as an estimate of fatness. They use the skin-fold pinch test, or may obtain a more precise measurement by using a caliper.

If your weight is less than 10 per cent over or under the desirable weight for your body frame, your weight is about what it should be. If you are between 10 and 20 per cent overweight, you should correct the situation before it gets more severe. If you weigh more than 20 per cent over or under your desirable weight, it would be a good idea to consult your physician about bringing your weight more nearly in line.

MEASURES AND WEIGHTS

Exceedingly small amounts of some nutrients such as vitamins are sufficient for good nutrition. For example, about 1/28,350 of an ounce—also written 0.000035 ounce—is your daily need for vitamin B_1. To express this amount as a fraction of an ounce, or to use its decimal equivalent, is extremely cumbersome. The metric system of weights and measures, once you become accustomed to it, is much easier to use. The following relationships are involved:

1 kg (kilogram) = 1000 gm (grams)
1 gm = 1000 mg (millograms)
1 mg = 1000 µg (micrograms)
1 liter = 1000 ml (milliliters); this is used for fluid measures

Become familiar also with the following equivalents:

1 kg = 2.2 pounds
1 gm = 0.035 ounces
1 mg = 0.000035 ounces

1 pound = 454 gm
1 ounce = 28.35 gm (for approximate calculations, 30 gm is often used as equivalent to 1 ounce)

RECOMMENDED DAILY DIETARY ALLOWANCES

You have learned that the body requires a great variety of nutrients so that it may be well nourished. Research workers have determined the amounts of each of these nutrients that people of various ages and activity require each day. Your needs will differ from those of others who are larger or smaller, older or younger, more active or less active than you.

TABLE 4–1   FOOD AND NUTRITION BOARD, NATIONAL ACADEMY OF SCIENCES— NATIONAL RESEARCH COUNCIL

RECOMMENDED DAILY DIETARY ALLOWANCES,* REVISED 1968
Designed for the Maintenance of Good Nutrition of Practically All Healthy People in the U.S.A.

	Age† Years From up to	Weight Kg	Weight (lbs)	Height cm	Height (in)	Kcalories	Protein gm	Fat-Soluble Vitamins Vitamin A Activity, I.U.	Vitamin D I.U.	Vitamin E Activity, I.U.
Infants	0–⅙	4	9	55	22	kg×120	kg×2.2‡	1500	400	5
	⅙–½	7	15	63	25	kg×110	kg×2.0‡	1500	400	5
	½–1	9	20	72	28	kg×100	kg×1.8‡	1500	400	5
Children	1–2	12	26	81	32	1100	25	2000	400	10
	2–3	14	31	91	36	1250	25	2000	400	10
	3–4	16	35	100	39	1400	30	2500	400	10
	4–6	19	42	110	43	1600	30	2500	400	10
	6–8	23	51	121	48	2000	35	3500	400	15
	8–10	28	62	131	52	2200	40	3500	400	15
Males	10–12	35	77	140	55	2500	45	4500	400	20
	12–14	43	95	151	59	2700	50	5000	400	20
	14–18	59	130	170	67	3000	60	5000	400	25
	18–22	67	147	175	69	2800	60	5000	400	30
	22–25	70	154	175	69	2800	65	5000	—	30
	35–55	70	154	173	68	2600	65	5000	—	30
	55–75+	70	154	171	67	2400	65	5000	—	30
Females	10–12	35	77	142	56	2250	50	4500	400	20
	12–14	44	97	154	61	2300	50	5000	400	20
	14–16	52	114	157	62	2400	55	5000	400	25
	16–18	54	119	160	63	2300	55	5000	400	25
	18–22	58	128	163	64	2000	55	5000	400	25
	22–35	58	128	163	64	2000	55	5000	—	25
	35–55	58	128	160	63	1850	55	5000	—	25
	55–75+	58	128	157	62	1700	55	5000	—	25
Pregnancy						+200	65	6000	400	30
Lactation						+1000	75	8000	400	30

* The allowance levels are intended to cover individual variations among most normal persons as they live in the United States under usual environmental stresses. The recommended allowances can be attained with a variety of common foods, providing other nutrients for which human requirements have been less well defined.

† Entries on lines for age range 22–35 years represent the reference man and woman at age 22. All other entries represent allowances for the midpoint of the specified age range.

The Food and Nutrition Board of the National Research Council is the recognized authority for setting standards of nutrition in the United States. This board has set up a table of Recommended Daily Dietary Allowances, which is revised from time to time as new research becomes available. (See Table 4–1.)

If you examine this table carefully, you will find recommendations listed for infants, preschool and school children, older boys and girls, men and women of varying ages, and for pregnancy and lactation. Thus the table is intended to be used as a guide for the entire healthy population.

For each age an individual of given size has been used as a standard. The "reference woman" is a person 22 years old, 64 inches tall, weighing 128 pounds, and is assumed to be normally active and to live in a temperate climate. Using this guide as a point of reference, one can decide what allowance might be suitable for a woman who is larger or smaller, who is younger or older, who lives in a warmer or colder climate, or who is more or less active.

Water-Soluble Vitamins							Minerals						
Ascorbic Acid, mg	Folacin,§ mg	Niacin, mg equiv.‖	Riboflavin, mg	Thiamine, mg	Vitamin B_6 mg	Vitamin B_{12} µg	Calcium, gm	Phosphorus, gm	Iodine, µg	Iron, mg	Magnesium, mg	Age† Years From up to	
35	0.05	5	0.4	0.2	0.2	1.0	0.4	0.2	25	6	40	0–⅙	Infants
35	0.05	7	0.5	0.4	0.3	1.5	0.5	0.4	40	10	60	⅙–½	
35	0.1	8	0.6	0.5	0.4	2.0	0.6	0.5	45	15	70	½– 1	
40	0.1	8	0.6	0.6	0.5	2.0	0.7	0.7	55	15	100	1– 2	Children
40	0.2	8	0.7	0.6	0.6	2.5	0.8	0.8	60	15	150	2– 3	
40	0.2	9	0.8	0.7	0.7	3	0.8	0.8	70	10	200	3– 4	
40	0.2	11	0.9	0.8	0.9	4	0.8	0.8	80	10	200	4– 6	
40	0.2	13	1.1	1.0	1.0	4	0.9	0.9	100	10	250	6– 8	
40	0.3	15	1.2	1.1	1.2	5	1.0	1.0	110	10	250	8–10	
40	0.4	17	1.3	1.3	1.4	5	1.2	1.2	125	10	300	10–12	Males
45	0.4	18	1.4	1.4	1.6	5	1.4	1.4	135	18	350	12–14	
55	0.4	20	1.5	1.5	1.8	5	1.4	1.4	150	18	400	14–18	
60	0.4	18	1.6	1.4	2.0	5	0.8	0.8	140	10	400	18–22	
60	0.4	18	1.7	1.4	2.0	5	0.8	0.8	140	10	350	22–35	
60	0.4	17	1.7	1.3	2.0	5	0.8	0.8	125	10	350	35–55	
60	0.4	14	1.7	1.2	2.0	6	0.8	0.8	110	10	350	55–75+	
40	0.4	15	1.3	1.1	1.4	5	1.2	1.2	110	18	300	10–12	Females
45	0.4	15	1.4	1.2	1.6	5	1.3	1.3	115	18	350	12–14	
50	0.4	16	1.4	1.2	1.8	5	1.3	1.3	120	18	350	14–16	
50	0.4	15	1.5	1.2	2.0	5	1.3	1.3	115	18	350	16–18	
55	0.4	13	1.5	1.0	2.0	5	0.8	0.8	100	18	350	18–22	
55	0.4	13	1.5	1.0	2.0	5	0.8	0.8	100	18	300	22–35	
55	0.4	13	1.5	1.0	2.0	5	0.8	0.8	90	18	300	35–55	
55	0.4	13	1.5	1.0	2.0	6	0.8	0.8	80	10	300	55–75+	
60	0.8	15	1.8	+0.1	2.5	8	+0.4	+0.4	125	18	450		Pregnancy
60	0.5	20	2.0	+0.5	2.5	6	+0.5	+0.5	150	18	450		Lactation

‡ Assumes protein equivalent to human milk. For proteins not 100 per cent utilized factors should be increased proportionately.

§ The folacin allowances refer to dietary sources as determined by *Lactobacillus casei* assay. Pure forms of folacin may be effective in doses less than ¼ of the RDA.

‖ Niacin equivalents include dietary sources of the vitamin itself plus 1 mg equivalent for each 60 mg of dietary tryptophan.

For each age category, specific allowances are listed for calories, protein, ten vitamins, and five minerals. The body requires other nutrients that are not listed, but the average, well-planned diet will furnish sufficient amounts of these.

Several points in the use of this table should be mentioned. Each person differs from all other individuals in his exact nutritional requirements. To ensure satisfactory nutrition for the population, the recommended allowances have been set up at levels above minimum requirements. For most people the listed allowances provide a "margin of safety." There is no practical way for you to determine whether you use nutrients more or less efficiently than the average. Your goal in dietary planning for yourself should be toward obtaining the full recommended allowances each day.

Another point concerns the interpretation of a diet against this table. A person who fails to get the full allowances cannot be said to be in poor nutrition; only a physician can judge his nutritional status. It seems less than wise, however, for normally healthy people to continue to eat diets that do not meet the recommended allowances. If you were catching a plane at a particular time, you would surely allow a little extra time to get to the airport in the event of a traffic tie-up. Why not allow yourself the margin of safety in your nutrition by meeting fully the recommended allowances each day?

TABLES OF FOOD COMPOSITION

In order to use the table of recommended allowances you need to know the nutritive values of the foods you eat. Table A–1 (Appendix) lists numerous foods and the values for many of the nutrients recommended in the table of allowances. The nutritive values are averages of many samples of food analyzed in laboratories. Many factors determine the nutritive values of the foods we eat: the conditions of growing; the handling from farm to market to consumer; the care given to food in the home; and the manner in which food is cooked. The study of the individual nutrients in the chapters that follow will point out some of the effects of food preparation.

Generally speaking, the values listed in Table A–1 are for household measures of food. Some measures may be greater than the usual serving portions—for example, a cupful of vegetables. Note that the foods in this table are grouped by classes such as Milk, Cream, Cheese; Meat, Poultry, Fish; Vegetables; and so on. This arrangement makes it easy to compare the nutritive value of one food in a group with another food in that same group.

Suppose you were going to calculate the nutritive value of your own diet for one day. You would need to list each meal in terms of the kinds and amounts of every food, not forgetting the sugar, butter, jelly, coffee, cream, and other incidentals. You should also record the kinds and amounts of every food that you eat between meals. For example, your breakfast might have included juice, toast, cereal, milk, and coffee. In order to look up the nutritive value you would need to have an exact record such as the following:

Grapefruit juice	1 small glass (4 oz)
Cornflakes	1 cup (1 oz)
Milk, whole	½ cup
Sugar on cereal	1 teaspoon
Raisin toast	1½ slices
Butter	2 pats
Cream for coffee	2 tablespoons

When your day's record is complete, it is a good idea to add up the daily total for all foods that are the same, such as milk, butter, sugar. You may wish to calculate the value of your diet for all nutrients listed in the table; or you might look up the values for only one nutrient at the time. As you study each of the chapters on the nutrients it is a good idea to calculate your own intake of that nutrient. In this way you begin to know the good and poor sources of the nutrients and you also learn how to improve your own diet.

When you have calculated the value of your diet, compare the totals with the recommended allowances for a person of your age. Does your diet add up to the allowances? There is no harm in being a little bit over, but if you are under the allowances, you should look for ways to improve your diet. For the correct calorie intake, your weight is your best guide: if you weigh too much, you are consuming too many calories; if you weigh too little, you are not eating enough to keep your weight at the desirable level.

FOUR FOOD GROUPS

If you have calculated the nutritive value of a diet for one day, you would agree that this is somewhat time-consuming. Fortunately, some short cuts have been developed. The Four Food Groups is one reliable and easily used guide. (See Fig. 4–1.) Each of the Four Food Groups contains a variety of foods that are important in obtaining an adequate diet each day. The milk group is excellent for calcium, riboflavin, and protein. The fruit-vegetable group is not especially outstanding for ribo-flavin and calcium, and gives very little protein; but this food group is excellent for iron and ascorbic acid, neither of which is provided in appreciable amounts by milk. By use of this simple guide, one can be reasonably certain of obtaining an adequate diet. As you progress in your

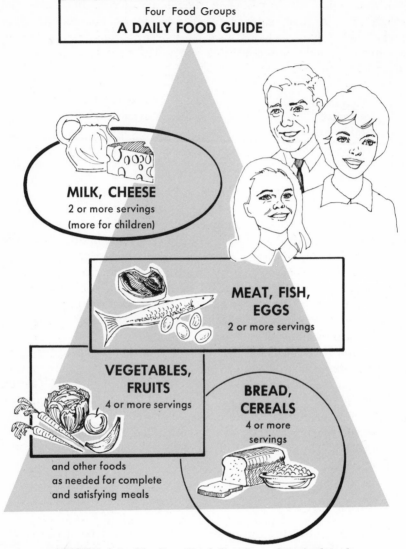

FIGURE 4-1 The Four Food Groups—a daily food guide.

study of nutrition, you will become thoroughly familiar with the nutritive contributions of foods in each group.

The food groups are:

Milk group
  2 cups for adults
  2 to 3 cups for children under 9 years
  3 cups or more for children 9 to 12 years

TABLE 4-2 NUTRITIVE VALUE OF A BASIC DIET PATTERN FOR THE ADULT IN HEALTH *

Food	Measure	Weight gm	Energy Calories	Protein gm	Fat gm	Carbohydrate gm	Minerals Ca mg	Minerals Fe mg	Vitamins A I.U.	Vitamins Thiamine mg	Vitamins Riboflavin mg	Vitamins Niacin mg	Vitamins Ascorbic Acid mg
Milk	2 cups	488	320	18	18	24	576	0.2	700	0.16	0.84	0.2	4
Meat group													
Egg	1	50	80	6	6	tr	27	1.1	590	0.05	0.15	tr	0
Meat, fish, poultry (lean cooked) †	4 ounces	120	240	33	10	0	17	3.6	35	0.32	0.26	7.4	0
Vegetable-fruit group													
Leafy green or deep yellow	¼–⅓ cup ‡	50	15	1	tr	3	14	0.5	3590	0.03	0.04	0.3	14
Other vegetable	¼–⅓ cup §	50	20	1	tr	4	13	0.5	300	0.04	0.03	0.4	9
Potato	1 medium	122	80	2	tr	18	7	0.6	tr	0.11	0.04	1.4	20
Citrus fruit ‖	1 serving	100	40	1	tr	10	18	0.2	150	0.07	0.02	0.3	42
Other fruit #	1 serving	100	60	1	tr	16	12	0.5	600	0.04	0.04	0.4	9
Bread-cereal group													
Cereal, enriched or whole grain **	¾ cup	30 (dry)	105	3	tr	22	10	0.8	0	0.12	0.04	0.8	0
Bread, enriched or whole grain	3 slices	69	180	6	3	36	57	1.8	tr	0.18	0.15	1.8	tr
Recommended Dietary Allowances		1140		72	37	133	751	9.8	5965	1.12	1.61	13.0 ††	98
Woman (18–35 years)			2000	55			800	18	5000	1.0	1.5	13	55
Man (18–35 years)			2800	65			800	10	5000	1.4	1.7	18	60

* Values for foods in the meat, vegetable-fruit, and bread-cereal groups are weighted on the basis of the approximate consumption in the United States.

† Calculations based upon an average weekly intake for meat of 11 oz beef, 7½ oz pork, 6½ oz poultry, 1½ oz lamb and veal, and 1½ oz fish. It is assumed that an average serving of ½ cup is eaten at least every other day.

‡ Dark-green leafy and deep-yellow vegetables include carrots, green peppers, broccoli, spinach, endive, and kale. It is assumed that an average serving of ½ cup is eaten at least every other day.

§ Other vegetables include tomatoes, lettuce, cabbage, snap beans, celery, peas, onions, corn, cucumbers, beets, and cauliflower. It is assumed that an average serving of ½ cup is eaten at least every other day.

‖ Citrus fruit includes fresh, canned, and frozen oranges, orange juice, grapefruit, and grapefruit juice.

Other fruit includes apples, peaches, pears, apricots, grapes, plums, and berries.

** Cereals include corn flakes, wheat flakes, rice, farina, macaroni, and oatmeal.

†† The protein in this diet furnishes about 720 mg tryptophan, equivalent to 12 mg niacin; thus, the niacin equivalent of this diet is 25 mg.

4 cups or more for teenagers
3 cups or more for pregnant women
4 cups or more for lactating women

Meat group

2 or more servings.　Count as one serving:
  2 to 3 ounces lean, cooked beef, veal, pork, lamb, poultry, fish—without bone
  2 eggs
  1 cup cooked dry beans, dry peas, lentils
  4 tablespoons peanut butter

Vegetable-fruit group

4 or more servings per day, including:
  1 serving of citrus fruit, or other fruit or vegetable as a good source of vitamin C, or 2 servings of a fair source
  1 serving, at least every other day, of a dark-green or deep-yellow vegetable for vitamin A
  2 or more servings of other vegetables and fruits, including potatoes

Bread-cereals group

4 or more servings daily (whole grain, enriched, or restored.) Count as one serving:
  1 slice bread
  1 ounce ready-to-eat cereal
  ½ to ¾ cup cooked cereal, corn meal, grits, macaroni, noodles, rice, or spaghetti

A BASIC DIET

The nutritive values for a basic diet pattern are shown in Table 4–2. This pattern includes the minimum amounts of foods listed for adults from each of the Four Food Groups. The nutritive values have been calculated on the basis of food consumption in the United States. From this calculation you can see that a young woman who chooses a variety of foods from the Four Food Groups would meet the recommended allowances for all nutrients except iron and calories. Additional foods from the Four Food Groups or desserts, fats, and sweets will easily bring the calories to the level to maintain desirable weight. Sufficient iron remains a special problem, which will be discussed further in Chapter 9.

REVIEW QUESTIONS AND PROBLEMS

1. Compare your present weight with your desirable weight. Calculate the percentage of overweight or underweight.

2. Look up the allowances recommended for you and become familiar with these as you learn more about the nutrients.

3. Keep a record of the foods you eat for one day. Check this against the recommended amounts from the Four Food Groups. Which foods should you add to your diet? Why?

4. Using Table A–1, list six foods that are especially rich in protein. How much of these foods would you be likely to eat in one meal?

5. Compare the ascorbic acid values for ½ cup grapefruit juice, 1 raw medium peach, 1 raw plum, 1 baked sweet potato, and ½ cup cooked spinach.

6. List the calorie values for 1 slice enriched bread, 1 tomato, 1 oz sweetened milk chocolate, 1 teaspoon sugar, 1 teaspoon butter, 1 cup buttermilk, and 1 pork chop.

7. Write a menu for one day including only the minimum amounts of foods recommended for adults in the Four Food Groups. What foods would you ordinarily add to this menu pattern?

8. From Table A–1 determine whether these statements are correct.

    a. A 4-oz glass of apricot nectar is not a good substitute for 4 oz of orange juice.

    b. Green peas and broccoli are about equal in value for vitamin A and ascorbic acid.

UNIT **II**

THE NUTRIENTS

5

PROTEINS AND AMINO ACIDS

Proteins are essential components of all living things—plants, animals, and even microorganisms. In fact, every tissue and fluid in the body except bile and urine contains proteins.

Most American diets provide an abundance of proteins, but certain groups of people even in this country may not get enough each day. Throughout the world, the shortage of protein is second to the shortage of calories.

NATURE AND PROPERTIES

Like carbohydrates and fats, proteins contain carbon, hydrogen, and oxygen. In addition, proteins contain about 16 per cent nitrogen. Sulfur, phosphorus, iron, and sometimes other elements such as iodine are found in small amounts. Proteins are built from 20 or so simpler building stones called *amino acids*. Just as the 26 letters of the alphabet can be combined in an amazing number of words, so the different amino acids can be joined to give an almost infinite variety of proteins. For example, the proteins found in bones, or teeth, or fingernails are quite different from those in hair, or muscle, or liver. The proteins in egg are different from those in milk, or wheat, or rice, and so on.

The amount of protein present in a food or in a tissue can be determined in the laboratory by an analysis for the nitrogen content. Each gram of nitrogen found in a food sample is equal to 6.25 gm protein.

Proteins coagulate when they are exposed to heat or to acid. Thus egg

41

white and meat coagulate when they are cooked; if too high heat is used, or if the food is cooked too long, the protein becomes dried out and tough. Perhaps at some time you have added a little vinegar to milk when you did not have the sour milk called for in a recipe. The milk thickens or curdles with the addition of the acid; in other words, the milk protein has been *coagulated*.

QUALITY OF FOOD PROTEINS

The body can manufacture some of the amino acids required by the tissues, but it is unable to make others. Those amino acids that cannot be manufactured by the body must be present in the protein of the diet, and are called *essential amino acids*. It is a good idea to be able to recognize the names of these essential amino acids when you see them. They are:

histidine (infants and children)	phenylalanine
isoleucine	threonine
leucine	tryptophan
lysine	valine
methionine	

Not all food proteins are of the same quality. When a food contains the amino acids in the proportions and the amounts needed by the body for tissue replacement and growth, it is said to provide *complete* protein, or a protein of *high biologic value*. Eggs, milk, cheese, meat, fish, and poultry are examples of such protein foods.

Some foods lack one or more of the essential amino acids in adequate amounts. Such foods would not meet the growth needs of the tissues, and so these food proteins are said to be *incomplete* or of *poor biologic value*. Generally speaking, plant foods—cereals, vegetables, and fruits—are in this group.

Fortunately, the same amino acids are not missing from all plant foods. When one food provides the amino acids that are missing in another, it is said to *supplement* the second food. Neither corn nor dry beans, when eaten at separate times, provide all the amino acids needed by the tissues. But if they are eaten at the same meal, as Mexicans often do, the two foods will supply all the amino acid needs of adults.

SOURCES

Most people immediately think of meat, fish, and poultry as good sources of protein. In the daily diet they do provide most protein per serving portion, but it is a mistake to assume that these are the only good sources of protein. The complete protein foods—meat, fish, poultry, eggs, milk, cheese—provide just over three fifths of all the protein in the average diet in the United States.

Legumes (dried peas and beans) are rich in protein, as are also nuts of many kinds. To be sure, beans do not form an important part of the American diet, but they are widely used in some parts of the world.

Breads and cereals contain relatively small amounts of protein per serving. However, the amount of bread and cereal may be sufficiently great to provide an important proportion of the total protein. For example, a boy of 16 who eats eight slices of bread in a day is thus obtaining 16 to 20 gm protein from this source alone.

Although the proteins in breads, cereals, and legumes do not provide enough of all the essential amino acids, we have seen that a proper supplementation of one with the other can "stretch" the supply of complete protein foods. Thus cereal and milk, baked beans and milk, bread and meat, as in a sandwich, are combinations that provide as good quality as that from larger servings of expensive meats and other animal protein foods alone.

The average serving of vegetable contributes 1 to 3 gm protein, and fruits are even lower in protein content. This food group accounts for only a small part of the protein in typical American diets.

The protein value for specific foods is listed in Table A–1 of the Appendix. The approximate amount of protein contributed by typical foods of the Four Food Groups is shown in Table 5–1 and Figure 5–1.

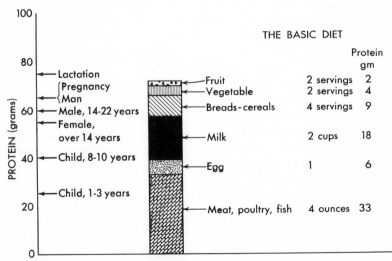

FIGURE 5–1 The Four Food Groups of the Basic Diet meet the recommended allowances for protein except for lactating women.

TABLE 5–1 AVERAGE PROTEIN COMPOSITION OF SOME FOODS

Food	Serving	Protein gm	Protein Quality
Milk group			
Milk, whole, skim, buttermilk	1 cup	9	Complete
Cheese, American, process	1 oz	7	Complete
Cheese, cottage	¼ cup	8	Complete
Cheese, cream	2 tablespoons	2	Complete
Ice cream	⅛ qt	3	Complete
Meat group			
Meat, fish, poultry	3 oz, fatty	15–20	Complete
	3 oz, lean	20–25	Complete
Egg	1 whole	6	Complete
Dried beans or peas	½ cup cooked	7–8	Incomplete
Peanut butter	1 tablespoon	4	Incomplete
Vegetable-fruit group			
Fruit juice	½ cup	Trace	
Fruits	1 serving	Trace–1	Incomplete
Vegetables	½ cup	1–3	Incomplete
Bread-cereal group			
Breakfast cereals	½ cup cooked	2–3	Incomplete
	¾ cup dry	2–3	Incomplete
Bread	1 slice	2	Incomplete
Macaroni, noodles, rice, spaghetti	½ cup cooked	2	Incomplete

FUNCTIONS

Proteins are digested to amino acids (see Chap. 3) and are absorbed through the walls of the small intestines into the portal blood circulation for delivery to the liver and the tissues of the body. The tissues and organs remove the kinds and amounts of amino acids required for a given function. The need for protein continues throughout life since there is a constant need for new cells to replace those that have broken down. For example, red blood cells have a life-span of 60 to 120 days. When they are broken down, there are equal numbers of new ones to take their places. So it is with every body tissue.

Throughout the period of pregnancy, and in infancy, childhood, and adolescence, protein is continuously required for the building of the marvelous variety of new tissues as well as for the replacement to take care of wear and tear.

Most of the regulatory materials of the body, including enzymes and hormones, are protein in nature. For example, thyroxine, which regulates energy metabolism, and insulin, which regulates the blood sugar level, contain specific kinds and amounts of certain amino acids. The red coloring matter of the blood, *hemoglobin*, is a protein that carries oxygen to the tissues so that the energy materials may be "burned" to supply energy. Other proteins in the blood are necessary to regulate osmotic pressure and to maintain water balance. The digestion of food requires certain enzymes that are constructed from amino acids. The body's defense against disease is brought about by antibodies that are composed of proteins.

Proteins also furnish 4 calories per gram. If the diet contains more protein than is needed, the nitrogen will be removed from the excess amino acids by the liver. The nitrogen is excreted in the form of urea by the kidney. The remainder of the amino acid molecule is then used as an immediate source of energy, or it may be stored in the form of fat. On the other hand, if the diet does not contain sufficient calories from fat and carbohydrate, the protein will be used for energy rather than for building or replacing tissues.

PROTEIN ALLOWANCES

The amount of protein required by the adult to maintain the tissues in good condition has been determined. Research workers have analyzed the nitrogen content of the food eaten by adults, and on the same days the nitrogen content of the urine and feces. By subtracting the total amount of nitrogen in the excretions from the total amount of nitrogen in the food, they were able to state whether the subjects were in "balance" or not. If the nitrogen in the food was exactly equal to the nitrogen in the excretions, the person was said to be in *nitrogen balance*. (See Fig. 5–2.)

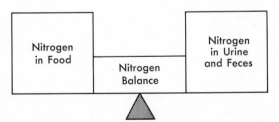

FIGURE 5–2 The healthy adult is in nitrogen balance. His intake of nitrogen from the protein in his foods and his excretion of waste nitrogen products are equal.

The protein need of the adult is based on body size, but it is not affected by the amount of exercise an individual takes. According to the Recommended Dietary Allowances, a woman of average size should include 55 gm protein daily, and the man of average size, 65 gm. This is 0.9 gm per kilogram, or 0.4 gm per pound of desirable body weight.

The minimum protein requirement for the adult may be as low as 25 to 40 gm daily, provided (1) that the individual is in good health, (2) that the quality of protein is excellent, and (3) that sufficient calories are available from carbohydrate and fat.

When new tissues are being built, the amount of nitrogen taken into the body through food must be greater than the amount of nitrogen in the excretions. Persons in such a circumstance are said to be in *positive nitrogen balance.* (See Fig. 5–3.) Greater amounts of protein will be

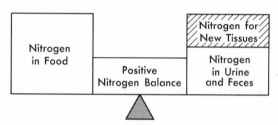

FIGURE 5–3 Protein in the diet furnishes enough nitrogen to build new tissues and to take care of waste nitrogen products. Positive nitrogen balance is normal for infants, children, adolescents, pregnant women, and convalescence from illness.

required in the diet to maintain this state. Infants, because of their rapid growth, should be given 2 gm protein per kilogram—about 1 gm per pound. A child of six to eight years, weighing 51 lb, should receive 35 gm protein a day, or about two thirds as much as a woman weighing over twice as much. A teen-age girl or boy will need 50 to 60 gm protein, depending on age and body size.

During the last half of pregnancy, when the fetus is developing rapidly, the pregnant woman should be given a daily increase of about 10 gm protein. To supply the nursing infant with sufficient protein, the lactating woman needs to include about 20 gm protein above her normal needs.

In planning diets, it is generally recommended that one third to one half of the protein in the day's diet for the adult be supplied from complete protein foods. During pregnancy and for infants and children about one half to two thirds of the protein intake should come from complete protein foods. It is also important to remember that each meal should contain some complete protein foods. Tissue building and repair do not take place if all the amino acids are not present in the blood circulation at the same time; this is sometimes referred to as the "all or none" law.

PROTEIN DEFICIENCY

Most people in America obtain an abundant intake of protein. An individual might be in *negative balance,* however. (See Fig. 5–4.) This

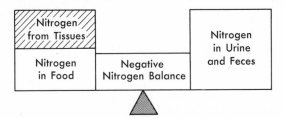

FIGURE 5–4 **When the diet does not supply enough protein for the body's needs, some body tissues are also broken down.**

means that his body is breaking down protein tissues faster than they are being replaced. Thus the excretions will contain more nitrogen than is being supplied by the diet. Just as overdrawing a bank account is not a good thing, so the excess removal of nitrogen from the tissue is also harmful. When negative nitrogen balance exists, the individual is less able to resist infections, he may withstand the stress of injury or surgery very poorly, and his general health will deteriorate.

Negative nitrogen balance exists when an individual does not eat enough protein or eats protein foods of poor quality. Some persons use crash diets for reducing weight and thus have a very low protein intake. Many elderly persons are unable to chew food well, and they may eat large quantities of bread and no meat, eggs, or milk; although the amount of protein may be sufficient, the quality is inadequate. Negative nitrogen balance occurs in many disease conditions and can be corrected only with a high-protein diet. See Chapter 23.

Infantile protein malnutrition, also called kwashiorkor, is rarely seen in the United States, but it is a major world health problem, most especially in Africa, Central and Latin America, and parts of the Orient. (See Fig. 5–5.) The condition usually appears shortly after the infant is weaned from the mother's breast and the food used is chiefly of a carbohydrate nature. The infants fail to grow, the muscles are poorly developed, the appetite is poor, the skin and hair change in texture and color, diarrhea follows, the tissues hold water (edema), and death finally results. Those children who do survive may suffer mental retardation because the brain has not had an opportunity to develop during the critical early years of life.

Kwashiorkor can be prevented or treated with inexpensive sources of protein-rich foods. Dry nonfat milk supplied through UNICEF to many infants and children has been highly effective. Many countries are now

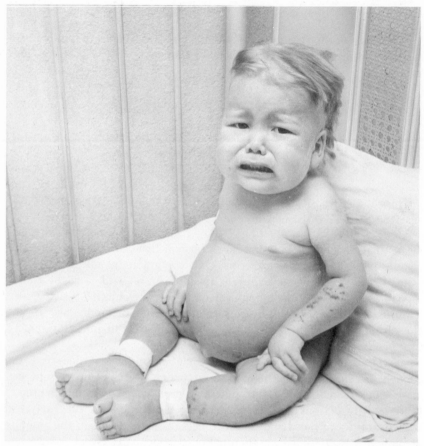

FIGURE 5–5 Child with kwashiorkor. Note swollen hands and feet, patchy hair, mottled skin, uncomfortable appearance. *(Courtesy, UNICEF. Photo by Nagata.)*

developing protein-rich foods by combining locally available plant foods. *Incaparina,* the best known of these, is a food powder that can be mixed with water for child feeding. It is made of corn, cottonseed, sorghum, and mineral-vitamin supplements. Fish protein concentrate, soybean protein, peanut protein, and others have been used in various mixtures.

SOME FALLACIES AND FACTS

1. *Fallacy.* Athletes need more protein than nonathletes.
   Fact. The protein requirement of the adult depends on the body size and not on the amount of exercise.
2. *Fallacy.* Older people need less protein than young adults.
   Fact. The need for replacing the protein of tissues continues through-

out life. Older people need the same amount of protein as the young adult of the same body size.

3. *Fallacy*. Gelatin is an excellent source of protein.

Fact. Although gelatin is useful in providing a variety of dishes in the diet, its protein contribution is not important. Dry gelatin is about 90 per cent protein, but the average gelatin dessert would furnish about 2 gm protein. Gelatin lacks some of the essential amino acids; as a sole source of protein it cannot maintain life or support growth.

4. *Fallacy*. Protein foods should not be eaten in the same meal as starches.

Fact. There is no reason to separate protein foods and starches. In fact, many common foods contain both protein and carbohydrate. The digestive tract efficiently digests protein, carbohydrate, and fat components of the diet at the same time. Each meal should contain one fourth to one third of the day's protein so that the amino acids will be most efficiently used for tissue synthesis.

REVIEW QUESTIONS AND PROBLEMS

1. Define amino acid, essential amino acid, complete protein, supplementary protein, biologic value, nitrogen balance, antibody, phenylalanine.

2. How do proteins differ from fats and carbohydrates?

3. Keep a record of the food you eat for one day. Using the approximate values on page 44, estimate the amount of protein in your diet. What foods provided you with complete protein?

4. Why should you include some complete protein at each meal?

5. What happens if you eat more protein than your tissues need for maintenance?

6. How does the protein need of a ten-year-old boy compare with your need?

7. How could you improve these meals for protein?

I	II
Large fruit salad	Baked beans
Roll with butter	Brown bread with butter
Cucumber–water cress sandwich	Sliced tomato salad
Iced tea	Jello with whipped cream

8. Name three substances in the body that are of a protein nature and that regulate body functions. Tell what each does.

9. What is kwashiorkor? How may it be prevented?

10. A 75-year-old woman refuses to drink milk or to eat meat because she thinks these foods are not good for her. How would you respond to this situation?

REFERENCES

Breeling, J. L. "Marketing Protein for the World's Poor," *Today's Health*, **47**:42, February 1969.

Cooley, D. G. "What's So Important About Proteins?" *Today's Health*, **43**:46, October 1965.

Robinson, C. H. *Proudfit-Robinson's Normal and Therapeutic Nutrition*, 13th ed. New York: The Macmillan Company, 1967, Chap. 5.

FATS

"The fat of the land." The word "fat" brings to mind such ideas as wealth, prosperity, and well-being; likewise, the word makes one think of such rich foods as pastries, cookies, cakes, ice cream, butter, cream, and oil. But fat is also associated with overweight and more recently with heart disease. *Lipid* is another term for fats and fatlike substances.

NATURE AND PROPERTIES

Fats are composed of three chemical elements: carbon, hydrogen, and oxygen. Fats contain much smaller proportions of oxygen than do carbohydrates. When they are oxidized they give more than twice as much energy as do carbohydrates and proteins.

Most fats are formed from three molecules of *fatty acids* attached to one molecule of *glycerol*. Each fatty acid consists of a short or long chain of carbon atoms joined to an acid group. Short-chain fatty acids contain 4 to 10 carbon atoms, and long-chain fatty acids contain 12 to 20 or more carbon atoms. Long-chain fatty acids may be saturated, monounsaturated, or polyunsaturated.

Saturated fatty acids are those to which no hydrogen can be added. Palmitic and stearic acid are two examples of such fatty acids; they are abundant in animal fats, including beef and mutton fat, butter, and others.

A *monounsaturated* fatty acid is one in which two of the carbon atoms are joined by a double bond. This means that a hydrogen atom could be added to each of the carbon atoms at the double bond. Oleic acid is the

51

most abundant monounsaturated fatty acid. Olive and peanut oils are especially high in oleic acid, but most fats contain generous amounts of this fatty acid.

A *polyunsaturated* fatty acid is one in which two or more double bonds are present. Thus, each of four or more carbon atoms could take up a hydrogen atom. *Linoleic* acid has two double bonds and is the most common of the polyunsaturated acids; it is abundant in most vegetable oils.

Hydrogenation is the addition of hydrogen to the carbon atoms in unsaturated fats to produce a solid fat. Regular margarines and many cooking fats are prepared from vegetable oils by this process. As might be expected, the addition of hydrogen increases the proportion of saturated fatty acids and decreases the proportion of unsaturated fatty acids.

The flavor and hardness of a food fat depend upon the kinds and amounts of the fatty acids that are present. Food fats are a mixture of saturated and unsaturated fatty acids, some with long chains and others with short carbon chains. For convenience a food fat is called *saturated* if it contains more saturated than polyunsaturated fatty acids; such fats are solid. If polyunsaturated fatty acids exceed the saturated fatty acids, the food fat is said to be *polyunsaturated*; such fats are liquid, such as oils, or very soft, such as some special type margarines.

Fats become rancid if they are exposed to air and light. The change is more rapid at high temperatures. Many manufacturers add antioxidants to fats to lengthen the time that they may be kept.

FOOD SOURCES

Some fats are "visible," as in butter, shortenings, and oils, whereas others are "invisible," as in milk, egg yolk, and food mixtures. The milk group and the meat group furnish about half of the fat in our diets. Visible fats and oils are the next important source of fats. The vegetable-fruit group (except olives and avocados) and the bread-cereal group are very low in fat. The fat content of the basic diet is shown in Figure 6–1.

The important way by which fats contribute to the calories of the diet is shown in Table 6–1.

The following classification of fat-rich foods indicates whether saturated fatty acids or polyunsaturated fatty acids predominate.

High in saturated fatty acids
   Whole milk, cream, ice cream, cheeses made from whole milk, egg yolk
   Medium fat or fatty meats: beef, lamb, pork, ham
   Bacon, beef tallow, butter, coconut oil, lamb fat, lard, regular margarine, salt pork, hydrogenated shortenings
   Chocolate, chocolate candy, cakes, cookies, pies, rich puddings

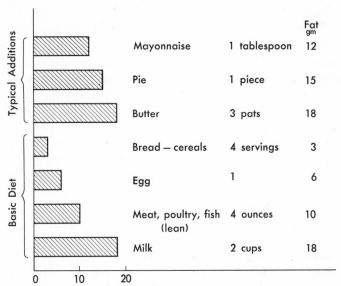

FIGURE 6-1 The fat content of a diet is rapidly increased with butter or margarine, salad dressings, and many desserts. See Table 4-2 for calculations of Basic Diet.

TABLE 6-1   COMPARISON OF FAT CONTENT AND CALORIES

	Total Fat gm	Calories
Skim milk, 1 cup	Trace	90
Whole milk, 1 cup	10	165
Half milk and half cream, 1 cup	29	330
Tossed salad	Trace	20
Tossed salad with 2 tablespoons blue cheese dressing	20	200
Bread, 1 thin slice	1	60
Bread, 1 slice with 1 pat butter	7	110
Baked potato, one	Trace	90
Baked potato with 2 tablespoons sour cream	6	160
Lamb chop, lean, one	6	140
Lamb chop, lean with fat, one	33	405

High in polyunsaturated fatty acids

Vegetable oils: safflower, corn, cottonseed, soybean, sesame, sunflower
Salad dressings made from the above oils: mayonnaise, French, and others
Special margarines: liquid oil listed first on label
Fatty fish: salmon, tuna, herring

FUNCTIONS

Normally, about 95 per cent of the fat in food is digested and absorbed. (See Chap. 3.) Fats, as we all know, are important sources of calories; each gram contributes 9 calories. It is quite normal for the body to have deposits of fat (adipose tissue) that serve as a continuing supply of energy each and every hour. In fact, if we had no reserves of fat in the body whatsoever, we would need to eat much more frequently in order to provide a continuous supply of energy. Fat is said to be *protein-sparing* because its availability reduces the need to burn protein for energy. Carbohydrates and proteins in excess of body needs are also changed into fatty tissue, just as fat in the diet contributes to these stores.

In addition to providing energy, fats are essential (1) to maintain the constant body temperature by providing effective insulation underneath the skin; (2) to cushion the vital organs, such as the kidney, against injury; (3) to facilitate the absorption of the fat-soluble vitamins A, D, E, and K; (4) to provide satiety and to delay the onset of hunger; and (5) to contribute flavor and palatability to the diet.

Essential fatty acids. Arachidonic acid, a long-chain polyunsaturated fatty acid, is essential for normal growth and skin health. This fatty acid occurs in only limited amounts in the food supply. However, linoleic acid occurs abundantly in foods that are high in polyunsaturated fatty acids and can be readily converted by the body to arachidonic acid. Linoleic acid is therefore considered to be a dietary essential.

Phospholipids are complex fats that also contain phosphorus and nitrogen. The diet supplies small amounts of these, and the body can make them. They are important in brain and nervous tissue. They also assist in the absorption of fat from the small intestine and in the transportation of fat in the blood.

DAILY ALLOWANCES

No specific recommendation for the level of fat intake has been made by the Food and Nutrition Board. The requirement for linoleic acid is low and is easily met. For infant formulas it is recommended that linoleic acid should supply 3 per cent of the calories.

Although fats account for about 40 per cent of the calories available in the United States, the actual intakes vary widely. Some people eat many fried foods, pastries, rich desserts, cream, and butter, whereas others rarely use such high-fat foods. Some people throughout the world, for example Asians and Africans, consume diets providing as little as 10 per cent of the calories from fat, whereas other people, such as Eskimos, eat large quantities of fat.

Many people today are concerned about the relationship of fat to heart disease. A large number of studies indicate that a diet high in poly-unsaturated fats and low in saturated fats is of value for people who have had a heart attack and also as a preventive measure for those who are classified as "high risks." (See Chap. 24.) Not all authorities are agreed that a drastic change in the type or amount of dietary fat is necessary for the general population. An adequate diet based upon the selection of a wide variety of foods from the Four Food Groups is still good advice. The American Heart Association recommends a moderate reduction in satu-rated fats and somewhat greater emphasis upon foods rich in poly-unsaturated fats. Any drastic changes in the diet should be made only upon the advice of a physician.

CHOLESTEROL

Cholesterol is a white, waxy substance related to fats but very different in chemical structure. It is abundant in certain foods, such as egg yolk, liver, kidney, brains, and shellfish. Other animal fats, including butter, cream, whole milk, whole-milk cheeses, ice cream, and meats, contain smaller amounts. Cholesterol is not found in plant foods.

Cholesterol is normally present in many tissues, but is especially im-portant in brain and nervous tissue and in the liver. It serves as a precursor of vitamin D; that is, cholesterol in the skin can be changed into active vitamin D by the ultraviolet light from the sunshine. Cholesterol is closely related to the sex hormones and the hormones of the adrenal gland. Excess cholesterol in the body is removed in the bile.

The amount of cholesterol in the diet may influence the amount of cholesterol in the blood. The body daily manufactures cholesterol to meet its needs from fats, carbohydrates, and even amino acids. Cholesterol sometimes accumulates abnormally in the gallbladder to form gallstones. Many Americans of middle age also have high blood cholesterol levels that appear to make them more prone to heart disease. These problems will be discussed in Chapter 24.

SOME FALLACIES AND FACTS

1. *Fallacy*. Fried foods are hard to digest.

Fact. Digestion of fried foods is as complete as that of other foods. However, because fat coats the food particles, the digestion of fried foods takes somewhat longer.

2. *Fallacy*. Mineral oil is a good substitute for regular oil in low-calorie salad dressings.

Facts. Mineral oil is not absorbed through the intestinal wall, but it also interferes seriously with the absorption of the fat-soluble vitamins A, D, E, and K. Therefore, it should never be used in food preparation.

3. *Fallacy*. Vegetable oils are less fattening than solid fats.

Fact. Oils and solid fats are equally high in calories; that is, 9 calories per gram of pure fat regardless of source.

4. *Fallacy*. All vegetable oils are high in polyunsaturated fatty acids.

Facts. Vegetable oils vary widely in their content of polyunsaturated fatty acids. Safflower, soybean, corn, cottonseed, and sesame oils are excellent sources. Peanut oil contains only about half as much linoleic acid as these oils. Olive oil is a poor source, and coconut oil contains only traces of polyunsaturated fatty acids.

5. *Fallacy*. Sour cream is lower in calories than sweet cream.

Fact. Weight for weight, sour cream contains the same number of calories as the sweet cream from which it was made. The sour cream usually available in markets and coffee cream are about 20 per cent fat.

REVIEW QUESTIONS AND PROBLEMS

1. What is meant by lipid, saturated fat, polyunsaturated fat, linoleic acid, hydrogenated fat?

2. What chemical elements are present in fats?

3. If a diet contains 90 gm fat, how many calories are provided by this fat?

4. List six functions of fats.

5. What precautions would you use in storing butter? An opened bottle of corn oil? A hydrogenated cooking fat? Give your reasons.

6. List the sources of fat you had in your diet yesterday. Which of these were good sources of linoleic acid?

7. A person complains that a meal that included fried chicken, French fried potatoes, and apple pie was "heavy." What does he probably mean by this? How do you explain it?

8. A person tells you that he has decided to eat no more eggs, milk, or butter because these foods are high in cholesterol. How would you respond to this?

REFERENCES

Coons, C. M. "Fats and Fatty Acids," in *Food, The Yearbook of Agriculture, 1959*. Washington, D.C.: U.S. Government Printing Office, 1959, pp. 74–87.

Dayton, S., *et al*. "Can Changes in the American Diet Prevent Coronary Heart Disease?" *J. Amer. Diet. Ass.*, 46:20, 1965.

Leverton, R. M. *Food Becomes You*, 3rd ed. Ames, Iowa: Iowa State University Press, 1965, Ch. 10.

7

UNIVERSAL ROLE | NATURE AND CLASSIFICATION | PROPERTIES |
SOURCES | FACTS ABOUT CARBOHYDRATE-RICH FOODS | FUNCTIONS |
DAILY NEEDS

CARBOHYDRATES

UNIVERSAL ROLE

All peoples of the world depend upon the carbohydrate-rich foods as the principal source of calories. In the United States carbohydrates furnish about half of the calories, whereas in some countries of the world as much as four fifths of the calories is obtained from carbohydrate. The carbohydrate-rich plants are easily grown, give a large yield of food per acre, keep rather well, and are thus inexpensive. The foods are highly acceptable in a great variety of ways and are easily digested and used in the body.

Cereal grains, legumes, roots, and sugars are the principal sources of carbohydrate. Rice is the leading staple food of the world, being especially prominent in Oriental diets. Wheat ranks second and is the staple cereal in parts of India, the Near East, Russia, western Europe, and America. Rye, oats, and millet are important cereals in some dietaries of the world. Corn and legumes such as beans are favored in Central and Latin America. Potatoes, sweet potatoes, taro, plantain, and cassava do not approach the cereal grains in importance; yet they furnish significant amounts of carbohydrate and calories to the diets of some peoples. Although sugars are universally liked, the highest consumption is found in the most highly developed and affluent countries.

In the United States the trend has been toward a steady decline in the use of cereal grains and potatoes, a gradual increase in the use of sugars, and a relatively limited use of legumes.

NATURE AND CLASSIFICATION

By a complex process known as photosynthesis all green plants use energy from the sun, water from the soil, and carbon dioxide from the air to make carbohydrate. All carbohydrates contain the chemical elements carbon, hydrogen, and oxygen. The hydrogen and oxygen are present in the same proportions as found in water. Carbohydrates may be classed as shown in Table 7-1.

TABLE 7-1 CLASSIFICATION OF CARBOHYDRATES

Class	Examples	Some Food Sources
Single sugars (monosaccharides)	Glucose (dextrose, grape sugar, corn sugar, blood sugar)	Fruits, honey, vegetables, corn syrup
	Fructose (fruit sugar, levulose)	Fruits, vegetables, honey, corn syrup
	Galactose	Occurs only from the digestion of lactose
Double sugars (disaccharides)	Sucrose	Cane, beet, maple sugar; small amounts in fruits, some vegetables
	Maltose	Malting of cereal grains; acid hydrolysis of starch
	Lactose	Milk only
Complex carbohydrates (polysaccharides)	Starch	Grains and grain foods, legumes, potatoes and other root vegetables, green bananas
	Glycogen	Liver and muscle of freshly killed animals; freshly opened oysters
	Dextrin	Partial breakdown of starch by heat or in digestion
	Cellulose	Bran of cereal grains, skins and fibers of fruits and vegetables
	Pectins	Ripe fruits

PROPERTIES

Carbohydrates may be ranked in decreasing order of sweetness: fructose, sucrose, glucose, lactose, dextrin, and starch. Regardless of their sweetness, all carbohydrates furnish 4 calories per gram. Only a small amount of honey, which is rich in fructose, can be eaten at one time. If one needs to increase the calorie value of a glass of lemonade, for example, one could use about twice as much glucose as sucrose. Lactose is only about one seventh as sweet as sucrose, and even more of it could be used in the lemonade.

Starches are bland in flavor and not sweet. When a banana ripens, the starch is changed into glucose, and the sweetness is thereby increased.

Sugars vary greatly in their solubility. Glucose is less soluble than sucrose; when making up a beverage it should be stirred well so that the sugar will not settle to the bottom. Lactose should be added to hot water because it dissolves poorly in cold water. Because of its poor solubility, its higher cost, and its tendency to irritate the intestinal tract when taken in large amounts, lactose is now seldom used in beverages.

The thickening property of starch is well known, as in the making of cornstarch pudding or the cooking of a breakfast cereal such as oatmeal. When mixed with water and cooked, the starch absorbs water, and the mixture thickens.

SOURCES

When planning diets one should consider the amount of carbohydrate in the food and also the contributions of other nutrients made by a given food. Of the Four Food Groups breads and cereals are the outstanding sources of carbohydrate. This group is important because the amounts of these foods eaten daily may be considerable, and because enriched or whole-grain breads and cereals provide substantial quantities of iron, B-complex vitamins, and some protein.

The whole grain is rich in iron, thiamine, niacin, and other nutrients. In the manufacture of white flour and refined cereals the germ and outer layers of the grain are removed. (See Fig. 7–1.) This refinement results in significant losses of iron and B-complex vitamins. Early in World War II a program of enrichment was initiated to replace the lost nutrients to cereal foods.

Enrichment is a legal term used by the Food and Drug Administration to apply specifically to the addition of thiamine, riboflavin, niacin, and iron. Enrichment of bread and flour is required in the majority of states and is voluntary in others. Some states in the South also require the enrichment of corn and rice. About 80 per cent of the white flour and bread in this country are now enriched, and also a substantial proportion of the macaroni, noodles, and spaghetti. When foods are labeled as enriched, they must contain the four nutrients within the ranges specified by the law.

Sweet potatoes and white potatoes are important contributors from the vegetable-fruit group to the carbohydrate intake, because they are daily

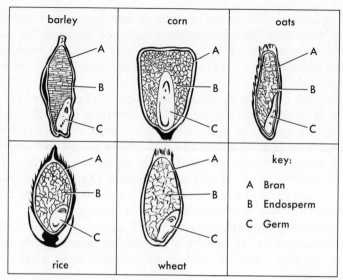

FIGURE 7-1   Structure of cereal grains. *(Courtesy, Cereal Institute, Inc.)*

items in many diets. Some fruits, such as bananas and dried fruits, and some vegetables, such as corn and Lima beans, are also relatively high in carbohydrate content. They are not usually daily items in the diet, and therefore the amount of carbohydrate realized from these foods is considerably less than that from potatoes.

Milk is unique in that it is the only dietary source of lactose. Each cup contains 12 gm; thus the daily intake from this source would be 24 to 48 gm lactose, depending upon the amount of milk consumed. Cheese contains only traces of lactose.

Meat, poultry, and fish contain no carbohydrate. The small amount of glycogen present in fresh liver and oysters has usually disappeared before the food reaches the consumer. Legumes and peanuts contain fair amounts of carbohydrate.

Next to breads and cereals, the sugars and sweets are important sources of carbohydrate. Cane and beet sugars are inexpensive, whereas honey, maple syrup, jellies and jams, and candies are moderately high in cost. Sugars and sweets are concentrated so that relatively small amounts will rapidly increase the carbohydrate and calorie intake. On the other hand, they do not contain important amounts of other nutrients; they are often referred to as "empty-calorie" foods. If too many sweets are included, they may take the place of foods that supply other nutrients, because they often destroy the appetite. Excessive amounts of sweets are sometimes irritating to the gastrointestinal tract. They may stick to the teeth so that tooth decay results. (See Fig. 7-2.)

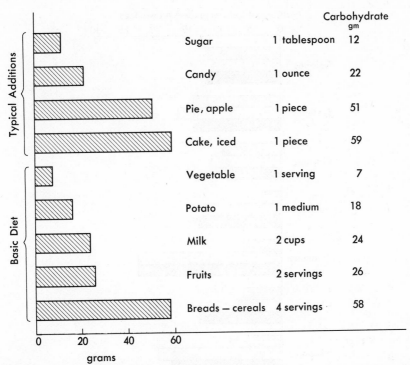

			Carbohydrate gm
Sugar	1 tablespoon		12
Candy	1 ounce		22
Pie, apple	1 piece		51
Cake, iced	1 piece		59
Vegetable	1 serving		7
Potato	1 medium		18
Milk	2 cups		24
Fruits	2 servings		26
Breads — cereals	4 servings		58

FIGURE 7–2 Desserts and sweets are typical additions to the Basic Diet for additional calories. Some additions provide few nutrients other than carbohydrate. See Basic Diet, Table 4–2, for calculations.

Cellulose, being the fibrous part of the plant, is supplied by the whole grains, raw fruits, and raw vegetables. During cookery some of the fibers disintegrate whereas others are softened.

FACTS ABOUT CARBOHYDRATE-RICH FOODS

1. Are honey, crude sugar, and brown sugar nutritionally better than cane or beet sugar?

Honey and brown sugar bring flavor variety to the diet. Like cane or beet sugar they are good sources of energy, but the amounts of minerals and vitamins are too small to make a worthwhile addition to the day's diet.

2. Are whole-grain breads more nutritious than white bread?

Cereal foods, whether whole grain or highly milled, are important and inexpensive sources of energy. They also furnish some protein. White breads that have been enriched are just as nutritious as whole-grain breads. (See Fig. 7–3.) Whole-grain breads contain appreciably more fiber than

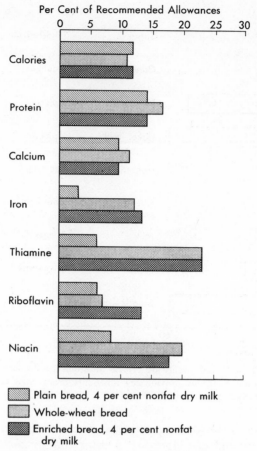

Per Cent of Recommended Allowances

Plain bread, 4 per cent nonfat dry milk
Whole-wheat bread
Enriched bread, 4 per cent nonfat dry milk

FIGURE 7–3 Enriched and whole-wheat bread are comparable in nutritive value.

white breads and the percentage of digestibility is, therefore, slightly lower. Unenriched white breads supply much lower amounts of iron and B-complex vitamins.

3. Are rice, macaroni, noodles, and spaghetti good substitutes for potatoes?

It depends upon the choices made. All these foods are high in starch and an average serving of each is similar in calorie and protein value. If the cereal foods are enriched, they would furnish about the same amounts of minerals and B vitamins as potatoes. Fresh potatoes contain some ascorbic acid not provided by cereal foods or dehydrated potatoes.

4. Is blackstrap molasses good for anemia?

Blackstrap molasses is relatively rich in iron but it does not have any special virtue over many foods that provide iron. Blackstrap molasses is widely used in livestock feeding. The treatment of anemia depends upon the type of anemia present and should be directed by a physician.

FUNCTIONS

Glucose, fructose, and galactose are the end products of carbohydrate digestion (see Chap. 3). These single sugars are absorbed from the small intestine into the portal circulation and are carried to the liver.

The form of sugar in the blood is glucose. Shortly after a meal the blood glucose will rise. This stimulates the production of the hormone insulin, which is necessary for (1) the utilization of glucose for energy by the tissues, (2) the conversion of glucose to glycogen in the liver, and (3) the conversion of glucose to fat. Thus insulin is a primary regulator of the level of the blood sugar.

The chief function of carbohydrate is to provide energy to carry on the work of the body and heat to maintain the body's temperature. Glucose is the only form of energy used by nervous tissue but other tissues also use fats for energy. Glucose and oxygen are carried by the blood to the tissues. In a complex manner involving many enzymes and intermediate reactions, glucose is oxidized to yield the following results:

$$\text{glucose} + \text{oxygen} = \text{energy} + \text{carbon dioxide} + \text{water}.$$

When tissues require much energy for their work, oxidation of glucose will proceed at a much more rapid rate. If you run, for example, you begin to breathe rapidly. You are then providing additional oxygen to combine with the extra glucose to meet this energy need. The carbon dioxide produced in this reaction is a waste product that is removed through the lungs. The water that results may be reused by the body in a number of ways or may be eliminated by the kidneys, skin, and lungs.

Carbohydrate spares protein. This means that the body need not burn protein from the diet or from body stores to meet energy needs when carbohydrate is available. Carbohydrates also furnish chemical elements that can be combined with nitrogen to manufacture nonessential amino acids.

Some carbohydrate is essential for complete oxidation of fat in the body. The diabetic patient, for example, cannot use carbohydrate as well as the normal individual. As a result, fats are used less effectively. Some acids from fat accumulate and produce the condition known as *acidosis* or *diabetic coma*. (See Chap. 22.)

The amount of carbohydrate in the body at any given moment is small —perhaps around ¾ lb or less. Some of this is present in the blood in the form of glucose, and the greater amount is stored in the liver and muscles as glycogen. Some body structures such as nervous tissues and cartilage contain small amounts of carbohydrate. Carbohydrate in excess of body needs is readily converted to fat, which serves as a reserve of energy.

Some cellulose is desirable, because it contributes bulk to the diet. It can absorb and hold water so that normal elimination occurs from the bowel.

Certainly the value of sugars and starches in providing variety and flavor in the diet should not be minimized. Jam on bread, strawberries on cereal, freshly baked dinner rolls, cake with frosting—all of these are taste-appealing and encourage food intake. To be sure, carbohydrates if eaten too liberally may well contribute to excessive caloric intake and thus to overweight.

DAILY NEEDS

Ordinarily the daily diet should contain not less than 100 gm carbohydrate. Note that the Basic Diet furnishes somewhat more than this. Some peoples of the world maintain vigorous health with high intakes of carbohydrate, and others are just as healthy on low-carbohydrate diets. The inclusion of four or more servings of enriched or whole-grain cereals and breads provides for important intakes of iron and the B-complex vitamins. Raw and cooked fruits and vegetables satisfy the fiber needs and bring bonus values for iron, ascorbic acid, and other vitamins.

REVIEW QUESTIONS AND PROBLEMS

1. Define these terms: photosynthesis, galactose, cellulose, dextrin, maltose, enrichment, legume, monosaccharide, carbohydrate, starch, glycogen.

2. List the foods you ate yesterday. Which of these are important sources of carbohydrate? Which are important sources of fiber? Which are "empty-calorie" foods?

3. Outline the steps in the digestion of a carbohydrate meal, including the names of the enzymes, the site of their activity, and the digestion products that result. (Review Chap. 3.)

4. You sometimes find that a glass of fruit juice quickly makes you feel better. How can you explain this?

5. List four functions of carbohydrates in the body.

6. How many calories would be provided by 250 gm carbohydrate?

7. Why is cellulose important? What foods would you increase in the diet for more cellulose?

8. Look up in Table A–1 the carbohydrate value of 1 piece of layer cake, 1 fresh peach, ½ cup cooked rice, 1 piece of apple pie, 1 sweet potato, 1 teaspoon sugar, 1 sweet roll, ½ cup spinach, 1 candy bar, 1 cup blueberries.

REFERENCES

Robinson, C. H. *Proudfit-Robinson's Normal and Therapeutic Nutrition*, 13th ed. New York: The Macmillan Company, 1967, Chap. 6.

Sebrell, W. H., Jr. "The Story of Enriched Bread," *Today's Health*, **39**:58, September 1961.

ENERGY METABOLISM

Fuel and Energy

Probably no aspect of nutrition is more discussed than that of calories. People say they "eat" too many calories or not enough calories. They associate calories with their weight. We need to know what we mean by calories, how many calories we need each day, and which foods are good and poor sources of calories.

Every engine requires fuel. The automobile runs only so long as it has .a supply of gasoline. The furnace heats the house only when oil, gas, or coal is fed into it. The human body, sometimes likened to an engine, requires fuel to carry on all of its activities and to keep it warm. Every moment of our lives some energy is being used by the body—for every breath we draw, every beat of the heart, the blinking of the eyelid, the lifting of the heavy weight, or any activity whatsoever. The carbohydrate, fat, and protein in the foods we eat are the potential sources of energy for all body activities.

CALORIE, A UNIT OF HEAT

Strictly speaking, we don't "eat" calories. When carbohydrates, fats, and proteins are oxidized in the body, heat is a by-product. Just as we can measure length in inches and weight in pounds or ounces, so we can measure the energy value of a food, or the heat production of the body, in heat units called *calories*. By definition, one large or kilocalorie is the

65

amount of heat required to raise the temperature of 1000 gm of water by 1°C. The large calorie is the unit always used in nutrition.

The energy value of a food is measured in the laboratory with an instrument called a *bomb calorimeter*. The caloric values for foods obtained with this instrument must be corrected to allow for some losses that occur in the feces and urine. In the body, these are the corrected values for pure carbohydrate, fat, and protein:

Carbohydrate	4 calories per gram
Fat	9 calories per gram
Protein	4 calories per gram

Thus 5 grams of sugar (1 teaspoon) would yield 20 calories, but 5 grams of fat would yield 45 calories.

If we know the carbohydrate, fat, and protein values for a food, we can easily calculate the calorie value of that food. For example, the calorie value of one cup of milk would be calculated thus:

$$12 \text{ gm carbohydrate} \times 4 \text{ calories} = 48$$
$$10 \text{ gm fat} \times 9 \text{ calories} = 90$$
$$8 \text{ gm protein} \times 4 \text{ calories} = 32$$

Total calories   170

You will see that this calculation, using figures for milk that have been rounded off, is quite close to the actual value listed in Table A–1 of the Appendix. Ordinarily, we don't need to make such calculations, because tables of calorie values are readily available.

Energy Needs of the Body

MEASURING ENERGY NEEDS

An individual uses oxygen to burn the carbohydrates, fats, and proteins in his body; the higher the rate of burning (oxidation) in his body, the more oxygen he will need. Therefore, the amount of oxygen used by an individual under certain conditions of rest or activity is measured to calculate the energy expended.

The total daily calorie requirement depends upon the basal metabolism, the amount of voluntary activity, the influence of food, the climate, and needs for growth.

BASAL METABOLISM

Basal metabolism, sometimes called "the cost of living," accounts for more than half of the calorie requirements of most people. It includes the involuntary activities of the body (activities over which we have no control) while resting but awake. The breathing, the beating of the heart, the circulation of the blood, the metabolic activities within the cells, the keeping of the muscles in good tone, and the maintenance of the body temperature require energy.

The basal metabolism may be measured in a number of ways. One of these consists in measuring the amount of pure oxygen a person breathes in for a given length of time under these conditions: (1) the individual is awake but lying quietly in a comfortable room; (2) he is in the *postabsorptive* state; that is, he has had no food for 12 to 16 hours; (3) his body temperature is normal; and (4) he is not tense or emotionally upset. When the test is performed the nose is clamped so that the person breathes through his mouth from a tank of oxygen. The amount of oxygen he uses is measured, and from that the number of calories is calculated.

For his basal metabolism, the adult requires about 10 to 12 calories per pound of body weight for a 24-hour period. The average woman has a basal metabolism around 55 calories per hour, or 1350 calories per day, and the average man has a basal metabolism of about 70 calories per hour, or 1700 per day.

Several factors affect the rate of basal metabolism. The first of these is *body size*. The larger a person is, the greater is the amount of lean muscle tissue and the greater is the skin surface area. Thus a tall, well-built man has a greater skin surface and will have a higher basal metabolism than a short, fat man of the same weight.

The amount of *muscle tissue* has an effect on the basal metabolism. An athlete with firm muscles has a higher rate than a nonathlete with poorly developed, flabby muscles. Usually men have a higher rate than women, because men, as a rule, have more muscle tissue, and women have more deposits of fat.

Rapid *growth* increases the basal metabolism greatly. Infants in proportion to body size have a very high rate of metabolism. The metabolism is also high during the rapid growth period of adolescence and the last trimester of pregnancy when the fetus is greatly increasing in size.

After the *age* of 25 years the metabolism declines gradually; thus the calories are reduced somewhat for every ten years. Many men and women become overweight during middle age because they fail to reduce their calories as their metabolism goes down.

The *thyroid* gland produces thyroxine, an iodine-containing hormone that regulates the rate of energy metabolism. If too much thyroxine is produced, the metabolism will increase; if too little thyroid hormone is manufactured, the metabolism will be correspondingly lower. The level of protein-bound iodine (PBI) in the blood is now widely used by physicians in place of the basal metabolism test to determine the activity of the thyroid.

VOLUNTARY ACTIVITY

Our daily work may well vary from sitting at a desk to bedside nursing, active housework, or hard manual labor. In our leisure time we might choose to watch television, take a leisurely walk, or go swimming or dancing. The kind of physical activity in which we engage, and the amounts of time spent in each activity, determine the amount of energy the body uses. It is difficult to assign exact values to any activity because individuals vary widely in the efficiency with which they use their bodies.

TABLE 8–1 CALORIE EXPENDITURE FOR VARIOUS TYPES OF ACTIVITIES *

Type of Activity	Calories per Hour
Sedentary activities, such as: Reading; writing; eating; watching television or movies; listening to the radio; sewing; playing cards; and typing, miscellaneous office work, and other activities done with sitting that requires little or no arm movement	80 to 100
Light activities, such as: Preparing and cooking food; doing dishes; dusting; handwashing small articles of clothing; ironing; walking slowly; personal care; miscellaneous office work and other activities done while standing that require some arm movement; and rapid typing and other activities done while sitting that are more strenuous	110 to 160
Moderate activities, such as: Making beds; mopping and scrubbing; sweeping; light polishing and waxing; laundering by machine; light gardening and carpentry work; walking moderately fast; other activities done while standing that require moderate arm movement; and activities done while sitting that require more vigorous arm movement	170 to 240
Vigorous activities, such as: Heavy scrubbing and waxing; handwashing large articles of clothing; hanging out clothes; stripping beds; other heavy work; walking fast; bowling; golfing; and gardening	250 to 350
Strenuous activities, such as: Swimming; playing tennis; running; bicycling; dancing; skiing; and playing football	350 and more

* Page, L., and Fincher, L. J., *Food and Your Weight*. Washington, D.C.: Home and Garden Bulletin No. 74, U.S. Department of Agriculture, 1964, p. 4.

Common activities have been placed in five groups in Table 8–1. The lower level of calories for each group is typical for the average woman, whereas the upper level of calories would more nearly apply to the average man. The figures include the calories for basal metabolism. One can readily see why a typist, classed as sedentary, requires fewer calories than the moderately active homemaker who might also do some gardening in addition to her housework.

Mental effort requires so few calories that it is hardly worth considering. If you are studying and nibbling foods all the while, it is certain that the calories you are consuming are far greater than are needed for your mental effort. Of course, if you are tense or squirm about quite a bit while you study, this would have some effect on increasing your calorie need.

INFLUENCE OF FOOD

The digestion, absorption, and metabolism of food increase the total calorie requirement slightly. It amounts to about 6 per cent of the total calories. This increase is sometimes referred to as *specific dynamic action.*

CALORIE ALLOWANCES

The recommended allowances for a 22-year-old man who weighs 154 pounds and who has average physical activity is 2800 calories. For the 22-year-old woman who weighs 128 pounds and who also has average physical activity, the calorie allowance is 2000. For persons who are lighter or heavier, and for older persons, calorie allowances are recommended in Table 8–2.

The calorie allowances for children are shown in Table 4–1. A rapidly growing infant, preschool and school child, and adolescent boy and girl must have sufficient calories to take care of building new tissues as well as their daily needs for basal metabolism and for voluntary activity. For example, children from six to eight years old require an average of 2000 calories, or as much as the woman of 22 years. Boys between 14 and 18 years need about 3000 calories, which is much more than the 2600 calories needed by a 45-year-old father.

Pregnant women need about 200 additional calories during the last trimester. The woman who nurses her baby needs an additional 1000 calories a day.

Ordinarily, no calorie adjustments need to be made for climate. Most Americans live in well-heated buildings in winter and wear warm clothing. Many people now also work in air-conditioned buildings in the summer.

Meeting Calorie Needs

CALORIE VALUE OF FOODS

In the United States about 45 to 55 per cent of the total calories in the diet come from carbohydrate; 35 to 45 per cent of the calories come from fat; and about 15 per cent of the calories come from protein.

TABLE 8–2   CALORIE ALLOWANCES FOR ADULT INDIVIDUALS OF VARIOUS BODY WEIGHTS AND AGES *

(At a mean environmental temperature of 20°C, assuming light physical activity)

Body Weight kg	lb	Resting Metabolism for Men † (age 22)	Men Total Calories		
			25 years	45 years	65 years
40	88				
45	99				
50	110	1540	2200	2000	1850
55	121	1620	2350	2150	1950
58	128				
60	132	1720	2500	2300	2100
65	143	1820	2650	2400	2200
70	154	1880	2800	2600	2400
75	165	1970	2950	2700	2500
80	176	2020	3050	2800	2600
85	187	2110	3200	2950	2700
90	198	2210	3350	3100	2800
95	209	2290	3500	3200	2900
100	220	2380	3700	3400	3100

* Adapted from Table 3 in *Recommended Dietary Allowances*, 7th ed. Pub. 1694. Washington, D.C.: National Academy of Sciences, National Research Council, 1968, p. 5.
† Resting metabolic rate is approximately 10 per cent above the metabolic rate measured under basal conditions.

The caloric value of many foods is given in Table A–1 of the Appendix. If you will examine this table you will find that you could draw some general conclusions about the caloric value of food groups. Some foods contain much water and some fiber and are low in calories. Vegetables and fruits, as a class, are in this group. The variation in calories between a tomato, for example, and a sweet potato lies in the much greater carbohydrate content of the sweet potato. Fresh fruits are much lower in calories than canned or frozen fruits, which have been packed in syrup.

Many foods contain little water but appreciable amounts of carbo-hydrate: flour, cereal foods, bread, sugar, candy, jellies, and others. Weight for weight these foods rank much higher in calories than vegetables and fruits.

The highest concentration of calories occurs in foods that contain much fat. Lean meat, poultry, and fish are moderate in calorie content, but fatty meats and fish are high in calories. Oils, butter, margarine, cooking fats, and cream are concentrated sources of calories because of their high fat content.

Many cooked foods are higher in calories because of the ingredients used and the method of preparation. Cakes, cookies, pies, and pastries contain much flour, sugar, shortening, eggs, and milk, and are, of course,

Resting Metabolism for Women † (age 22)	Women Total Calories			Body Weight	
	25 years	45 years	65 years	kg	lb
1280	1550	1450	1300	40	88
1380	1700	1550	1450	45	99
1460	1800	1650	1500	50	110
1560	1950	1800	1650	55	121
1620	2000	1850	1700	58	128
1640	2050	1900	1700	60	132
1740	2200	2000	1850	65	143
1830	2300	2100	1950	70	154
				75	165
				80	176
				85	187
				90	198
				95	209
				100	220

high in calories. A piece of lean meat may be only moderately high in calories if it is broiled, but if it is dipped in egg, crumbs, and then fried, the calorie value could be twice as high. Deep-fat fried foods are, gen-erally speaking, high in calories.

CALORIE FALLACIES AND FACTS

1. *Fallacy.* Potatoes, bread, meat, and milk are fattening. Grapefruit is not fattening.

Facts. No single food can be called fattening or nonfattening. A calorie from one food is the same as a calorie from another food. Some foods provide more calories than others. One becomes fat only if the total calorie intake is greater than the calorie expenditure of the body.

2. *Fallacy.* Boiled potatoes are more fattening than baked potatoes.

Facts. Potatoes of the same weight will have the same number of calories whether boiled or baked. The "hidden" calories in the form of butter or cream would rapidly increase the number of calories.

3. *Fallacy.* Margarine has fewer calories than butter.

Facts. One tablespoon of margarine or of butter contains 100 calories and equal amounts of fat and vitamin A. One tablespoon of whipped margarine will have somewhat less calories because air has been beaten in and the volume is greater; but gram for gram, or pound for pound, whipped margarine would be equal to regular margarine or butter in calories.

4. *Fallacy.* Toast has fewer calories than bread.

Facts. A slice of bread loses some weight when it is toasted because it dries out. The calorie content of that slice of bread does not change with toasting.

CALORIE VALUE OF THE BASIC DIET

The minimum number of servings of the Four Food Groups supplies a little more than half of the calorie needs of the average woman. Note in Figure 8–1 that the milk and meat groups are roughly equal in their

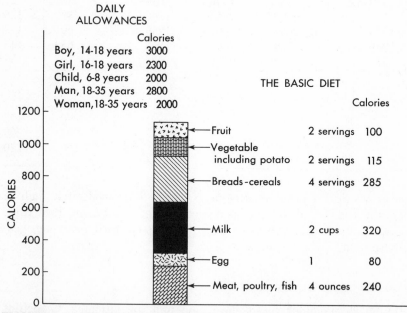

FIGURE 8–1 The Basic Diet furnishes a little more than half of the energy requirements for girls and women. The full energy requirement is met by eating additional foods from the Four Food Groups and by including fats and sugar. See Table 4–2 for complete calculation.

calorie contribution; likewise, the vegetable-fruit group and the bread-cereal group are about equal in their contribution.

CALORIE BALANCE AND BODY WEIGHT

For the adult the best guide to the calorie requirement is the body weight. If the amount of energy needed by the body is less than the amount of energy supplied by the diet, the extra energy will be stored as fat, and the individual will gain weight. This is the problem that many men and women face. On the other hand, insufficient energy in the diet to meet body needs means that the adipose tissue will be used up, and thus weight is lost.

The adult in good health and who has a desirable body weight should aim to keep his weight constant. If people will weigh themselves regularly and will learn to avoid many hidden calories, to refuse second servings, to select low-calorie snacks, and to engage in a regular program of exercise, the maintenance of weight is not difficult. If a pound is gained, the effort should be made to lose it promptly so that there is no accumulation from month to month and year to year. (See also Chap. 21.)

REVIEW QUESTIONS AND PROBLEMS

1. What is meant by a calorie? What is a bomb calorimeter?

2. What is measured when a person is having a basal metabolism test? What conditions are necessary for such a test? What would be your approximate basal metabolism?

3. List ten foods you especially like. Without looking up the calorie values, which would you rate as high in calories? Check your classification with the actual calorie values in Table A–1 of the Appendix.

4. Keep a record of your food intake for one day. Calculate the calorie value of these foods. Does the total compare with the allowance stated for you in Table 8–2?

5. Keep a record of your activities for 24 hours. Classify these activities according to the groups in Table 8–1 and calculate your approximate calorie expenditure. For each hour of sleep assume that you need 0.4 calorie per pound of body weight.

6. What is the best guide for determining whether you are obtaining your calorie requirement?

REFERENCES

Leverton, R. M. *Food Becomes You*, 3rd ed. Ames, Iowa: Iowa State University Press, 1965, Chaps. 4 and 5.

Page, L., and Fincher, L. J. *Food and Your Weight*. Home and Garden Bulletin No. 74. Washington, D.C.: U.S. Department of Agriculture, 1964.

Robinson, C. H. *Proudfit-Robinson's Normal and Therapeutic Nutrition*, 13th ed. New York: The Macmillan Company, 1967, Chap. 8.

WATER AND MINERAL ELEMENTS

Next to oxygen, water is most immediately important for life. We can survive, at best, for only a few days without water; persons who have been lost in the desert have sometimes perished within 24 hours. The body fluids contain precise amounts of a number of mineral elements combined as *salts*. The maintenance of delicate balances of fluids and the concentrations of the mineral elements in them is essential for numerous functions that will be mentioned in this chapter. It is appropriate that water and mineral elements be considered together.

Water

DISTRIBUTION

About two thirds of the total body weight is made up of water. The proportion varies somewhat, with fat persons having less body water than lean persons. Infants and young children have more body water than older persons.

About three fourths of the water in the body is within the cells; this is referred to as *intracellular* fluid. The remaining water is in the blood and lymph circulation and in the fluids around the cells and tissues. This is called *extracellular* fluid.

FUNCTIONS

Every cell in the body contains water. Muscle tissue contains as much as 80 per cent, fat tissue about 20 per cent, and bone about 25 per cent water.

Water is the solvent for materials within the body. The foods we eat are digested by enzymes in an abundance of digestive juices; the nutrients are carried in solution across the intestinal wall; the blood transports nutrients to all body tissues; materials dissolved in water are transported across the cell membranes; chemical reactions take place in the presence of water; and body wastes are carried by the blood for elimination by the kidneys, lungs, skin, and bowel.

Water is also a lubricant, for it avoids friction between moving body parts. Water regulates the body temperature through its evaporation from the skin, thus giving a cooling effect. On very humid days we feel uncomfortable because water does not evaporate very readily.

NORMAL WATER LOSSES

Water is lost from the body through the kidneys, skin, lungs, and bowel. Usually, most of the water is lost in the urine. The amount of urine is related to the daily intake of water and other fluids, and varies from about 500 to 2000 ml. Because the nitrogenous and other materials must be kept in solution, about 500 ml urine is the minimum excretion.

An appreciable amount of water is lost through the skin by *insensible* and *visible* perspiration. Insensible perspiration is so called because one is not aware of it; it evaporates as rapidly as it is formed. On the other hand, with vigorous activity, especially in warm weather, we lose much additional water through visible perspiration. A baseball player, for example, might lose 3 to 5 qt of fluid through perspiration. Appreciable amounts of urea, salts, and traces of other mineral elements are also lost in the visible perspiration. When we perspire a great deal, the urine volume is reduced.

The adult loses about 350 ml water in the air exhaled through the lungs. The amount of water lost in the feces is small, averaging about 100 to 150 ml daily.

WATER REQUIREMENT

The daily water requirement is about 1 ml per calorie; thus a caloric requirement of 2000 necessitates a water intake of 2000 ml. Infants have proportionately greater water losses, and should be allowed about 150 ml (5 oz) water for each 100 calories. Thirst is a good guide for adequate fluid intake, except for sick persons and for infants.

SOURCES OF WATER

The fluids we drink account for the chief intake of water. There is no harm in drinking water with meals provided it is not used to wash foods down without chewing them.

Foods contribute a fair amount of water, as may be seen from Table 9–1.

TABLE 9–1   WATER CONTENT OF FOODS

	Water Per Cent		Water Per Cent
Milk	87	Fruits and vegetables	70–95
Egg	74	Bread	35
Cooked meat, poultry, fish		Dry cereals, crackers	3–7
Well done	40–50	Cooked cereals	60–85
Medium to rare	50–70	Nuts, fats, sweets	0–10
Cheese, hard	35–40		

Water also results from the oxidation of carbohydrates, fats, and proteins. The amount of water produced in the body from metabolism is about 300 to 450 ml daily.

WATER BALANCE

Ordinarily the water sources to the body and the water losses from the body are in balance, as the following example shows:

Sources of Water		Losses of Water	
Water, tea, coffee	1100	Urine	1200
Milk (2 cups)	420	Feces	100
"Solid" foods	480	Skin and lungs	1000
Metabolic water	300		——
	——		2300
	2300		

Dehydration results when the intake is less than the body needs. This can occur when, for some reason, there is no food or fluid intake, or when the losses from the body are abnormally high: excessive perspiration because of marked activity in hot weather; severe diarrhea; vomiting; fever with increased losses through the skin; hemorrhage; severe burns with the accompanying water losses from the skin; uncontrolled diabetes with frequent urination. Dehydration is a serious medical problem requiring prompt attention. Fluids are given by mouth when possible; intravenous fluids are given when the patient is unable to take sufficient fluid by mouth.

Edema is the accumulation of water in the body. It may occur when the body is unable to excrete sodium in sufficient amounts. This is not unusual in diseases of the heart, when the circulation is impaired, or when the kidneys are unable to excrete wastes normally. Edema also occurs following prolonged protein deficiency, because the tissues are no longer able to maintain normal water balance.

Mineral Elements

NATURE AND DISTRIBUTION

Mineral elements are inorganic substances, as contrasted to such organic compounds as proteins, fats, and carbohydrates. The mineral elements do not exist as such in foods, but are combined in salts; for example, sodium chloride, or table salt. They may be combined with organic compounds; for example, iron in hemoglobin and sulfur in almost all proteins. Unlike carbohydrates, fats, and proteins, mineral elements cannot be used for energy. They are found in all body tissues and fluids.

It is often said that valuable things come in small packages. About 15 or more mineral elements account for only 4 per cent of the body weight. They vary in amount from calcium, which alone accounts for one half of all mineral matter in the body, to iodine, of which only $\frac{1}{1000}$ ounce is in the body, to cobalt, which in traces is not readily measured. Yet the absence of any one of these elements can cause serious problems. An excess of some of them can be toxic.

Table 9–2 provides a summary of the kinds and average amounts of mineral elements in the body. The *major* elements are those that occur in the largest amounts, whereas *trace* elements are found in very small amounts indeed.

FOOD CHOICES FOR MINERAL ELEMENTS

If one burns a sample of food, the mineral matter or ash remains. The ash can be analyzed for the kinds and amounts of each mineral element present. Tables of food composition show the values for various elements found in foods. You should become thoroughly familiar with the dietary sources of calcium and iron. Recommended servings from the Four Food Groups furnish sufficient amounts of all the minerals needed by humans, except possibly iron, iodine, and fluorine. Sources of these elements will be discussed later in this chapter. Usually, only calcium and iron need to be calculated for normal diets. Occasionally, calculations are made for

TABLE 9–2   MINERAL ELEMENTS IN THE ADULT BODY *

	Per Cent of Body Weight	Man 154 lb gm	Principal Locations in Body
Major elements			
Calcium (Ca)	1.5–2.2	1050–1540	99% in bones and teeth
Phosphorus (P)	0.8–1.2	560– 840	80–90% in bones, teeth
Potassium (K)	0.35	245	Fluid inside cells
Sulfur (S)	0.25	175	Associated with protein
Chlorine (Cl)	0.15	105	Fluid outside cells
Sodium (Na)	0.15	105	Fluid outside cells
Magnesium (Mg)	0.05	35	70% in bones and teeth
Trace elements			
Iron (Fe)	0.004	2.8	Chiefly in hemoglobin; stores in liver and other organs
Manganese (Mn)	0.0003	0.21	
Copper (Cu)	0.00015	0.11	
Iodine (I)	0.00004	0.02	Thyroid gland
Fluorine (F)			Bones and teeth
Zinc (Zn)			
Molybdenum (Mo)			
Selenium (Se)			
Cobalt (Co)			Part of vitamin B_{12} molecule
Chromium (Cr)			

Present but not known to be essential: aluminum, arsenic, barium, boron, bromine, lead, nickel, silicon, strontium

* Calculations based on elementary composition of the body as stated by H. C. Sherman, *Chemistry of Food and Nutrition*, 8th ed. (New York: The Macmillan Company, 1952), p. 227.

other mineral elements in certain therapeutic diets, for example, sodium-restricted diets. (See Chap. 25.)

GENERAL FUNCTIONS

For convenience mineral elements are often discussed separately. However, within the body they function together in building body tissues and in the regulation of body metabolism. Some of the important ways in which mineral elements function together are discussed below. Specific functions will also be listed under the headings for each element.

Bone formation. Bone consists of a soft, pliable, but tough protein material into which minerals are deposited. Most of the calcium, phosphorus, and magnesium, and smaller amounts of other mineral elements, are deposited in the bones and teeth. During the last two months of pregnancy most of the ossification of the bones of the fetus occurs. The infant at birth has a well-formed skeleton, but the bones are still quite soft. Throughout childhood, adolescence, and into the early twenties the bones continue to harden as well as to grow in length and in diameter. The individual who has ample calcium, phosphorus, and protein in his diet during the growing years will be taller than the one who is poorly nourished.

As well as providing the framework for the body, bones serve as a storehouse for the mineral elements they contain. They are never fixed for life. The blood can withdraw mineral elements from the bone according to the daily soft-tissue and fluid needs of the body. These withdrawals are ordinarily replaced from the diet. However, an individual who has a poor diet for a long time may have very weak, thin bones because of the day-to-day withdrawals. As much as 10 to 40 per cent of the calcium can be removed from the bones before it will show up on x-ray.

Tooth formation. Teeth, like bones, contain a ground substance of protein. The tooth enamel and dentine are hard substances containing appreciable amounts of calcium and phosphorus. The first teeth form in the fetus at the fourth to sixth week of pregnancy and begin to calcify by the twentieth week. The permanent teeth calcify soon after birth up to about three years of age. Wisdom teeth may calcify as late as eight to ten years of age. The teeth are fully mineralized before they erupt. A decayed tooth cannot repair itself, so that proper care of the teeth once they have erupted is vital.

Soft tissues contain many mineral elements in their structure, including potassium, sulfur, phosphorus, iron, and others. In fact, every cell in the body contains iron and phosphorus as part of its structure.

Nerve irritability and muscle contraction. Body fluids contain exact amounts of sodium, potassium, calcium, and magnesium. These elements control the passage of materials into and out of the cell. They regulate the transmission of the nerve impulses and the contraction of muscles. If, for example, the amount of calcium is lowered, the individual might have twitching and cramping of the muscles and convulsions, and the rhythm of the heart might be affected. This condition is known as tetany. Potassium in too small or great concentration will also affect the contraction of the muscles and the work of the heart.

Water balance. The balance of fluid between the inside and the outside of each cell depends upon the correct concentrations of sodium and potassium. Sodium occurs primarily in the extracellular fluid, and potassium is found chiefly in the intracellular fluid. These balances are upset in edema or dehydration. (See pp. 77, 78.)

Acid-base balance. In chemistry *pH* is used to express the degree of acidity or alkalinity. A pH of 7 is neutral; a pH below 7 indicates acidity; a pH above 7 indicates alkalinity. The pH of the blood normally ranges between 7.3 and 7.5; thus the blood is slightly alkaline.

The body maintains a relatively constant pH at all times. Mineral elements, especially sodium and phosphate compounds, contribute to the maintenance of the normal pH of the blood. They are not the only means for controlling acid-base balance.

Some foods are potentially *alkali-producing* because they contain important amounts of calcium, sodium, potassium, and magnesium. Other foods are *acid-producing* because they contain greater amounts of sulfur, chlorine, and phosphorus than they do of the alkali-producing elements. Still other foods are low in mineral elements and are considered to be neutral.

Acid-producing: meat, poultry, fish, eggs, cheese, legumes, cereal foods, corn, almonds, chestnuts, coconut, prunes, plums, cranberries
Alkali-producing: fruits, vegetables, milk, peanuts, walnuts, Brazil nuts
Neutral: butter, margarine, oils, cooking fats, sugar, syrup, starch, tapioca

The individual who eats a normal diet need have no concern about whether his diet is acid or alkaline. The kidneys, lungs, skin, and various mechanisms in the blood all assist in the regulation of acid-base balance. Only in disease conditions when the food intake is inadequate, or the kidney is failing, or the water balance is upset, is there a concern about acid-base balance. These are medical problems beyond the scope of this text.

Other regulatory functions. Mineral elements function in numerous ways to regulate metabolism. Some of them activate enzymes. Many enzymes, hormones, vitamins, and other compounds contain minute amounts of mineral elements in their molecules.

CALCIUM

Functions. About 99 per cent of the body calcium is found in the bones and teeth where it is combined with phosphorus and other elements to give rigidity to the skeleton. The bones also serve as the storehouse for calcium needed for a number of cellular functions. Calcium is required for the complex process of blood coagulation. Together with other elements it regulates the passage of materials into and out of cells; controls the transmission of nerve messages; and brings about the normal contraction of muscles, including the heart.

Utilization. Calcium absorption from the gastrointestinal tract is regulated according to the body needs for maintenance and growth. A child who is growing rapidly would therefore absorb a greater proportion of the calcium in his diet than the adult who simply needs to maintain the proper levels of calcium in the bones and soft tissues. The average daily absorption is about 30 to 40 per cent.

Since calcium salts are more soluble in acid solution, most of the absorption takes place from the upper small intestine. Vitamin D is essential for efficient absorption. Lactose from milk also improves the uptake of calcium.

The parathyroid hormone governs the correct amount of calcium in the blood. When the blood level of calcium is low, calcium is removed from the bones. When the blood level goes up, calcium is deposited in the bones or is excreted in the urine. Vitamin D is also essential for the normal deposit of calcium and phosphorus in the bones and teeth.

Calcium is excreted in the feces and the urine. Much of the calcium in the feces comes from the insoluble salts that could not be absorbed.

Daily allowances. The calcium allowance for adults throughout life is 800 mg. During periods of rapid growth in boys and girls and during pregnancy and lactation the calcium allowances are about 50 per cent higher. (See Table 4–1, p. 31.)

Food sources. Any kind of milk—fresh whole, skim, evaporated, dry, or buttermilk—is an equally good source of calcium. Hard cheeses such as American and Swiss are excellent. You would need to eat quite a bit of ice cream or cottage cheese to get the same amount of calcium as that in one cup of milk. Cream cheese and butter, although dairy products, are not sources of calcium. (See Fig. 9–1.)

Kale, turnip greens, mustard greens, and collards are good sources of calcium. Broccoli, cabbage, and cauliflower rate as fair sources. Such other greens as spinach, chard, and beet greens contain oxalic acid, which combines with calcium in the intestines to form an insoluble salt. This insoluble compound cannot be absorbed into the blood. Therefore, these greens should not be counted on for calcium, but they do not affect the utilization of calcium from other foods.

Among the fruits oranges contribute some calcium, although oranges cannot take the place of milk. Canned salmon is a fairly good source of calcium if the tiny bones are eaten. Clams, oysters, lobster, dried beans, and peas are moderate sources, but these foods are not eaten often enough to make an appreciable contribution. (See Fig. 9–2.)

Deficiency. Calcium deficiency becomes evident only after years of inadequate intake. Therefore, an adequate diet becomes a kind of insurance against future problems. Osteoporosis is a frequent bone disease observed principally in older women. The posture is poor, the bone mass is reduced, the bones break readily, and healing is slow. The causes of the condition are complex, but nonmilk drinkers are more frequently susceptible than those who drink milk throughout life.

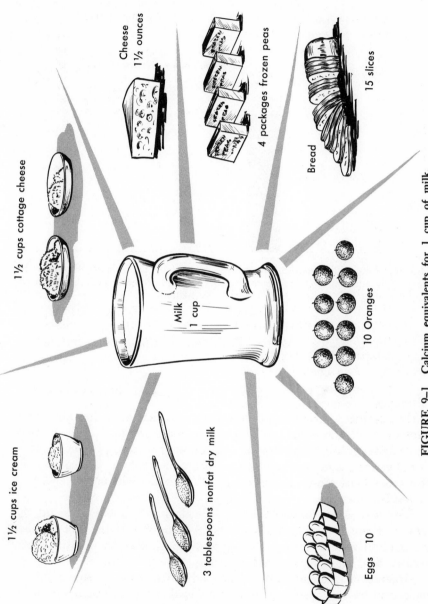

Cheese
1½ ounces

4 packages frozen peas

Bread

15 slices

1½ cups cottage cheese

Milk
1 cup

10 Oranges

1½ cups ice cream

3 tablespoons nonfat dry milk

Eggs   10

FIGURE 9–1   Calcium equivalents for 1 cup of milk.

83

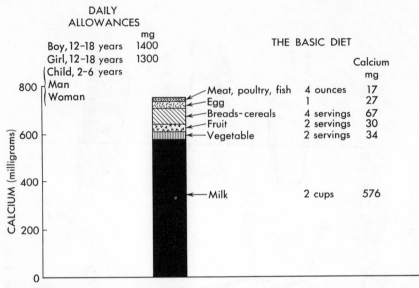

DAILY
ALLOWANCES
mg
Boy, 12–18 years   1400
Girl, 12–18 years   1300
Child, 2–6 years
Man
Woman

THE BASIC DIET

		Calcium mg
Meat, poultry, fish	4 ounces	17
Egg	1	27
Breads-cereals	4 servings	67
Fruit	2 servings	30
Vegetable	2 servings	34
Milk	2 cups	576

CALCIUM (milligrams)

FIGURE 9–2 Milk furnishes about three fourths of the calcium allowance for adults. The addition of 1 to 2 cups for boys and girls supplies their greater needs during growth. See Table 4–2 for complete calculation.

Rickets, infrequently seen in infants and toddlers in the United States, is a deficiency related to vitamin D, calcium, and phosphorus metabolism. (See Chap. 10.)

PHOSPHORUS, MAGNESIUM, SODIUM, AND POTASSIUM

Phosphorus. Probably no mineral element has more functions than phosphorus. It is essential for (1) building bones and teeth, (2) phospholipids that regulate the absorption and transport of fats, (3) nucleic acids of all cells, (4) enzymes involved in energy metabolism, (5) compounds that bring about muscle contraction, and (6) buffer salts in the regulation of acid-base balance.

The phosphorus allowances for individuals of various ages are the same as those for calcium. (See Table 4–1, p. 31.) If the diet supplies enough calcium and protein, it will furnish enough phosphorus. Milk, meat, poultry, fish, egg yolk, legumes, and nuts are rich sources.

Magnesium. About half of the body magnesium is found in the bones and teeth. Together with other mineral elements, magnesium regulates nervous irritability and muscle contraction. Magnesium activates many enzymes including those involved in energy metabolism. Like calcium, the salts of magnesium are rather insoluble, and much of the dietary magnesium is not absorbed. Most absorption occurs from the upper gastrointestinal tract.

The adult allowance for magnesium is 300 to 350 mg per day. Magnesium is a constituent of the chlorophyll of plants; so one would expect green leaves to be rich in this mineral element. Nuts, cereal grains, and seafoods are especially rich in magnesium. Recommended amounts of the Four Food Groups will furnish the daily needs.

Dietary deficiency of magnesium is not likely. However, some disease states give rise to symptoms of deficiency. Patients with diabetic acidosis, chronic alcoholism, kwashiorkor, and severe malabsorption diseases sometimes show the characteristic symptoms of tremor and nervous irritability.

Sodium is found principally in the extracellular fluid. It helps to maintain the fluid and acid-base balance of the body.

Sodium in the diet is almost completely absorbed from the gastrointestinal tract. Any excess is rapidly excreted in the urine. A person who is perspiring heavily will also lose much sodium through the skin. The amount of sodium that is excreted is regulated by adrenal hormones that exert their control over the kidneys. When the sodium intake is high, the excretion of the kidneys is increased; but if the body stores of sodium, or the dietary supply, are low, only traces of sodium will be excreted by the kidneys.

No recommendations have been made for the daily sodium requirement. The daily diet provides far more than is needed, chiefly from salt used in cooking and at the table. Other sodium compounds used in food processing and preparation—baking powder and baking soda, for example—are also important sources. Milk, meat, poultry, fish, and eggs are well supplied with sodium.

When the kidney or heart is not functioning normally, sodium may accumulate in the tissues and water will also be held (edema). The need for diets restricted in sodium is fully discussed in Chapter 25. Dietary deficiency of sodium does not occur. However, excessive perspiration, severe vomiting or diarrhea, or diseases of the adrenal gland may lead to depletion of body sodium.

Potassium. Just as sodium is the principal mineral element in fluids surrounding the cells, so potassium is the principal mineral element within the cell. Potassium is essential for the synthesis of proteins, for enzyme functions within the cells, and for maintenance of the fluid balance. A small amount of potassium is also found in the extracellular fluid, and aids in the regulation of muscle contraction and nervous irritability.

No recommendation has been made for the daily intake of potassium. Most foods supply liberal amounts and dietary deficiency does not occur.

Problems of potassium deficiency are sometimes seen following severe vomiting and diarrhea and diabetic acidosis. Excessive potassium is a problem in renal failure.

IRON

Functions. The amount of iron in the body is about 3 to 5 gm. Most of the body iron is found in hemoglobin, the red-colored compound consisting of the iron-containing *heme* and a protein called *globin.* Copper is required for its synthesis. *Myoglobin,* which is similar to hemoglobin, is found in muscle tissue. It holds oxygen in the cell until it is needed for muscle contraction. A number of enzymes contain iron as part of the molecule.

Utilization. Iron salts are relatively insoluble and the amount absorbed from the gastrointestinal tract varies widely. The amount absorbed depends upon the body's need for iron. The well-nourished adult may absorb only 10 to 20 per cent of the iron in the diet, but larger percentages are absorbed by children during rapid growth periods and by people who have anemia.

Iron salts are more soluble in acid so most of the absorption takes place from the upper part of the small intestine. Vitamin C improves the absorption of iron. The iron in animal foods is probably absorbed somewhat better than that from plant foods.

Iron is used very economically by the body. When the red blood cells are destroyed after their normal life-span of about 120 days, the hemoglobin is broken down. The iron that is released is used over and over again. Small daily losses amounting to about 1.0 mg do occur in the urine and from the skin. On the average, the menstrual losses account for 15 to 30 mg per month or 0.5 to 1.0 mg per day.

Daily allowances. The well-nourished woman should receive 18 mg iron per day, whereas the healthy man needs 10 mg. Infants and children need liberal amounts of iron to take care of the expanding blood circulation as they grow. (See Table 4–1, p. 31.)

Food sources. Foods in the meat group are all good sources of iron, any kind of liver or organ meat being especially rich. (See Fig. 9–3.) Oysters and clams are rich in iron, but other seafoods are somewhat lower than meat. Egg yolk is an excellent source of iron, but egg white contains only traces. Legumes and nuts are fairly rich in iron. When dry beans are baked with molasses, the iron contribution is good.

Dark-green leafy vegetables of all kinds are especially rich in iron. Fruits are fair contributors. Dried prunes, apricots, peaches, and raisins are rich in iron, but again their infrequent use means that the daily diet is not importantly affected.

The enrichment program for flours, breads, and cereals has had a significant effect on the iron intake during the last 25 years (see p. 59). Of the foods not included in the Four Food Groups, dark molasses is the only good source of iron, although it is used infrequently. Molasses in gingerbread or in baked beans, or the addition of one tablespoon molasses

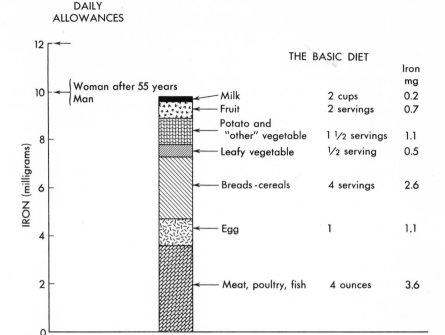

FIGURE 9-3 The Basic Diet supplies sufficient iron for the adult male. For women and children, additional foods from the meat, vegetable-fruit, and bread-cereal group are necessary to meet the iron allowance. See Table 4-2 for complete calculation.

to milk (some children like this for variety), can make an important contribution to the iron intake.

From Figure 9-3 it becomes evident that the Basic Diet including recommended amounts of the Four Food Groups does not furnish enough iron for the girl or woman. In fact, typical American diets that are adequate in all other nutrients furnish about 6 mg iron per 1000 calories. The Food and Nutrition Board has stated that fortification of the food supply with iron is desirable.

Deficiency.   Iron-deficiency anemia is believed to be widespread in the United States, most especially in infants and in young women. Such anemia is considered to result from diets which have long been deficient in iron. Anemia can also result from hemorrhage following an accident or surgery or from chronic blood loss as from a bleeding ulcer.

In an anemia the blood is unable to supply the full oxygen needs of the tissues. With even a little physical effort the person becomes very tired, looks pale, and may have a poor resistance to infection. When anemia is suspected, the diagnosis should be made by a physician because there are many kinds of anemia and likewise a variety of causes. Iron-deficiency anemia is most effectively treated with iron salts and an adequate diet.

High-iron diets are impractical, since it is very difficult to obtain dietary intakes of more than 15 to 20 mg. Such levels would not appreciably treat the anemia.

IODINE

Iodine is a trace element stored chiefly in the thyroid gland. It is an essential constituent of two hormones, thyroxine and triiodothyronine, that regulate energy metabolism.

The adult allowance for iodine ranges from 100 to 140 µg. Foods grown along the seacoast, salt water fish, and shellfish are good sources. With the wide distribution of foods all over the country, people cannot be certain that the foods they eat are good sources of iodine. Therefore, the most reliable source is iodized salt.

When there is a lack of iodine, the thyroid gland enlarges in an attempt to produce more thyroxine. The condition is called simple or endemic goiter. Aside from detracting from the appearance of the normal neckline, few if any symptoms are detectable in mild deficiency. However, if the condition persists, the woman who has a simple goiter and who fails to get iodine during pregnancy will be unable to supply the fetus; thus the baby is more severely affected than she was. When the deficiency is severe, growth is retarded and the mentality is dulled.

Recent studies show that more people in the United States have simple goiter than was true some years ago. Continuing emphasis must be given to the use of iodized salt. Endemic goiter is still a major problem in some Central and South American countries, Asia, and Africa. In some areas the most severe form of deficiency is seen, namely, *cretinism*. A cretin is stunted in growth and does not progress in mentality beyond the early preschool years.

FLUORINE

Fluorine exists in the body in compounds called fluorides. Minute traces of fluoride are decidedly beneficial in protecting the teeth from decay. They may also be useful in maintaining the bone structure. To be of most value, fluorides must be supplied to the young child before the permanent teeth have erupted. In communities where fluoridation of the water supply has been used for some years, tooth decay has decreased up to 50 per cent or more.

Fluoride is best provided in the water supply. In a few communities the natural content in water is sufficient to protect the teeth. Many major cities and hundreds of smaller communities now add 1 part fluoride to 1 million parts water (about 1 mg per quart). This inexpensive, safe, and effective public health measure for protection of the teeth deserves the fullest public support.

In some parts of the world natural supplies of drinking water contain excessive amounts of fluoride (over 1.5 parts per million of water). People who live in these areas have *mottled* teeth; that is, their teeth have a chalky white appearance, and later become discolored. Such teeth are resistant to decay, and no signs of other health changes have been found in these people.

OTHER TRACE ELEMENTS

A number of trace elements function primarily as parts of enzyme or vitamin molecules, or as catalysts for chemical reactions. They include:

Chromium: involved in carbohydrate metabolism
Cobalt: a constituent of vitamin B_{12}
Copper: a catalyst for hemoglobin formation
Manganese: enzyme systems; normal bone structure; blood formation
Molybdenum: enzyme systems
Selenium: related to activity of vitamin E
Zinc: a constituent of insulin and some enzymes

The amounts of these elements required by the body are not known, but at any rate they are very small. The mixed diet supplying adequate amounts of other nutrients will furnish sufficient amounts of these elements.

SOME FALLACIES AND FACTS

1. *Fallacy.* A diet low in calcium leads to nervousness.

Fact. When the diet is inadequate, calcium is readily withdrawn from the bones to supply the minute amounts needed to regulate the response of the nerves. There is no evidence that a low-calcium intake leads to nervousness.

2. *Fallacy.* Grapefruit, oranges, and peaches cause an "acid" stomach.

Fact. Most fruits contain organic acids that account for their acid taste. These acids are weak and they do not increase the acidity of the stomach. The stomach contents are normally acid because of the presence of hydrochloric acid, a strong acid that is useful in the digestive process. The organic acids of fruits are completely oxidized in a manner similar to carbohydrates.

3. *Fallacy.* Cocoa and chocolate interfere with the absorption of calcium.

Fact. The amounts of cocoa and chocolate normally eaten do not interfere with the absorption of calcium. Although they contain some oxalic acid, one would need to eat abnormally large amounts of chocolate and cocoa to have any noticeable effect. Hot cocoa, chocolate pudding, and chocolate milk are quite appropriate in the menus of children as well as adults. However, the child should not be given these foods so often that he refuses to take regular milk.

4. *Fallacy.* Foods purchased in American markets are likely to be lacking in important trace elements.

Fact. The wide variety of foods used in the diet supplies ample amounts of all trace elements known to be needed except iodine and fluorine. See discussion on pages 88 and 89. Farmers use chemical and organic fertilizers in order to realize high yields of foods that are excellent in nutritive quality. Present-day techniques of food processing retain most of the nutritive values.

TABLE 9–3 SUMMARY OF MINERAL ELEMENTS

Element	Function	Utilization	Daily Allowances Food Sources
Calcium	99% in bones, teeth Nervous stimulation Muscle contraction Blood clotting Activates enzymes	About 40% absorbed Aided by vitamin D and lactose; hindered by oxalic acid Parathyroid hormone regulates blood levels	RDA, adults: 800 mg Milk, cheese, ice cream Mustard and turnip greens Cabbage, broccoli Clams, oysters, salmon
Phosphorus	80–90% in bones, teeth Acid-base balance Transport of fats Enzymes for energy metabolism	Vitamin D favors absorption and use by bones Dietary deficiency unlikely	RDA, adults: 800 mg Milk, cheese, ice cream Meat, poultry, fish Whole-grain cereals, nuts, legumes
Magnesium	50% in bones, teeth Transmit nerve impulses Muscle contraction Enzymes for energy metabolism	Salts relatively insoluble Acid favors absorption Dietary deficiency unlikely	RDA, adults: 300–350 mg
Sodium	Extracellular fluid Water balance Acid-base balance Nervous stimulation Muscle contraction	Almost completely absorbed Body levels regulated by adrenal; excess excreted in urine and by skin	No recommended intake Table salt Baking powder, soda Milk, meat, poultry, fish, eggs
Potassium	Intracellular fluid Protein synthesis Water balance Transmit nerve impulse Muscle contraction	Almost completely absorbed Body levels regulated by adrenal; excess excreted in urine	No recommended intake Ample amounts in meat, cereals, fruits, fruit juices, vegetable

Element	Function	Utilization	Daily Allowances Food Sources
Iron	Mostly in hemoglobin Muscle myoglobin Oxidizing enzymes	10–20% absorption Acid and vitamin C aid absorption Daily losses in urine and feces Menstrual losses Anemia is common	RDA, men: 10 mg women: 18 mg Organ meats, meat, fish, poultry, eggs Whole-grain and enriched cereal Green vegetables; dried fruits
Iodine	Form thyroxine for energy metabolism	Chiefly in thyroid gland Deficiency leads to endemic goiter	RDA: 100–140 ug Iodized salt Shellfish, saltwater fish
Fluorine	Prevent tooth decay		Fluoridated water

REVIEW QUESTIONS AND PROBLEMS

1. Define these terms: insensible perspiration, water balance, ossification, pH, osteoporosis, fluoridation, cretinism.

2. List the ways in which water assists in making the nutrients of food available to the cells of the body.

3. Record your fluid intake for one day. Include water, tea, coffee, soft drinks, milk, fruit juices, and soup.

4. What reasons might account for edema? For dehydration?

5. Which mineral elements are listed in the Recommended Dietary Allowances? What are your daily allowances? How do these compare with those of a 14-year-old girl?

6. What other mineral elements are known to be essential for human nutrition? Why are there no allowances listed in the table of Recommended Dietary Allowances?

7. What is meant by intracellular fluid? By extracellular fluid? What mineral elements would you expect to find in each?

8. What mineral elements are especially important for each of the following: building hemoglobin; construction of bones and teeth; function of the thyroid gland; maintenance of water balance; release of energy from fats, carbohydrates, and proteins.

9. A woman patient asks you why it is important to drink milk. What would you tell her?

10. Write a menu for one day, including foods from the Four Food Groups. Do not use liver. Calculate the iron content of your menu. Adjust the menu so that it includes 18 mg iron.

11. What is meant by anemia? What lack in the diet may cause it?

12. Of what importance is fluorine? How is it best supplied?

13. List three acid-producing foods; three alkali-producing foods.

REFERENCES

Carlisle, N. "Water, Thirst, and Your Health," *Today's Health*, **40**:26, August 1962.

Council on Foods and Nutrition. "Iron Deficiency in the United States," *J. Amer. Med. Ass.*, **203**:119, 1968.

Goulding, P. C. "Why Doctors Vote Yes to Fluoridation," *Today's Health*, **43**:8, October 1965.

Knutson, J. W. "Fluoridation," *Amer. J. Nurs.*, **60**:196, 1960.

Robinson, C. H. *Proudfit-Robinson's Normal and Therapeutic Nutrition*, 13th ed. New York: The Macmillan Company, 1967, Chaps. 9 and 44.

Snively, W. D., Jr., and Brown, B. J. "In the Balance," *Amer. J. Nurs.*, **58**:55, January 1958.

Swanson, P. *Calcium in Nutrition*. Chicago: National Dairy Council, 1963.

VITAMINS: INTRODUCTION AND FAT-SOLUBLE VITAMINS

Introduction to Vitamin Study

Undoubtedly the discovery of vitamins in the twentieth century will go down in history as one of the major factors in the improvement of health of people throughout the world. The fact that these substances in such small amounts affect the course of health in so many ways has also led to widespread abuse of them. Many people, lacking full understanding of how vitamins function, place emphasis upon vitamin intake from one source or another, while ignoring other equally important nutrients. Other people somehow expect that a vitamin pill will solve many nutritional problems. Let us now look at some of the facts concerning vitamins.

DEFINITIONS

Vitamins are chemical compounds of an organic nature that occur in minute quantities in foods and are necessary for life and growth. They do not provide energy, but they facilitate the use of the energy nutrients. Nor are vitamins important constituents of major body structures; yet they regulate the building of such structures. In other words, vitamins function, for the most part, as constituents of enzymes.

Precursors or *provitamins* are compounds that can be changed into the active vitamin.

Avitaminosis means "without vitamins." It denotes a deficiency or lack of sufficient vitamin to carry out normal body functions. Some defi-

93

ciencies are so mild that a diagnosis can be made only by biochemical test of the blood and urine. As deficiencies become more severe, clinical signs typical of the specific vitamin lack begin to appear.

Hypervitaminosis is an excessive accumulation of a vitamin in the body leading to toxic symptoms. Excessive intakes of vitamins A, D, and K can be toxic.

Vitamin *antagonists* or *antivitamins* are substances that interfere with the functioning of a vitamin.

NOMENCLATURE AND MEASUREMENT

Vitamins were initially known by letter names, vitamin A having been identified first. As the nature of vitamins was determined, more appropriate names were adopted. The following list indicates the commonly used names for the fat-soluble and water-soluble vitamins.

Fat-soluble

Vitamin A—precursors are alpha-, beta-, and gamma-carotene and crypto-xanthin

Vitamin D—precursors are 7-dehydrocholesterol in the skin and ergosterol in plant foods; irradiated ergosterol is known as calciferol or viosterol

Vitamin E—alpha tocopherol

Vitamin K—menadione is the synthetic form

Water-soluble

Ascorbic acid—vitamin C

Thiamine—vitamin B_1

Riboflavin—vitamin B_2

Niacin—nicotinic acid, niacinamide; tryptophan is a precursor

Folacin—folic acid; folinic acid is the active form

Vitamin B_{12}—cyanocobalamin, anti-pernicious anemia factor, extrinsic factor

Vitamin B_6—three forms: pyridoxine, pyridoxal, pyridoxamine

Pantothenic acid

Biotin

Choline

Vitamins A, D, and E are measured in international units (I.U.). The unit is based upon the response, such as growth, that a test animal makes when it is fed a standard dose of the vitamin.

Ascorbic acid, choline, thiamine, riboflavin, and niacin values are recorded in milligrams. Vitamin B_{12} values are expressed in micrograms ($1 \ \mu g = \frac{1}{1000}$ mg). Other B-complex vitamin values are sometimes expressed in milligrams and sometimes in micrograms.

MEETING DAILY NEEDS

The recommended allowances for all age-sex categories for three fat-soluble and five water-soluble vitamins are listed in Table 4–1. No recommended allowances have been established for vitamin K, biotin, choline, and pantothenic acid. As you study each of the vitamins, you should refer to the table of allowances so that you become familiar with the range for the various age-sex groupings.

The rapidly growing child needs proportionately more of the vitamins than the mature adult. The recommended allowances in each instance provide a generous margin of safety. The classic deficiency diseases can probably be prevented with half or less of the daily allowances. However, these lower levels would not encourage optimum nutrition.

SELECTION OF FOODS

Values for five vitamins are given for commonly used foods in Table A–1 in the Appendix. Most foods are poor sources of vitamin D and hence no values are published. Analyses have been made for a number of B-complex vitamins not included in Table A–1, but the nurse is rarely required to refer to these data. The diet that supplies sufficient thiamine, riboflavin, and niacin will also furnish enough of the other B factors.

In selecting food sources for vitamins we should keep in mind (1) how much of a given food we would ordinarily eat, (2) how often the food is eaten, and (3) how stable the vitamin may be after processing or cooking. Parsley may be an excellent source of vitamin A, but it will make little difference in the average diet, because it is so often left on the plate or, when eaten, is consumed in such small amounts. A raw fruit might be a good source of ascorbic acid but might contain little of the vitamin after drying or canning.

Wheat germ, dried yeast, and fish-liver oils are rich sources of several vitamins but are generally regarded as dietary supplements rather than basic items of the diet. Liver and other organ meats are outstanding sources of vitamin A and B-complex vitamins; yet their contribution to the diet will be important only if these foods are included on a fairly regular basis—for example, once a week.

STABILITY IN FOODS

Some vitamins are quickly destroyed by heat, light, and oxidizing agents; others are relatively stable. Some vitamins are highly soluble in water; others dissolve in water slowly or not at all. Although the properties of no two vitamins are exactly alike, it is possible to set up practical guides for the care and preparation of foods that will ensure maximum vitamin values. Thus, by preventing losses of vitamin A, ascorbic acid, and thiamine in foods, losses of other vitamins will also be avoided.

Vitamin A is oxidized in air, so that wilted vegetables will contain less of the vitamin than crisp vegetables. Vitamin A is rapidly destroyed in rancid fats, but we are unlikely to eat such spoiled fats. In ordinary cooking procedures vitamin A is not subject to much loss.

Ascorbic acid is the most easily destroyed of the vitamins, and thiamine is almost as easily lost. Both these vitamins are very soluble in water and are easily destroyed by heat or dehydration. The losses are greatly increased in the presence of alkali or traces of copper or iron. Enzymes that are present in raw foods are activated when the food is cut, and hasten the destruction of the vitamins.

Other B-complex vitamins are more stable to processing and cooking procedures than is thiamine. Therefore, if food preparation methods take into account the solubility in water and the effects of temperatures and other agents on the retention of ascorbic acid and thiamine, the retention for other vitamins will be good. Riboflavin is especially sensitive to light, and a bottle of milk that stands for an hour or two in the sun may lose much of its riboflavin. See Chapter 17 for principles of food preparation.

Fat-Soluble Vitamins

VITAMIN A

Function. Vitamin A is important (1) for the normal structure of the bones and teeth; (2) for the maintenance of the epithelium or outer layer of the skin, and the mucous membranes that line the nose and respiratory tract, the mouth and gastrointestinal tract, the eyes, the genito-urinary tract, and the glands of secretion; and (3) for the formation of *visual purple,* which enables the retina of the eye to adapt to dim light.

Bile is essential for the absorption of carotenes from the intestines. Mineral oil can seriously interfere with the absorption of vitamin A; if it is used as a lavative, it should not be taken near mealtimes. The liver stores vitamin A, and well-nourished individuals usually have a sufficient supply to last for several months.

Deficiency. Night blindness (nyctalopia) is a form of vitamin A deficiency sometimes seen in this country. It is experienced when the visual purple is slowly produced in the eye because of lack of vitamin A. The affected person has difficulty in adjusting to the glare of automobile highlights or in trying to find a seat in a darkened theater, for example.

Skin changes and infections caused by lack of vitamin A are rarely seen in the United States, but are fairly prevalent in the Far East. With the lack of the vitamin the skin becomes *keratinized* (dry and scaly). Soft, moist epithelium normally offers protection against bacteria, but when it becomes dry and hard, infections of the respiratory tract, the mouth, the eye, and the genitourinary tract occur easily. Additional vitamin A does not provide further protection against infection to individuals who are well nourished, but it would be indicated for those persons whose vitamin A has become depleted. *Xerophthalmia* is the severe eye disease caused by changes in the epithelium of the eye and is the cause of some blindness in the Orient.

Meeting daily needs. The allowance for vitamin A from 12 years throughout life is 5000 I.U. During pregnancy and lactation 6000 and 8000 I.U. are recommended. Intakes of 1500 I.U. for infants and 2000 to 4500 I.U. for children are recommended.

The animal stores most of its vitamin A in the liver; hence the liver of any animal—beef, veal, pork, lamb, chicken—is a rich source of the vitamin. Fish-liver oils are excellent sources, but are considered supplements rather than foods. Liver once a week or every ten days will go far toward ensuring the full weekly allowance. Many people, however, do not like liver. However, with many other good sources of vitamin A, there is little excuse for an inadequate intake.

Whole milk, cream, butter, and whole-milk cheeses are good sources of vitamin A. One egg yolk furnishes one tenth of the daily allowance of the adult. Fortified margarine contains the same levels as butter.

Dark-green leafy vegetables and deep-yellow vegetables and fruits are rich in carotene, which can be converted into vitamin A by the intestinal wall. Among the carotene-rich foods are carrots, sweet potatoes, pumpkin, yellow winter squash, cantaloupe, yellow peaches, apricots, spinach, kale, turnip greens, dark salad greens, broccoli, and green asparagus. (See Fig. 10–1.)

Toxicity. Vitamin A given in doses of 25,000 to 50,000 I.U. daily for several months has led to loss of appetite, failure to grow, fretfulness, drying and scaling of the skin, thinning of the hair, swelling and tenderness of the long bones, joint pains, and enlargement of the liver and spleen. These symptoms may also occur in adults after a somewhat longer period of excessive intake. The intakes far in excess of needs result when infants are given the wrong dosages of supplements, or when individuals persist in taking vitamin pills of high potency for prolonged periods of time without medical indication for need. The condition is corrected when the individual stops taking the supplement.

VITAMIN D

Function. Vitamin D is essential for the normal absorption of calcium and phosphorus from the gastrointestinal tract and for the normal calcification of the bones and the teeth.

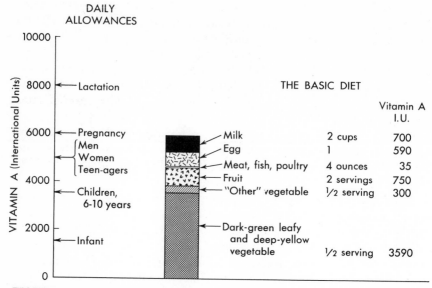

FIGURE 10-1 The Four Food Groups of the Basic Diet provide a liberal allowance of vitamin A. Note the contributions made by dark-green, leafy, and deep-yellow vegetables. Breads, cereals, and white potato do not provide vitamin A. See Table 4-2 for complete calculation.

Deficiency. Rickets is the deficiency disease seen in children who fail to get enough vitamin D. Calcium and phosphorus are inadequately deposited in the bones. The soft, pliable bones yield to pressure, the joints enlarge, and there is delayed closing of the skull bones. The child may have an enlarged skull, chest deformities, spinal curvature, and bowed legs. (See Fig. 10-2.)

Rickets is rarely seen in the United States because of the widespread use of supplements for infant feeding and the trends in dress that permit exposure of the skin to sunlight. Premature infants are more susceptible to rickets than full-term infants. Insufficient calcium and phosphorus intakes may also be responsible for rickets.

Osteomalacia is adult rickets sometimes seen in women of the Orient who have had a grossly inadequate intake of calcium, phosphorus, and vitamin D and have had several pregnancies.

Meeting daily needs. An allowance of 400 I.U. vitamin D is recommended for infants, children, adolescents, young men and women to age 22 years, and pregnant or lactating women. Adults probably get enough vitamin D through exposure of the skin to sunlight. However, clothing, soot, fog, and window glass cut off the ultraviolet light and prevent the change of the precursor in the skin to the active vitamin. People who work at night and sleep in the day, invalids who do not get out in the sun, and people who wear religious habits may require a vitamin D supplement.

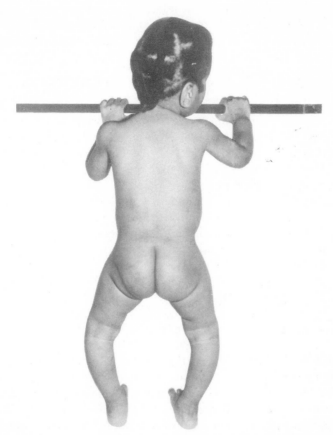

FIGURE 10-2 Early skeletal deformities of rickets often persist throughout life. Bowlegs that curve as shown here indicate that the weakened bones have bent as the result of standing. (*Courtesy, Dr. Rosa Lee Nemir and the Upjohn Company.*)

Foods are not good sources of vitamin D, except when they are fortified. Each quart of fresh milk or each tall can of evaporated milk may be fortified with 400 I.U. vitamin D, thus providing for the daily needs during growth and in pregnancy and lactation. Instead of fortified milk, some pediatricians recommend calciferol or a fish-liver-oil source such as cod, halibut, or percomorph oil.

Toxicity. Large doses of vitamin D—20,000 to 100,000 I.U.—have severe effects including loss of appetite, vomiting, diarrhea, fatigue, growth failure, and drowsiness. The blood calcium level is increased, and calcium salts are deposited in the soft issues, including the blood vessels, heart, and kidney tubules. Kidney stones may form.

More recently it has been found that as little as 1800 I.U. of vitamin D given daily may be mildly toxic, with some of the symptoms listed above being observed. Thus, if an infant is receiving vitamin D concentrate, it is important to measure the intake carefully, and also to avoid the use of fortified milk or other foods that might contain vitamin D.

VITAMINS E AND K

Vitamin E. Although vitamin E has been known since the 1920's its functions are still poorly understood. It protects vitamin A by preventing the oxidation in the intestine. It likewise prevents the rapid oxidation of unsaturated fatty acids. It protects the red blood cell against hemolysis. Vitamin E is required by animals, and presumably by humans, for the normal reproductive processes.

Deficiency of vitamin E in humans is unlikely except when diets are grossly lacking in many other nutrients. Many claims have been made for vitamin E as a treatment or cure for muscular dystrophy, rheumatic fever, heart disease, and reproductive disorders in humans. No sound evidence to date supports any of these claims.

The vitamin E requirement is related to the fat intake, especially the level of polyunsaturated fatty acids. The recommended allowance for men and women, respectively, is 30 I.U. and 25 I.U. This assumes a food pattern in which about 40 per cent of the calories are from fat and about 35 gm polyunsaturated fatty acids is ingested daily.

Vitamin E is widely distributed in foods, with salad oils, shortening, and margarines furnishing about two thirds of the day's intake. Whole-grain cereals, legumes, nuts, and dark-green vegetables are also good sources.

Vitamin K. Vitamin K is needed for the formation of prothrombin, a substance necessary for blood clotting. Intestinal bacteria normally synthesize a substantial amount of vitamin K. Because vitamin K is a fat-soluble vitamin, absorption is facilitated by the presence of bile. Anything that interferes with the absorption of fat will likewise interfere with the absorption of vitamin K. Only a limited amount of the vitamin is stored in body tissues.

Hemorrhage is the principal finding in vitamin K deficiency. It results from failure to synthesize vitamin K in the intestine or inability to absorb the vitamin. Some newborn infants have a tendency to hemorrhage because their intestinal bacteria are not sufficiently developed for synthesis of the vitamin. The hemorrhagic tendency may also develop in patients who have been treated with oral sulfa drugs or antibiotics, or in whom there is interference with the production or flow of bile.

The requirement for vitamin K is not known. Green leaves are an excellent source of the vitamin; cereals, fruits, and nonleafy vegetables are rather poor sources. Vitamin K preparations are sometimes given to the newborn infant to protect against hemorrhage.

Dicoumarol is a vitamin K antagonist. It counteracts the effect of vitamin K in the formation of prothrombin and thus prevents blood clotting. It has been an effective aid in treating heart diseases in which blood clots tend to form and that might endanger the patient's life.

TABLE 10–1   SUMMARY OF FAT-SOLUBLE VITAMINS

Vitamin	Metabolism and Function	Deficiency or Excess	Meeting Body Needs
Vitamin A precursors: Carotenes	Bile needed for absorption of carotenes. Mineral oil prevents absorption. Stored in liver. Bone and tooth structure. Healthy skin and mucous membranes. Vision in dim light	Night blindness. Lowered resistance to infection. *Severe:* drying and scaling of skin; eye infections; blindness. Overdoses are toxic: skin, hair, and bone changes	Adult: 5000 I.U. Liver, kidney. Egg yolk, butter, fortified margarine. Whole milk, cream, cheese. Dark-green leafy and deep-yellow vegetables. Deep-yellow fruits
Vitamin D precursors: Ergosterol in plants 7-Dehydro-cholesterol in skin	Some storage in liver. Aids absorption of calcium and phosphorus; Calcification of bones, teeth	*Rickets* Soft bones. Enlarged joints. Enlarged skull. Deformed chest. Spinal curvature. Bowed legs. *Osteomalacia* in adults (infrequent in U.S.) Even small excess is toxic	Infants, children, adolescents, and pregnant women: 400 I.U. Fortified milk. Concentrates: calciferol, viosterol. Fish-liver oils. Exposure to ultraviolet rays of sun
Vitamin E tocopherols	Prevents oxidation of vitamin A in intestine. Protects red blood cells. Limited stores in body. Requirement increased for high-fat diets	Deficiency not a problem in humans	Men: 30 I.U. Women: 25 I.U. Salad oils, shortenings, margarines. Whole grains, legumes, nuts, dark leafy vegetables
Vitamin K	Forms prothrombin for normal blood clotting. Dicoumarol is an antagonist	Hemorrhage, especially in newborn infants, and biliary tract disease	No recommended allowances. Synthesis by intestinal bacteria. Dark-green leafy vegetables

REVIEW QUESTIONS AND PROBLEMS

1. Explain the meaning of each of these terms: antagonist, antivitamin, avitaminosis, calciferol, carotene, ergosterol, keratinization, menadione, precursor, provitamin, rickets, tocopherol, viosterol, xerophthalmia.

2. If an individual is on a very low-fat diet, what effect might this have on the fat-soluble vitamins?

3. State the vitamin most directly concerned with each of the following items and indicate the relationship of the vitamin: visual purple, blood clotting, healthy skin, formation of bones and teeth, normal mucous membranes, carotene, ergosterol.

4. If your intake of vitamins A and D is more than you need, what happens to the excess?

5. Keep a record of your own diet for two days. Which foods provided you with vitamin A? What improvements are needed, if any?

6. Examine the labeling on fresh milk, evaporated milk, nonfat dry milk, and margarines. What information do you find concerning vitamins A and D?

7. What problems may arise if an individual uses vitamin A and D supplements in addition to an adequate diet?

REFERENCES

Cooley, D. G. "What Is a Vitamin?" *Today's Health*, **41**:20, January 1963.
Council on Food and Nutrition. "Vitamin Preparations as Dietary Supplements and Therapeutic Agents," *J. Amer. Med. Ass.*, **169**:41, 1959.
Elvehjem, C. A. "Why Vitamins?" *Today's Health*, **36**:18, February 1958.
Flynn, H. *Venture, Voyages and Vitamins*. Chicago: National Dairy Council.
Robinson, C. H. *Proudfit-Robinson's Normal and Therapeutic Nutrition*, 13th ed. New York: The Macmillan Company, 1967, Chap. 10.

WATER-SOLUBLE VITAMINS

ASCORBIC ACID

Functions. Ascorbic acid is essential for building the "cementing" material that holds cells and tissues together. The effect of this material is to provide firm tissues of all kinds: strong blood vessels, teeth firmly held in their sockets, and bones firmly held together.

Ascorbic acid aids in the absorption of iron from the intestines; it is needed to convert folacin to folinic acid (see p. 110); it participates in the metabolism of certain amino acids; it is required by the adrenal gland for the synthesis of hormones; it protects against infections; and it is essential for wound healing. The body tissues maintain a normal saturation of vitamin C, but excessive intakes are excreted in the urine.

Deficiency. Severe deficiency of ascorbic acid leads to *scurvy*. This was the disease that figured so importantly in the sea journeys of explorers in the sixteenth century and accounted for the death of so many sailors. Scurvy is characterized by easy bruising and hemorrhaging of the skin, loosening of the teeth, bleeding of the gums, and disruption of the cartilages that support the skeleton.

Scurvy is occasionally seen in infants who have had a cow's milk formula for several months without vitamin C supplements. One of the outstanding symptoms found in the infant is the extreme tenderness of the skin to touch. (See Fig. 11–1.)

Meeting daily needs. A minimum intake of 10 mg ascorbic acid daily will prevent scurvy, but higher intakes are recommended for optimum

103

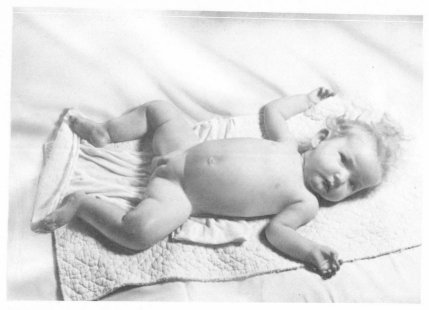

FIGURE 11–1 Infants who have been bottle-fed but who have no supplement of vitamin C will have scurvy. They assume this position because of the pain and tenderness of the skin. *(Courtesy, Dr. Bernard S. Epstein and the Upjohn Company.)*

health. The recommended allowance for men and women is 60 and 55 mg, respectively; for infants, 35 mg; and for children, 40 mg. (See also Table 4–1, p. 31.)

Ascorbic acid is sometimes called the "fresh-food" vitamin. It occurs in the growing parts of the plant, but it is absent from the dormant seed. Only the vegetable-fruit group contributes to the vitamin C intake. (See Fig. 11–2.) Human milk from a healthy mother supplies sufficient amounts for the young infant. Pasteurized milk contains only traces.

Raw fresh fruits and vegetables all contain vitamin C, but some foods are more outstanding than others. Oranges, grapefruit, tangerines, limes, and lemons are especially rich. Cantaloupe, strawberries, guava, and fresh pineapple are good sources. Blueberries, peaches, apples, pears, and banana are lower in vitamin C; if they are eaten in large amounts, they may be important for this vitamin.

The dark-green leafy vegetables so rich in carotene are also important for ascorbic acid. Tossed salad, or freshly prepared cabbage slaw, or fresh tomatoes are excellent sources. Broccoli is one of the outstanding sources; one serving, even after cooking, is equal in vitamin content to that of an orange.

Potatoes and sweet potatoes contain much less vitamin C, but it is sometimes said that "the lowly potato has prevented more scurvy than the lordly orange." This statement applies, of course, to those people who

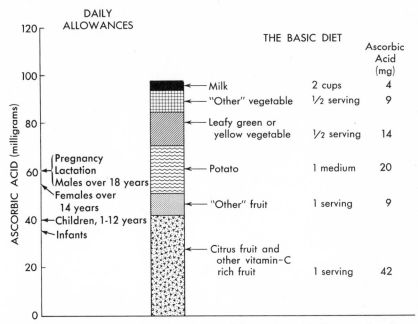

FIGURE 11–2 The Basic Diet furnishes the full ascorbic acid allowance for all age categories. Note the absence of the meat group and the bread-cereal group. For complete calculations of the Basic Diet see Table 4–2.

include appreciable amounts of fresh potato in the daily diet and who exercise care in proper preparation so that the vitamin is retained.

Canned and frozen citrus juices and fruits and tomato juice contain almost as much ascorbic acid as the fresh fruit. Cooked or canned non-acid fruits and vegetables lose more of the ascorbic acid. Frozen vegetables and fruits contain most of the vitamin C of the fresh product. On the other hand, dried foods contain only traces; thus, the widespread use of dehydrated potatoes by many homemakers and in institutions means that one should not rely on any vitamin being present.

THIAMINE

Functions. Thiamine is a coenzyme for an enzyme known as *carboxylase.* This enzyme is required for one of the many steps in the breakdown of glucose for energy. The adequate functioning of thiamine maintains healthy nerves, a good mental outlook, a normal appetite, and good digestion.

Deficiency. Thiamine deficiency may account for signs of fatigue, irritability, a feeling of depression and moodiness, poor appetite, a tingling and numbness of the legs, and constipation because of poor tone of the gastrointestinal tract. As you know, many other reasons could also explain such symptoms, and a diagnosis of thiamine deficiency could be made only with laboratory tests. *Beriberi,* sometimes called "rice-eater's disease" because it is often seen in people whose chief diet is refined rice, is the severest form of thiamine deficiency. It is still seen frequently in the Orient. The symptoms include polyneuritis (disease of the nerves, especially of the legs and hands), heart disease, and edema. Severe thiamine deficiency is sometimes seen in alcoholics who fail to get enough thiamine over long periods of time.

Meeting daily needs. The thiamine allowance is 0.5 mg per 1000 calories. Thus, an adult whose calorie allowance is 2000 would need 1.0 mg thiamine daily. For older adults 1.0 mg is allowed even though the calorie intake may be less than 2000.

Each of the Four Food Groups contributes importantly to the daily thiamine intake. (See Fig. 11–3.) Meats, especially pork and liver, are

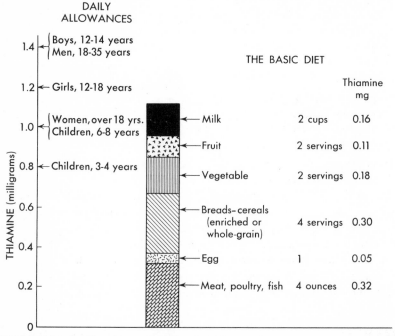

FIGURE 11–3 The thiamine needs of children and women are met by the Basic Diet. Additional foods from any of the Four Food Groups to satisfy the calorie requirement will also fulfill the thiamine need. See Table 4–2 for complete calculation.

rich in thiamine and account for about one fourth of the average intake. Dry beans and peas, peanuts, peanut butter, and eggs are good sources.

Enriched and whole-grain breads and cereals supply about one third of the daily thiamine intake. Although individual foods of the fruit-vegetable and milk groups contain lower concentrations of thiamine, the intake of recommended amounts of foods from these groups accounts for about 40 per cent of the daily thiamine need.

RIBOFLAVIN

Functions. Like thiamine, riboflavin is concerned with the break-down of glucose for energy. It is a component of many enzymes that are essential for a healthy skin and for good vision in bright light. If the individual ingests riboflavin in excess of his body needs, the urinary excretion will increase; if the intake is inadequate, the body conserves its supply very carefully and the urinary excretion will be practically stopped.

Deficiency. Riboflavin deficiency leads to *cheilosis,* a cracking of the skin at the corners of the lips and scaliness of the skin around the ears and nose. There may be redness and burning as well as itching of the eyes and extreme sensitivity to strong light.

Meeting daily needs. The requirement for riboflavin is related to the calorie and protein intake of the individual. The recommended allowance for the reference woman is 1.5 mg and for the reference man is 1.7 mg. The allowances are somewhat higher in proportion to body size for growing children and during pregnancy and lactation.

About half of the intake of riboflavin daily is furnished by milk alone. Cheese is a good source, although some of the vitamin has been lost in the whey. Important but smaller contributions are made by meat, especially organ meats, dark-green leafy vegetables, and enriched cereal foods. (See Fig. 11–4.)

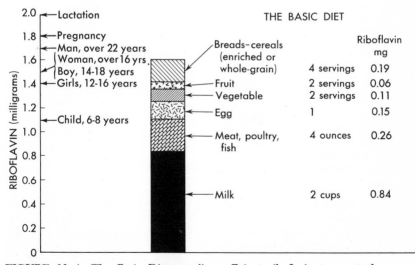

FIGURE 11–4 The Basic Diet supplies sufficient riboflavin to meet the recommended allowances for all groups except men and pregnant or lactating women. Note the importance of milk and meat groups. See Table 4–2 for complete calculation.

NIACIN

Functions. Niacin also is required for the stepwise breakdown of glucose in metabolism. Thus, if niacin, or thiamine, or riboflavin is missing in the diet, the metabolism will fail at the point of the missing enzyme. Moreover, each of these vitamins is needed for a specific step and cannot be replaced by any other. Niacin is essential for a healthy skin, normal function of the gastrointestinal tract, and maintenance of the nervous system.

Deficiency. Pellagra, the deficiency disease resulting from lack of niacin, is less prevalent than it was in this country early in the century. Nevertheless, in areas of poverty where the diet is low in both niacin and protein, some cases of pellagra are still seen. Dermatitis, especially of the skin exposed to the sun, soreness of the mouth, swelling of the tongue, diarrhea, and mental changes including depression, confusion, disorientation, and delirium are typical of the advancing stages of the disease, which ends in death if not treated.

Meeting daily needs. The recommended niacin allowance is 6.6 mg equivalents per 1000 calories. A niacin equivalent is 1 mg preformed niacin or 60 mg tryptophan. Tryptophan, one of the essential amino acids, can be changed to niacin in the body. Each 6 gm of protein in the diet will supply about 60 mg tryptophan equivalent to 1 mg niacin.

The Basic Diet (see Fig. 11–5) supplies 13 mg niacin from food. In addition, the protein of the diet furnishes 720 mg tryptophan or 12 mg niacin; thus, the diet is equal to 25 mg equivalents.

The meat group, especially organ meats and poultry, is the chief source of preformed niacin. Dark-green leafy vegetables and whole-grain or enriched breads and cereals are fair sources. Milk contains little preformed niacin. All good sources of complete proteins, including milk, cheese, eggs, meat, poultry, and fish, are good sources of the precursor tryptophan.

OTHER B-COMPLEX VITAMINS

Vitamin B_6. The functions of vitamin B_6 are closely related to protein metabolism: the synthesis or breakdown of amino acids; the production of antibodies; the conversion of tryptophan to niacin; the formation of heme in hemoglobin; and others. More vitamin B_6 is required when diets are high in protein than when they are low in protein. The adult allowance is 2.0 mg per day. See also Table 4–1 for other categories.

The symptoms of vitamin B_6 deficiency include loss of appetite, nausea, vomiting, dermatitis, soreness of the lips and tongue, nervous irritability, and anemia. Some years ago vitamin B_6 deficiency was observed in infants who had received a formula in which the vitamin B_6 had been inadvertently destroyed by high heat. These infants experienced a reduced

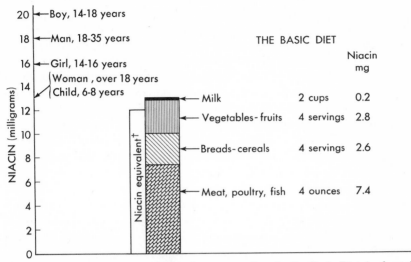

DAILY ALLOWANCES

THE BASIC DIET

		Niacin mg
Milk	2 cups	0.2
Vegetables-fruits	4 servings	2.8
Breads-cereals	4 servings	2.6
Meat, poultry, fish	4 ounces	7.4

NIACIN (milligrams)

Niacin equivalent†

20 ←—Boy, 14-18 years
18 ←—Man, 18-35 years
16 ←—Girl, 14-16 years
Woman, over 18 years
14 Child, 6-8 years

FIGURE 11-5 The niacin available from tryptophan in the Basic Diet is about 12 mg. The preformed niacin especially from the meat and bread-cereal groups brings the total well above the needs for all age groups. See Table 4-2 for complete calculation.

growth rate, nervous irritability, anemia, and convulsions; they recovered promptly when adequate vitamin B_6 was provided.

Diets that include recommended levels of the Four Food Groups will meet the requirements for vitamin B_6. Meats, organ meats, whole-grain cereals, soybeans, peanuts, and wheat germ are rich sources. Milk and green vegetables supply smaller amounts.

Vitamin B_{12}. Of all vitamins, vitamin B_{12} is the most complex. The trace element cobalt is an essential part of the molecule. Vitamin B_{12} is required for the production of red blood cells in the bone marrow, for the synthesis of proteins, and for the metabolism of nervous tissue. A protein substance, known as *intrinsic factor*, is produced in the stomach, and is essential for the absorption of vitamin B_{12}.

Pernicious anemia is the disease resulting from vitamin B_{12} deficiency. It is caused by lack of intrinsic factor in the stomach and not by dietary deficiency. Since the vitamin present in the diet cannot be absorbed without intrinsic factor, the normal functions of the vitamin cannot be performed. Patients with pernicious anemia have a macrocytic type of anemia; that is, the red blood cells are large and reduced in number. The patients frequently have a sore mouth, poor appetite, and gastrointestinal disturbances. The nervous system is affected so that the individual shows poor coordination in walking, for example; his mental processes may also be affected. Parenteral injections of vitamin B_{12} effectively control the condition; they must be used throughout the life of the patient. Macrocytic anemia also develops in patients with severe malabsorption as in sprue, or in those whose stomach has been removed.

For adults 5 μg vitamin B_{12} is recommended daily; 1 to 2 μg for infants, 2 to 5 μg for children, and 8 and 6 μg during pregnancy and lactation. Milk, eggs, cheese, and meat supply ample vitamin B_{12} even though the intakes of these animal foods may be relatively low. Plant foods supply practically no vitamin B_{12}, and use of an exclusively vegetarian diet for a long period of time will lead to some of the symptoms of deficiency.

Folacin. The formation of red blood cells and the metabolism of protein are important functions of folacin, but it must be remembered that folacin and vitamin B_{12} are both needed; they cannot replace each other. Folacin is converted to its active form, *folinic acid*, by ascorbic acid. Some folacin is synthesized in the small intestine.

Folacin deficiency occurs from (1) its lack in the diet, or (2) failure to absorb the vitamin in diseases such as sprue. It is not uncommon to find folacin deficiency in pregnancy; apparently the fetus has a high requirement for folacin. The principal characteristic of folacin deficiency is a macrocytic anemia. A sore mouth and diarrhea are usually present.

The recommended allowance for folacin is 0.4 mg for adults and 0.05 to 0.3 mg for children. The word "folacin" is derived from *folium*, meaning green leaf, and thus indicates that green, leafy vegetables are a good source. Organ meats, meat, fish, and whole-grain cereals are excellent sources.

Biotin occurs in extremely minute amounts in the body and in foods. It is required for many enzymes that participate in the metabolism of carbohydrates, fats, and amino acids. It is closely related to folacin and pantothenic acid in its activities.

No recommended allowances have been set for biotin. Average diets supply 100 to 300 μg daily. A protein, *avidin*, found in raw egg white is an antagonist to biotin. The protein combines with biotin in the small intestine and prevents absorption of the vitamin. However, the amount of egg white that needs to be ingested is far in excess of the number of eggs that would be eaten in a day. No deficiency of biotin has been observed on typical diets.

Pantothenic acid is an essential constituent of a complex enzyme known as *coenzyme* A. This enzyme is a key, as it were, to the breakdown of carbohydrates and fats to produce energy. It is also involved in the synthesis of cholesterol and of steroid hormones.

No recommended allowance has been set for pantothenic acid. The word "pantothenic" means "from everywhere," and the vitamin is widely distributed in foods. Deficiency of pantothenic acid occurs only when the diet is markedly deficient in other vitamins. Meat, whole-grain cereals, and legumes are rich in the vitamin, and milk, fruits, and vegetables are moderate sources.

SOME FALLACIES AND FACTS

1. *Fallacy.* Supplements of vitamins, especially vitamins A and C, will help to prevent colds and other infections.

TABLE 11–1 SUMMARY OF WATER-SOLUBLE VITAMINS

Vitamins	Metabolism and Function	Deficiency	Meeting Body Needs
Ascorbic acid Vitamin C	Strong blood vessels Teeth firm in gums Hormone synthesis Resistance to infection Improve iron absorption	*Scurvy:* Bruising and hemorrhage Bleeding gums Loose teeth	Men: 60 mg Women: 55 mg Citrus fruits Strawberries, cantaloupe Tomatoes, broccoli Raw green vegetables
Thiamine Vitamin B₁	Healthy nerves Good digestion Normal appetite Good mental outlook Breakdown of glucose for energy	Fatigue Poor appetite Constipation Mental depression Neuritis of legs *Beriberi:* Polyneuritis Edema Heart failure	0.5 mg per 1000 calories Pork, liver, other meats, poultry Dry beans and peas, peanut butter Enriched and whole-grain bread Milk, eggs
Riboflavin Vitamin B₂	Enzymes for protein and glucose metabolism Healthy skin Normal vision in bright light	*Cheilosis:* Cracking lips Scaling skin Burning, itching, sensitive eyes	Men: 1.7 mg Women: 1.5 mg Milk, cheese Meat, poultry, fish Dark-green leafy vegetables Enriched and whole-grain breads
Niacin Nicotinic acid	Enzymes for energy metabolism Normal digestion Healthy nervous system Healthy skin Tryptophan a precursor: 60 mg = 1 mg niacin	*Pellagra:* Dermatitis Sore mouth Diarrhea Mental depression Disorientation Delirium	6.6 mg equivalents per 1000 calories Meat, poultry, fish, Dark-green leafy vegetables Whole-grain or enriched breads, cereals Tryptophan in complete proteins

Facts. A normal diet based upon the Four Food Groups will furnish enough of all vitamins to maintain good health. It is true that some of the functions of vitamins include the maintenance of normal mucous membranes, the synthesis of antibodies, and healthy body tissues. But this does not mean that "if a little bit is good, more is better." In fact, if too much vitamin A is taken over several months, toxic effects may result (see p. 97). An excess of vitamin C would be excreted in the urine and would be of no value in building up additional resistance to an already healthy tissue.

2. *Fallacy.* Vitamin concentrates should never be used.

Facts. Sometimes vitamin concentrates are prescribed by a physician because of various disease conditions that may be present. Someone who is ill may have a very poor appetite and may be unable to eat the kinds and amounts of foods for an adequate diet. Other persons may have a disease of the gastrointestinal tract that reduces the absorption of the vitamins present in a normally adequate diet. Still other persons may have a deficiency disease because they did not understand what foods are necessary for health, or because they did not have enough money to buy a satisfactory diet. Once a deficiency disease is present, the most rapid way to cure it is to give large doses of vitamins in addition to improving the quality of the diet. Of course, these are all situations requiring a physician's diagnosis and prescription.

3. *Fallacy.* Vitamins from food sources are better than those from pills.

Facts. Each vitamin has a definite chemical composition. Thus, 1 mg of vitamin from a food source or from a concentrate may be expected to have the same value. But if the foods you eat for energy, protein, and minerals also furnish the vitamins you need, why spend additional money for vitamin pills that you do not need?

REVIEW QUESTIONS AND PROBLEMS

1. Define each of the following terms: anti-pernicious anemia factor, beriberi, biotin, cheilosis, cyanocobalamin, dermatitis, extrinsic factor, folacin, folinic acid, macrocytic, niacin equivalent, pellagra, pyridoxine, scurvy.

2. Which vitamins are most directly concerned with each of the following: scurvy, wound healing, healthy skin, pellagra, normal red blood cells, breakdown of glucose for energy, intercellular substance for firm skeletal structure, tryptophan, bleeding gums?

3. If your daily intake of ascorbic acid, thiamine, riboflavin, or niacin is greater than your body needs, what happens to the excess?

4. What vitamins are added to flours and cereal foods through the enrichment program? Collect labels of several enriched foods and evaluate them according to your daily need for these vitamins.

5. Suppose a person is allergic to citrus fruits. What foods could you recommend to meet the day's needs for ascorbic acid?

6. Record your own food intake for two days. Which foods in your diet

are providing you with riboflavin; niacin; thiamine; ascorbic acid? What changes do you need to make to improve your intake?

7. Normally you do not need to be concerned about the food sources for B-complex vitamins other than thiamine, riboflavin, and niacin. Explain why this is true.

8. Vitamin B_{12} must be given by injection to patients who have pernicious anemia. Explain why this is true.

REFERENCES

Dodds, M. L. "Vitamin C" in *Foods, The Yearbook of Agriculture 1959*. Washington, D.C.: U.S. Department of Agriculture, 1959, p. 150.

Goldsmith, G. A. "Vitamins of the B Complex" in *Foods, The Yearbook of Agriculture 1959*. Washington, D.C.: U.S. Department of Agriculture, 1959, p. 139.

Martin, E. A. *Nutrition in Action*, 2nd ed. New York: Holt, Rinehart and Winston, 1965, Chap. 7.

Robinson, C. H. *Proudfit-Robinson's Normal and Therapeutic Nutrition*, 13th ed. New York: The Macmillan Company, 1967, Chaps. 11 and 12.

Stare, F. J. "Good Nutrition from Food, Not Pills," *Amer. J. Nurs.*, **65**:86, February 1965.

PRACTICAL PLANNING
FOR GOOD NUTRITION

12

MEAL PLANNING FOR ADULTS

A family may sit down, day by day, at the same table and partake of the same choice of food with apparently different results. A six-year-old boy seems to grow slowly, the teen-age boy may be a foot taller and 15 lb heavier in a year's time, one parent may gain weight, and the other maintains constant weight. The six-year-old may be finicky about his food, the teen-ager never seems to get filled up, and the parent whose weight never changes appears to have a hearty appetite. If there are toddlers, preschool children, or grandparents at this table, it may be that the homemaker makes particular adaptations for them and yet tries to keep the meal as uniform as possible.

The ideas expressed above suggest that meal planning and food service may be individualized within a unified pattern. The purposes of this unit are to consider the particular emphases on nutritional requirements that must be made in each phase of the life cycle, to study ways by which food habits can be improved, and to learn something about meal planning, purchase, sanitary handling, and basic principles of food preparation. These are practical aspects of nutrition that will be of equal value to you either in your personal and family life or in your professional career.

Factors in Meal Planning

FOUR FOOD GROUPS IN MEAL PLANNING

Preceding chapters have emphasized why you need protein, minerals, and vitamins as well as calories, and have shown how your needs are met by using the Four Food Groups as a basis for planning. To satisfy the nutritional needs, one should first set up a skeleton plan for the day that includes the stated minimum amounts of foods from each of the four groups. See Table 12–1 for an example of such a plan.

TABLE 12–1 FOUR FOOD GROUPS IN A BASIC MENU PLAN

Skeleton Menu Plan Based on Four Food Groups	Sample Menu	Typical Additions for Calories
Breakfast		
Citrus fruit	Orange juice	
Cereal	*	
Egg	Egg, fried	Butter for egg
Bread	Whole-wheat toast	Butter for toast
		Jelly for toast
Milk	Milk	Sugar, cream for coffee
Luncheon		
Meat, poultry, fish— small serving	Sandwich 2 slices bread	
Bread	1 ounce bologna	Butter or mayonnaise
	1 ounce cheese	for sandwich
Milk	Milk	
Fruit	Stewed plums	Sugar for plums
		Cookie
Dinner		
Meat, poultry, fish— small serving	Baked meat loaf	Gravy
Potato	Mashed potato	
Dark-green or deep- yellow vegetable	Parslied carrots	Butter on carrots
Bread	Hard roll	Butter for roll
		Tossed green salad
		Russian dressing
		Chocolate cake with icing

* Note that cereal was omitted in the sample menu and used as a slice of bread for the sandwich.

Additions for the pregnant woman: 1 cup milk at dinner; 1 cup milk at bedtime. The teen-age mother-to-be should include 5 to 6 cups milk daily.

When you examine the skeleton outline, you realize that not enough food is listed to meet the calorie needs of the man and the calorie and iron allowances of the woman. The man may, therefore, add any foods he desires so that he maintains normal weight: fats, such as butter or margarine for bread and vegetables, or salad dressings; sugar for cereals and fruits, jam, jellies, or marmalade on breads and rolls; desserts of many kinds, some of which add appreciable amounts of protein, minerals, and vitamins. Fruits are low in calories but increase the mineral and vitamin intake; puddings and ice cream add to the level of calcium, and somewhat to the amount of protein, as well as being somewhat higher in calories; cakes, cookies, pies, and pastries are high in calories and contribute in a variable way to protein, minerals, and vitamins, depending upon the specific ingredients used.

Because of the high iron requirement, the teen-age girl or woman needs to select her foods carefully for additional calories to supplement the Basic Diet. A serving of liver weekly, whole-grain or enriched breads and cereals, frequent use of dried fruits, molasses, and legumes should represent a substantial portion of the additional foods selected to maintain weight.

MEAL PATTERNS

Breakfast. Far too many people skip breakfast, giving such excuses as not being hungry, wishing to lose weight, or not having enough time. Appetite for breakfast is largely a matter of habit; for many people breakfast is the most enjoyable meal of the day. It breaks the night's fast, helps to ensure energy for the morning's work, and reduces irritability. A light breakfast will provide one fourth of the day's calories even if one is reducing. (See Fig. 12–1.) As a matter of fact, people who do not eat breakfast often eat more frequently during the rest of the day, choosing high-calorie snacks, such as pretzels, soft drinks, candy, and so on. Each meal of the day should include some protein food for satiety value and for optimum use of amino acids. Breakfast is a good time to include fruit that is rich in vitamin C, whereas other fruits may be included at lunch and dinner. A good breakfast need take little time to prepare. Two examples of quickly prepared breakfasts are:

Orange juice (frozen)	Stewed prunes
Wheat flakes *with*	Scrambled eggs
Whole or skim milk and sugar	Enriched toast
Toasted English muffin *with*	Butter
Butter and orange marmalade	Coffee
Coffee, if desired	

Luncheons. Good lunches need not be elaborate. The following examples could be adapted to a carried lunch, one purchased in a cafeteria, or one prepared at home.

Fresh fruit salad with cottage cheese	Baked custard with caramel sauce
Crisp roll with butter	Milk

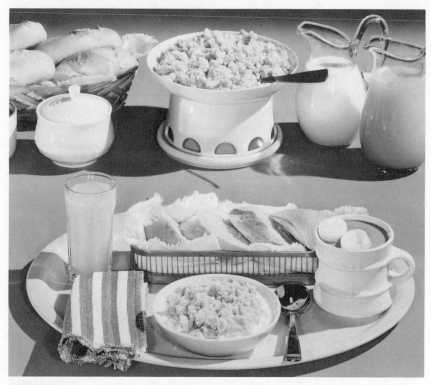

FIGURE 12–1 A basic breakfast for adult or child; citrus fruit, hot or cold cereal, bread, milk for children, coffee. *(Courtesy, Cereal Institute, Inc.)*

Split-pea soup (canned)
Sandwich
    Rye bread—2 slices
    Baked ham
    Lettuce
    Mustard, mayonnaise
Sliced tomato and cucumber on
    lettuce

Fresh peach
Milk

Dinner. The dinner meal customarily includes meat, poultry, or fish. Cheese, eggs, or legume dishes may occasionally be substituted. White or sweet potato plus another vegetable, rolls or bread, butter, dessert, and beverage complete the meal. The vegetable should be deep-yellow or dark-green leafy at least every other day. If a salad is not served at luncheon, one should be included in the evening meal. The dessert may be light and simple with a heavy meal, or it may be elaborate as for some company meals.

ACHIEVING ATTRACTIVE, PALATABLE MEALS

In addition to planning meals for good nutrition, the following should also be kept in mind:

1. Select appealing color combinations. A dinner of baked fish with mushroom sauce, mashed potato, and creamed cabbage is lacking in color. Some minced parsley and pimento on the fish, and the substitution of broccoli for the cabbage, would greatly improve the appearance of this meal.

2. Include some soft and chewy foods. The tossed salad adds crispness to the sample meal shown in Table 12–1. Crisp crunchy rolls would also be suitable with this meal.

3. Vary the shapes of food portions. Several round mounds of food on the same plate are monotonous to the eye.

4. Provide satiety but avoid meals that are so heavy as to give one a feeling of fullness and discomfort. A meal with a hearty soup, meat, potatoes, and vegetables may end with fruit for dessert, for example.

5. Consider the flavor and odor of foods. Rubbing a salad bowl with garlic lends some interest to a salad, but a heavy hand with onion, garlic, pepper, and other seasonings is objectionable. Cabbage and onions in the same meal are poor choices, because they are both strongly flavored vegetables. Combine, then, some bland and spicy, sweet and tart flavors.

6. Adapt meal patterns to the family pattern of living. It makes little difference whether dinner is served at noon or night or whether breakfast is light or substantial in size. When the members of the family are engaged in much activity, the caloric needs are much greater, and the meals will be correspondingly heavier.

7. Prepare foods in a variety of ways. Any good cookbook will give numerous ways to cook meats, eggs, fruits, vegetables, cereal foods. Ground meat, for example, may appear in meat loaf, in chili con carne, in spaghetti sauce, in a macaroni casserole, as well as in hamburgers.

8. Good meals need not require a great deal of preparation time. Today's homemaker makes use of canned soups, frozen and canned fruits and vegetables, mixes, and many other convenience foods to save time. With careful selection, such foods do not cost much more than home-prepared products and may save much time.

SNACKS

The coffee break and eating between meals are a well-established custom. (See Fig. 12–2.) Snacks should be planned as part of the daily meals. They should not replace breakfast or lunch. Some people eat snacks to gain weight; others find it easier to lose weight if they have five or six small meals a day rather than three larger meals; still others realize only too

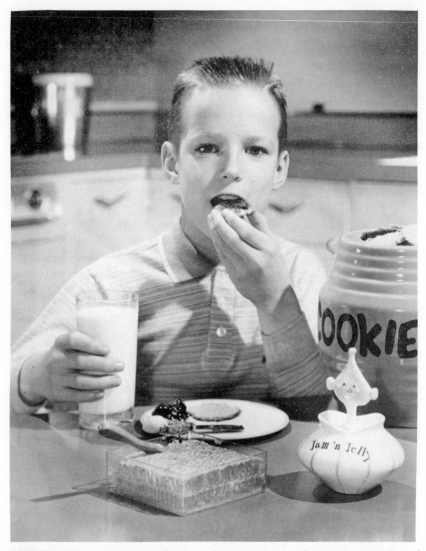

FIGURE 12–2 Active boys and girls need snacks that provide protein, minerals, and vitamins as well as energy. (*Courtesy, American Dairy Association.*)

late that snacks can be the undoing of effective weight control. Soft drinks, doughnuts, cakes, sweet rolls, pretzels, potato chips, and the like may be a liability, because the additional calories are appreciable although the nutrient contribution is small. More nutritious snacks in increasing order of caloric value are:

Raw vegetables—celery and carrot sticks; tomato juice
Fresh fruits and fruit juices

Milk, skim or whole
Milk beverages
Ice cream, plain or with sauce
Hamburger on bun, pizza

Nutrition for Older Persons

Geriatrics is that branch of medicine especially concerned with the prevention and treatment of diseases in older people. There is, of course, no specific age that characterizes a person as "old"; some people are "old" at 50 years, and others are "young" at 70 years. About 20 million people in the United States today are over 65 years of age. The majority of these people are productive, live in their own homes, and enjoy good health. Good nutrition, heredity, and environment play dominant roles in the maintenance of health. (See Fig. 12–3.)

NUTRITIONAL NEEDS

As you well know, it is altogether too common for people to gain weight as they become older. This weight gain is explained in part by a progressively lower basal metabolism after 25 years of age. In addition, older men and women are usually less active than they were in their youth. The recommended energy allowance at 55 to 75 years for men is 2400 calories, and for women, 1700 calories. For persons in this age group who are extremely inactive because of illness the calorie requirement may be even less. The allowances for protein, calcium, vitamin A, and ascorbic acid are the same as those for young adults. Provided that she does not have anemia, the woman who reaches 55 years of age can meet her iron needs with 10 mg daily. See Table 4–1 (p. 31) for recommended allowances.

PROBLEMS OF FOOD INTAKE

People over 65 years of age are no more like one another than teenagers are like one another. The nurse is likely to encounter a great variety of problems concerned with adequate nutrition of older persons. She needs to be alert to these problems and to use ingenuity, patience, and kindness in solving them.

1. Inability to chew is a frequent source of difficulty because of poorly fitting dentures or absence of teeth.

2. Appetite usually declines in later years because the senses of smell and taste are less acute, the secretion of gastric juices may be reduced, and the satisfactions of sociability with family and friends may be lacking. Chronic disease and medications may also interfere with the appetite.

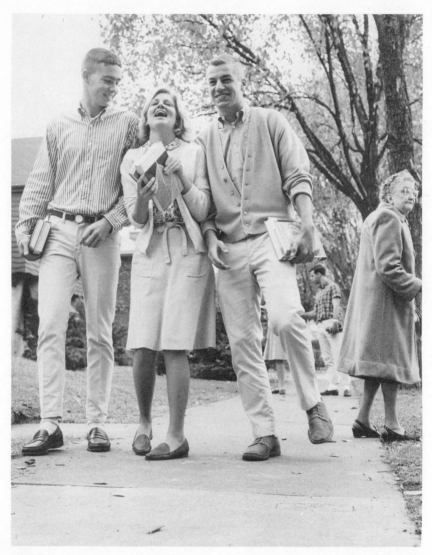

FIGURE 12–3 Calcium—a stitch in time? Good food habits in youth and through-out life may help to prevent bone diseases in later years. (*Courtesy, National Dairy Council.*)

3. Complaints of heartburn, belching, indigestion, and flatulence are frequent. Specific foods are often blamed for these effects, but no firm rules can be given that apply to all persons. Thus, one individual may experience discomfort every time he eats onions, and another enjoys onions and tolerates them well. Concern for the individual would omit onion for the former and include them for the latter. See also discussion on fiber and flavor in Chapter 19.

4. Constipation is a common problem of the older individual and is related to the reduction of muscle tone of the gastrointestinal tract and to lessened activity. It is aggravated by eating too many soft, low-fiber foods and failing to drink sufficient fluid.

5. Chronic diseases of the heart, kidney, circulatory system, gastrointestinal tract, and joints impose needs for modified diets (see Unit IV) or interfere with tolerance for foods and ability to manage one's own diet.

6. Poor dietary habits in the past may have contributed to various signs of nutritional deficiency including fatigue, anemia, fragility of bones, poor wound healing following injury or surgery, and reduced resistance to infection.

7. Living alone, physical handicaps, poor cooking facilities, low income, frustration, boredom, and fear of the future all reduce the desire to eat or the capacity to prepare adequate meals.

8. Faddism and misinformation are responsible for much poor nutrition. Because many older people believe that their nutritional needs are small, they tend to consume less meat, eggs, milk, and vegetables and more high-carbohydrate foods that are ready to eat. They are especially likely to fall prey to the food quack who makes promises of good health, vigor, and even cure of disease.

DIETARY PLANNING

The lifetime pattern of eating is not easily changed, and the older woman who has always liked rich desserts or the man accustomed to eating hearty rich foods will find it difficult to adjust to the lower calorie requirements. The Four Food Groups still furnish the basis for meal planning because they provide all the nutrients needed by the older man and woman. (See Table 12–1.) Since the Basic Diet provides 1140 calories (see Table 4–2, p. 35), the woman of 55 to 75 years or older will need to restrict her intake of calorie-rich foods lest she rapidly gain weight. Some useful points to keep in mind when planning meals for older persons are noted below.

1. Consider the food likes and dislikes of the individual. Learn to use essential foods in dishes acceptable to the person. For example, milk may be disliked as a beverage but well accepted in puddings, custards, cream soups, and cream sauces, on cereals, and so on.

2. Fried foods, rich desserts, highly seasoned foods, and strongly flavored vegetables need not be omitted, but they should be used with discretion and according to the patient's tolerance. (See also Chap. 19.)

3. If chewing is difficult, adjust the meals to include finely minced or chopped meats, soft breads, fruits, and vegetables. (See "Mechanical Soft Diet," Chap. 19.)

4. Four or five small meals may be better than three meals when the appetite is poor.

5. Breakfast is the meal most enjoyed by many older persons, and every effort should be made to provide pleasing variety.

6. Dinner at noon rather than in the evening is preferred by some.

7. If coffee and tea produce insomnia, they should be restricted to meals early in the day.

8. Encourage a liberal fluid intake daily. Adjust the fiber content of the diet if constipation is a problem. (See "High-Fiber Diet," Chap. 19.)

Pregnancy

The orderly sequence of fetal development and growth, the mechanisms for nourishment of the fetus, the storage of nutrients in anticipation of labor and delivery, and the development of the mammary glands represent a level of anabolism unequaled in any other time of life. All these needs can be met only through a diet planned to meet these increased requirements.

NUTRITION BEFORE PREGNANCY

The young woman who is in good health prior to conception and who maintains good nutrition has the best chance of a pregnancy without complications, a healthy baby, and the ability to nurse. During early pregnancy, often before the woman is even aware that she is pregnant, critical development of the fetus takes place. A woman poorly nourished prior to pregnancy is much more subject to the complications of pregnancy, including toxemia, hypertension, anemia, and premature birth.

Two of every five first babies are born to young women under 20 years of age. These young women must still meet the growth needs of their own maturing bodies as well as the nutritional demands of the fetus. Yet, girls in their late teens have, far too often, had diets that were inadequate in calcium, iron, and protein. Therefore, it should be a special concern that these young women receive nutrition education in their early teens in order that they may recognize the value of good diet.

DEVELOPMENT DURING PREGNANCY

During the first two weeks after conception the embryo is fixed in its position in the uterus. The placenta, which is the organ that transfers nutrients from the maternal blood circulation to the fetus, is well developed early in pregnancy. During the second to eighth weeks there is rapid development of the skeleton and the organs so that the tiny fetus is a clearly distinguishable human being. By the twelfth week the fetus still weighs only about 1 oz.

The pregnant woman will normally gain 16 to 24 lb. The lower level may be more desirable for women who are overweight, but the higher level is more suitable for women who are slightly underweight. Of this weight, very little should be gained during the first trimester, about 6 to 8 lb during the second trimester, and 10 to 12 lb during the third trimester.

The weight gain is accounted for by fetus, 7½ lb; uterus, 2 lb; placenta and membranes, 2½ lb; and breast tissue, 2 lb. The blood volume increases by about 25 per cent toward the latter part of pregnancy. In addition, much nitrogen, calcium, and phosphorus are stored in preparation for delivery and lactation.

NUTRITIONAL ALLOWANCES

The recommended allowances for girls and women prior to and during pregnancy and lactation are shown in Table 12–2. If one compares these allowances with the value of the basic diet (see Table 4–2, p. 35), it becomes evident that calcium, iron, and vitamin D are the nutrients that require particular emphasis.

TABLE 12–2 RECOMMENDED DIETARY ALLOWANCES FOR WOMEN BEFORE AND DURING PREGNANCY AND LACTATION

Nutrient	Girl 16–18 Years	Woman 18–35 Years	Pregnancy	Lactation
Calories	2300	2000	+200	+1000
Protein, gm	55	55	65	75
Calcium, gm	1.3	0.8	+0.4	+0.5
Iron, mg	18	18	18	18
Vitamin A, I.U.	5000	5000	6000	8000
Thiamine, mg	1.2	1.0	+0.1	+0.5
Riboflavin, mg	1.5	1.5	1.8	2.0
Niacin, mg	15	13	15	20
Ascorbic acid, mg	50	55	60	60
Vitamin D, I.U.	400		400	400

DIETARY PLANNING

By adding 1½ cups milk to the basic diet pattern (see Table 12–1), the woman can meet her increased calcium need during pregnancy. The 16-to-18-year-old girl, however, would need to consume 5 to 5½ cups milk daily to meet her calcium allowance. The addition of milk to the basic pattern will also supply the additional vitamin A and B-complex vitamins that are recommended.

Milk may be flavored with chocolate, coffee, molasses, or puréed fruit such as strawberries or apricots. Part of the milk may be used on cereal or in soups, puddings, or cream sauces. One ounce of American or Swiss cheese supplies about the same amount of protein and calcium as 1 cup of milk. If calories are restricted, skim milk may be substituted for part or all of the whole milk. Such a substitution, however, will lower the vitamin A intake unless the skim milk is fortified with vitamin A.

The iron allowance, as pointed out before, is not easily met. See page 119 and Chapter 9. Iron supplements, usually prescribed by the physician, constitute a safeguard during pregnancy. But the pregnant woman should also make every effort to select iron-rich foods. Liver including liverwurst, molasses in beverages, in baked beans, and in desserts, dried fruits, and legumes enhance the iron content of the diet.

During pregnancy 400 I.U. vitamin D is essential. This is provided by 1 qt vitamin D milk. It is important that iodized salt be used.

Excessive weight gain must be avoided during pregnancy. Simple desserts such as fruit and milk puddings need to be substituted for calorie-rich pastries and other desserts. The intake of sugars, candies, butter, cream, and fried foods must often be reduced.

COMPLICATIONS

Anemia. Iron-deficiency anemia during pregnancy increases the likelihood of premature birth. The baby at birth is less well supplied with hemoglobin and thus is likely to become anemic during the first year of life. This type of anemia is best treated with iron supplements. Macrocytic anemia is occasionally seen in pregnant women and is treated with supplements of folacin.

Mild nausea. The discomfort of early-morning nausea during the first trimester can usually be overcome by eating some high-carbohydrate food, such as dry toast, crackers, or hard candy, before arising. Several small meals a day, rather than three large meals, may be more desirable. Fluids should be taken between meals rather than at mealtimes.

Constipation is rather common during the latter part of pregnancy. It can usually be avoided by placing more emphasis upon raw fruit and vegetables, some whole-grain breads and cereals, a liberal intake of liquids, and a regular program of exercise.

Toxemia of pregnancy is characterized by high blood pressure, swelling of the ankles, and protein in the urine. It occurs especially in women who are overweight or who gain weight too rapidly but who have had a diet poor in nutritive quality. A sodium-restricted diet of about 1000 mg is sometimes ordered. (See Chap. 25.)

Weight control. When weight is gained too rapidly the physician may recommend a 1500-calorie to 1800-calorie diet. The low-calorie diets described in Chapter 21 may be adjusted by including additional skim milk.

Lactation

The lactating woman will produce 20 to 30 oz of milk each day, representing 20 to 30 gm protein and 400 to 600 calories. In order to produce this milk, her nutritive allowances are increased as shown in Table 12–2. You will note that the greatest increase beyond that of the pregnant woman is in the calorie allowance. The further need for calcium is met by increasing the milk intake by ½ to 1 cup daily beyond that taken during pregnancy. The calorie needs are met by choosing any foods desired in addition to the basic diet.

REVIEW QUESTIONS AND PROBLEMS

1. Write a menu for one day that is satisfactory for the healthy young man or woman. How would you change this menu for a 25-year-old pregnant woman? What further changes are necessary for the teen-age mother-to-be?

2. Why is good nutrition so important prior to pregnancy?

3. Compare the nutritional needs of a woman of 25 years and of 65 years. How would you adapt the menu you wrote for the older woman?

4. As a nurse, what problems might you find in feeding the elderly patient?

5. What is meant by toxemia of pregnancy? What are some common causes? What change in diet may be required?

6. List five ways to increase milk intake by a person who does not like milk.

REFERENCES

Beck, J. "Guarding the Unborn," *Today's Health*, **46**:38, January 1968.

Eating Is Fun—For Older People Too. Chicago: American Dietetic Association, 1952.

Gordon, B. M. "A Feeding Plan for Geriatric Patients," *Hospitals*, **39**:92, April 16, 1965.

Keller, M. D., and Smith, C. E. "Meals on Wheels," *Geriatrics*, **16**:237, 1961.

Lane, M. M. "The Ideal Geriatric Diet," *Nurs. Homes*, **16**:27, January 1967.

Prenatal Care. Pub. No. 4. Washington, D.C.: Children's Bureau, 1962.

Rasmussen, S. *Foundations of Practical and Vocational Nursing*. New York: The Macmillan Company, 1967, Chaps. 41, 47, 48, 49.

Robinson, C. H. *Proudfit-Robinson's Normal and Therapeutic Nutrition*, 13th ed. New York: The Macmillan Company, 1967, Chaps. 14, 22, 25.

Rust, H. "Food Habits of Pregnant Women," *Amer. J. Nurs.*, **60**:1636, 1960.

Sebrell, W. H. "It's Not Age That Interferes with Nutrition of the Elderly," *Nutr. Today*, 1:15, June 1966.

Stare, F. J. "Good Nutrition from Food, Not Pills," *Amer. J. Nurs.*, 65:86, February 1965.

United States Department of Agriculture: *Food for the Young Couple*. Home and Garden Bulletin No. 85, 1962. *Food Guide for Older Folks*. Home and Garden Bulletin No. 17, 1963.

NUTRITION FOR GROWTH AND DEVELOPMENT

Infant Feeding

GROWTH AND DEVELOPMENT

Infants vary widely in their growth patterns, and it is not wise to compare one infant with another; yet, there is some value in being familiar with typical patterns of development and growth. On the average, infants gain 5 to 8 oz per week during the first five months, and double their birth weight in this time. For the remainder of the year the weight increase is about 4 to 5 oz per week; the birth weight is tripled by the age of 10 to 12 months. The initial height of 20 to 22 in. has increased to 30 in. or more by the end of the first year.

The body content of water at birth is high and that of fat is low. The relative lack of subcutaneous fat and the proportionately high surface area explain why additional precautions may be taken to keep infants warm. The bones are comparatively soft in the newborn baby, but they will continue to add mineral substance throughout childhood and adolescence. Teeth begin to erupt at five to six months. By the end of the year the infant will have five to ten teeth.

The baby is born with a large head and short arms and legs. In the first years of life the nervous system continues to develop rapidly so that the brain will have reached 90 per cent of adult size at the age of four years. Severe malnutrition during these years leads to inadequate development of the central nervous system, and cannot be corrected later in life.

Thus, the poorly nourished infant and child can never reach his full mental potential.

The newborn infant's stomach has a capacity of about 1 oz, and at one year can hold about 8 oz. The ability to digest protein, simple sugars, and emulsified fats is present at birth in the full-term infant. During the early months of life the production of digestive enzymes increases so that starchy foods and fats may be gradually included.

BREAST FEEDING

No one would deny that breast feeding, whenever possible, is best for the infant. Human milk provides benefits of easy digestion, desirable rates of growth and development, and protection against infections. Most women can nurse their babies if they desire to do so and if they eat the foods necessary to build up the stores of nutrients for milk production.

About ½ to 1½ oz of a thick, yellowish fluid called *colostrum* is produced during the first few days after delivery. Although this small amount of milk does not provide much nutrient intake, it is believed that it does provide the infant greater protection against infection. Placing the infant at the breast early also helps to stimulate the milk flow.

Self-demand feeding permits the baby to nurse when he is hungry, rather than according to an arbitrary time schedule. The mother soon learns to recognize when the baby is hungry and not crying for relief of some other discomfort. Infants may nurse as often as every two hours during the first few weeks, but soon regulate to an approximate three- or four-hour schedule. About the second month the baby begins to sleep through the 2 or 3 A.M. feeding. By five months he usually does not awaken for a feeding at 10 to 11 P.M.

Breast-fed babies should be weaned about the fifth month or later. A bottle or cup feeding may be substituted at a convenient feeding time. When the baby has become accustomed to this—after about a week or two—a second bottle or cup is offered. As much as two or three months may be needed for full weaning. Breast-fed babies, like bottle-fed babies, require the addition of foods from time to time as discussed later in this chapter.

PLANNING FORMULAS

In spite of the fact that most women could breast-feed their babies, bottle feeding is now used for about four fifths of all babies. With present standards of sanitation, most babies thrive well on formulas. (See Fig. 13–1.)

Nutritional needs. The calorie, protein, mineral, and vitamin needs of the infant are very high in proportion to body size. (See Recommended

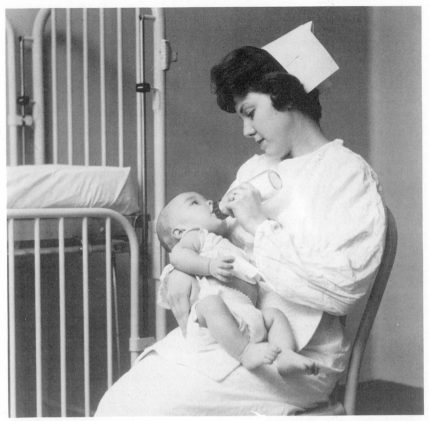

FIGURE 13–1 The baby should always be held while he is being fed. (*Courtesy, Ross Laboratories.*)

Dietary Allowances, Table 4–1, p. 30.) Per pound of body weight the infant requires 45 to 55 calories, and 0.9 to 1.0 gm protein. He needs 0.4 to 0.6 gm calcium and 35 mg ascorbic acid. During the early months his formula will provide the protein, calorie, and calcium needs, but other foods will be gradually introduced to meet the iron, ascorbic acid, and vitamin B-complex requirements.

Cow's milk. Most infants are given cow's milk formulas. Cow's milk contains almost three times as much protein and more than three times as much calcium as human milk. It contains about the same amount of fat and somewhat less lactose. (See Table 13–1.) Ounce for ounce, cow's milk and human milk contain about 20 calories.

In order to make cow's milk more comparable to human milk, several changes are made for infant feeding: (1) formulas are sterilized to ensure a safe supply of food for the baby and reduce the size of the curd that forms in the stomach; (2) the milk is diluted with water so that the protein

TABLE 13-1 COMPOSITION OF HUMAN AND COW'S MILK *
(PER 100 GM OF MILK)

Nutrient	Human Milk	Cow's Milk	Nutrient	Human Milk	Cow's Milk
Calories	77	66	Vitamin A, I.U.	240	150
Protein, gm	1.1	3.5	Thiamine, mg	0.01	0.03
Fat, gm	4.0	3.7	Riboflavin, mg	0.04	0.17
Carbohydrate, gm	9.5	4.9	Niacin, mg	0.2	0.1
Calcium, mg	33	117	Ascorbic acid, mg	5	1
Phosphorus, mg	14	92			
Iron, mg	0.1	trace			

* Watt, B. K., and Merrill, A. L. *Composition of Foods—Raw, Processed, Prepared*, Handbook No. 8. Washington, D.C.: U.S. Department of Agriculture, 1964, p. 39.

concentration will be somewhat lower; and (3) some form of carbohydrate is added. Sometimes milk is acidified with lactic acid to produce a finer curd for babies who have a tendency to vomit.

Planning the formula. Fresh whole milk, preferably homogenized, evaporated milk, and dried whole milk are used for most infant formulas. Cane sugar, corn syrup, and dextrimaltose are widely used for additional carbohydrate. A formula of evaporated milk and cane sugar is the least expensive. Also, evaporated milk is sterile and requires no refrigeration until the can is opened. An example of a formula for an infant weighing 12 lb and four months old is shown here.

Feedings: 5 (approximately 6 and 10 A.M., 2 and 6 and 10 P.M.)
Size of feedings: 6 oz each (age in months + 2)
5 × 6 ounces = 30 ounces of formula required
Whole milk: 1.5 to 2 oz per pound of body weight
          12 lb × 1.75 oz = 21 oz whole milk
                    (10.5 oz evaporated milk)
Sugar: 1 oz
Water: 30 − 21 = 9 oz, for fresh-milk formula
     (30 − 10.5 = 19.5 oz, for evaporated-milk formula)

STERILIZATION OF FORMULAS

These simple steps should be followed in the preparation and *terminal sterilization* of the formula. (See Fig. 13-2.)

1. Scrub bottles, nipples, saucepan, and measuring equipment with a detergent and water. Rinse well. Squeeze water through nipples to be sure they are not clogged.

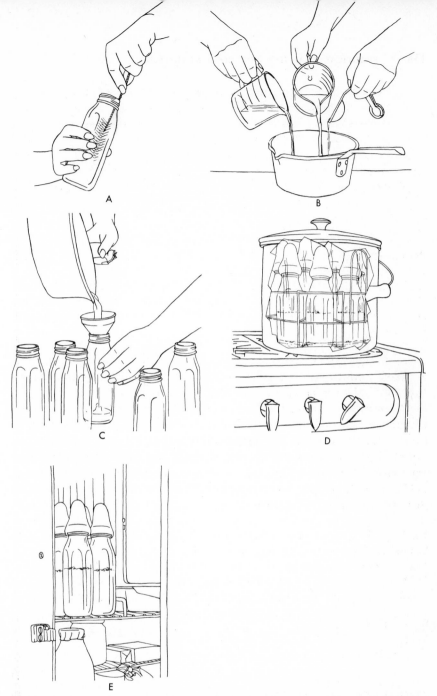

FIGURE 13–2 Steps in preparation and terminal sterilization of infant's formula. (*Courtesy, Children's Bureau, U.S. Department of Health, Education, and Welfare.*)
A. Scrub bottles, nipples, and equipment.
B. Measure and mix milk, sugar, and water in pan with pouring lip.
C. Pour mixture into bottles.
D. Place bottles on rack in sterilizer. Boil gently for 25 minutes.
E. Store capped bottles in refrigerator.

2. Measure milk, sugar, and water into saucepan, and mix well.

3. Divide formula equally into number of bottles needed for 24 hours.

4. Put nipples on bottles. Cover loosely with nipple covers.

5. Set bottles in rack of sterilizer. Include also one or two bottles of drinking water. Pour water until it reaches halfway up on the bottles. Cover sterilizer.

6. Bring water to boil. Continue boiling gently for 25 minutes.

7. Remove sterilizer from heat and let stand until bottles are cool enough to handle.

8. Press nipple covers down firmly. Cool bottles to room temperature. Refrigerate bottles.

Standard clean technique or aseptic technique consists in sterilizing bottles, nipples, and equipment first. The formula is boiled for three minutes and then poured into the bottles; nipples are put in place and covered. There is greater danger of contamination with this technique.

COMMERCIAL FORMULAS

Pediatricians may choose from a wide variety of commercial formulas that have been developed to resemble the composition of human milk. Cow's milk is the usual base for these formulas, but it has been modified in one or more of the following ways: to reduce the protein content; to reduce the calcium level and increase the lactose content; to increase the essential fatty acids by substituting vegetable oils for butterfat; to adjust the mineral and vitamin content; and to produce a soft, flocculent curd.

Special formulas are also available for therapeutic purposes. For infants who are allergic to milk, nutritionally adequate formulas of soybean or meat base may be substituted. Enzyme deficiency such as galactosemia or lactose intolerance requires meat base or amino acid formulas. A low-phenylalanine formula (Lofenalac *) is used for phenylketonuria, an inborn error of metabolism.

Many of the commercial formulas in dry powder form or canned evaporated require only the addition of water. Some formulas are fully prepared and packaged in disposable bottles. A home delivery service of ready-prepared formulas is available in some communities, but this is usually too expensive for most families.

SUPPLEMENTARY FEEDINGS

Neither human nor cow's milk will meet the full nutritive needs of the infant during the first year of life. Foods are added gradually to supplement the nutrient needs and to accustom the baby to the textures and flavors of solid foods. (See Tables 13–2 and 13–3.)

* Mead Johnson and Company, Evansville, Indiana.

TABLE 13–2   SEQUENCE FOR FOOD ADDITIONS TO INFANT'S DIET

Age	Food Addition and Its Nutritive Contribution
2–4 weeks	400 I.U. vitamin D from vitamin D milk or from a prescribed supplement
2–4 weeks	Orange or grapefruit juice or other source of vitamin C; twice as much tomato juice needed; start with 1 teaspoon diluted with boiled water; increase gradually to 3 oz full strength by 3 months
2–3 months	Cereal for iron, thiamine, calories; mix precooked cereal with formula; give thin consistency at first; increase to 2 to 5 tablespoons by 7 to 8 months
3–4 months	Mashed ripe banana, applesauce, strained pears, apricots, prunes, or peaches; start with 1 teaspoon and increase to 3–4 tablespoons by one year
3–5 months	Strained asparagus, green beans, carrots, peas, spinach, squash, or tomatoes; start with 1 teaspoon, increasing to 3–4 tablespoons by end of the year
4–6 months	Egg yolk for iron, vitamin A, thiamine, protein; mash hard-cooked egg with a little formula; use ¼ teaspoon at first
5–7 months	Strained meats for protein, iron, B complex; sometimes prescribed as early as 6 weeks of age
5–8 months	Crisp toast, zwieback, arrowroot cookies, teething biscuits
7–8 months	Baked or mashed potato or enriched pastas for calories and some additional iron and B complex
9 months	Peeled raw apple
8–10 months	Chopped vegetables and fruits
10 months	Whole egg; plain puddings, such as custard, Junket

Practices vary considerably on which foods are added first and on the age of introducing these foods. Some babies need supplements earlier than others; some are ready for changes in texture sooner than others. Techniques for introducing new foods and establishing good food habits, are discussed in Chapter 14.

Well-cooked cereals may be prepared in the home, sieved if they are coarse, and mixed with part of the formula to a suitable consistency. Cooked, blandly flavored, and lightly salted vegetables, and cooked or canned fruit may also be pressed through a sieve for infant feeding.

TABLE 13–3   TYPICAL SCHEDULES FOR FIVE-MONTH AND YEAR-OLD INFANTS

Five-Month Infant	Year-Old Infant
6 A.M. Formula, 6–7 oz	6:00 A.M. Orange juice, 3 oz Zwieback
8 A.M. Orange juice, 3 oz Vitamin D supplement *	7:30 A.M. Cereal, 2–5 tablespoons Milk, 8 oz Chopped fruit, 1–2 table- spoons Vitamin D supplement *
10 A.M. Formula, 6–7 oz Cereal, 2–3 tablespoons	11:30 A.M. Chopped meat, ½–1 oz *or*
2 P.M. Formula, 6–7 oz Egg yolk, ½–1 Vegetable, ¼ to 2 table- spoons	Egg, 1 Potato, 2–4 tablespoons Chopped vegetable, 2–4 tablespoons Milk, 8 oz
6 P.M. Formula, 6–7 oz Cereal, 2–3 tablespoons	5:30 P.M. Cereal or potato, 2–5 tablespoons Milk, 8 oz
10 P.M. Formula, 6–7 oz	Chopped fruit, 1–2 table- spoons Toast or zwieback

* If vitamin D milk is used, a supplement is not needed.

Strained baby foods were among the first convenience foods to be introduced on the market. They possess many advantages over home-prepared products: (1) newer techniques of processing result in maximum retention of nutritive value; (2) some infant foods, such as cereals, are enriched to meet more easily the iron and vitamin requirements; (3) much time is saved; and (4) these products are economical, because much food is often wasted when fruits and vegetables are sieved at home.

Preschool and School Children

NUTRITIONAL NEEDS

Any table of allowances must be interpreted according to the growth pattern of the individual child, the activity, the appetite, and the amount of musculature or body fatness. The growth patterns of children vary widely. Some children, by heredity, are destined to be short and stocky; others, tall and thin. Some children will have their rapid growth spurts at an earlier age than others. If a child does not have a satisfactory nutrient intake he may not reach the full growth of his hereditary pattern. The amount of physical activity varies widely and influences the calorie requirements.

During the second year the baby gains 8 to 10 lb. Following the second birthday and to the ninth year, the increase in height and weight is at a much slower rate; the annual gain in weight is about 4 to 7 lb. The muscles increase in size, the baby fat is lost, the legs become longer, and the bones becomes harder. There is great development in motor coordination, in changing body proportions, and in mental development.

The daily allowances for children of one to ten years are relatively high for all nutrients, when the size of the child is taken into account. See Table 4–1 for a complete list of recommended allowances. Six- to ten-year-old children have calorie needs equal to those of their mothers, and they need even more calcium. Because of the possibility of anemia, additional iron is recommended in the preschool years.

FOOD SELECTION AND HABITS

The Four Food Groups provide the basis for planning the diet for young children. Each child should receive 2 cups of milk daily. The size of servings from the other three groups is scaled according to the age of the child and his appetite. See Table 13–4 for a guide.

Few foods need to be omitted entirely from the diet of children, but some discretion in food selection is necessary. The appetite falls off during the preschool years, corresponding to the slower rate of growth. The appetite is ordinarily a good guide, but parents have a responsibility to provide a choice of foods within the framework of the Four Food Groups. When the child is permitted to eat freely from sweets and other empty-calorie foods, he will not obtain sufficient nutrients.

Young children prefer plain, blandly flavored foods that are only lightly seasoned. Mixtures, as in casseroles, are well accepted only as the child becomes older. Some foods that require chewing are essential, but meats that are not chopped or ground may be too tough for the preschool child. Lukewarm, rather than hot, foods are preferred. Vegetables are least well liked of all food groups. Strongly flavored vegetables may not be accepted until late school years; some children never learn to like them.

Children sometimes go on food jags; that is, they will eat only certain foods—for example, peanut-butter-and-jelly sandwiches. Usually these diversions of appetite do not last too long if the parents make no particular point of them. Milk may be refused as a beverage, but can often be given in puddings, or will be accepted if it is occasionally flavored or even colored with vegetable color! American cheese may be used as a substitute.

Children require snacks to provide for their relatively high energy needs and to avoid excessive hunger at mealtimes. The snacks should be

Food	Approximate Quantity Needed Daily	Average Size of Serving for Each Age		
		1 Year	2 and 3 Years	4 and 5 Years
Milk, to drink and in or on foods	2 to 3 measuring cups	½ to 1 cup	½ to 1 cup	1 cup
Eggs	1	1	1	1
Meat, poultry, fish, cottage cheese	1 to 4 tablespoonfuls †	1 tablespoonful	2 to 3 tablefuls	4 tablespoonfuls
Potatoes, white or sweet	1 serving	2 tablespoonfuls	3 tablespoonfuls	4 tablespoonfuls
Other cooked vegetables (mostly green leafy or deep-yellow ones)	1 to 2 servings	2 tablespoonfuls	3 tablespoonfuls	3 to 4 tablespoonfuls
Raw vegetables (carrots, cabbage, tomatoes, lettuce, etc.)	1 serving	Small portion (such as, ¼ medium-sized carrot)		
Fruit for vitamin C	1 medium orange or ⅓ cup citrus fruit juice or ⅔ cup tomato juice	⅓ to ½ cup	⅓ to ½ cup	⅓ to ⅔ cup
Other fruit (apples, apricots, bananas, pears, peaches, prunes, most berries, etc.)	1 serving	¼ cup	⅓ cup	½ cup
Bread, whole-grain or enriched	1½ to 3 slices	½ to 1 slice	1 slice	1 to 1½ slices
Cereal, whole-grain, enriched, or restored	1 serving	¼ cup	⅓ cup	½ cup
Butter or fortified margarine—Spread on bread, and used to season vegetables				
Fish-liver oil or vitamin D concentrate or vitamin D milk	400 units	(A quart of vitamin D milk contains 400 units.)		

* Children's Bureau, U.S. Department of Health, Education, and Welfare. "Your Child from One to Six," publication 30, revised 1956. Washington, D.C.

† One tablespoon means a level tablespoonful. A rounded tablespoonful is equal to 2 level ones.

selected largely from the Four Food Groups and may include fruits and fruit juices; milk; occasionally ice cream; crackers and peanut butter; molasses or peanut butter cookies; small sandwiches.

By the time a child is ready for school his food likes have increased, but he may face other problems relative to maintaining good nutrition. Mornings in many homes are too often rushed, so that breakfast is a hurried meal or may be skipped entirely. A child who is ill at ease at school may eat poorly at lunch. A short lunch period may be upsetting to the slow eater. Children of this age who are extremely active may become unduly tired before meals.

THE SCHOOL LUNCH

About one third of all school children participate in the school lunch. In a few cities breakfast programs are being tested. The type A school lunch provides about one third of the daily nutritive needs of the child. It includes:

½ pt fluid whole milk
Protein-rich food: 2 oz meat, fish, poultry, or cheese; 1 egg; ½ cup cooked beans or peas; or 4 tablespoons peanut butter
2 servings or more (at least ¾ cup) of vegetables and fruit (this must include a rich source of ascorbic acid daily and a rich source of vitamin A at least twice a week)
1 slice whole-grain or enriched bread or rolls, muffins, corn bread, or biscuits
2 teaspoons butter or fortified margarine

The school lunch does more than feed the child. The program helps the child to learn to like nutritious foods and to become familiar with food selection of an adequate diet. It gives an opportunity to strengthen nutrition education in the classroom.

The American Medical Association, the American Dietetic Association, and the National Congress of Parents and Teachers oppose the sale of candy and soft drinks within the schools. These foods contribute little to the nutritional needs of the child, and may divert the child from spending his money for the school lunch.

Preadolescent and Adolescent Youth

NUTRITIONAL NEEDS

Table 13–5 lists the allowances for calories and four nutrients for boys and girls from 10 to 18 years and for men and women of 45 years. The calorie and calcium needs of boys and girls considerably exceed those of their parents, and the protein and ascorbic acid allowances are only slightly below those for adults. Iron requires especial emphasis in the diet of boys and girls. Throughout the growing years 400 I.U. vitamin D should be included daily. Likewise, iodized salt should be used. For other mineral and vitamin allowances of boys and girls, see Table 4–1.

TABLE 13–5   SOME NUTRITIVE ALLOWANCES FOR BOYS AND GIRLS AND THEIR PARENTS

Age-Sex Group	Calories	Protein gm	Calcium gm	Iron mg	Ascorbic Acid mg
Boy, 10–12 years	2500	45	1.2	10	40
Boy, 12–14 years	2700	50	1.4	18	45
Boy, 14–18 years	3000	60	1.4	18	55
Man, 35–55 years	2600	65	0.8	10	60
Girl, 10–12 years	2250	50	1.2	18	40
Girl, 12–14 years	2300	50	1.3	18	45
Girl, 14–16 years	2400	55	1.3	18	50
Girl, 16–18 years	2300	55	1.3	18	50
Woman, 35–55 years	1850	55	0.8	18	55

The girl is especially vulnerable in iron nutrition. Her needs for iron are considerably increased because of the expanding blood circulation and to compensate for the monthly losses through menstruation.

Early marriage is the pattern in today's society, and the teen-age girl not infrequently becomes a mother at a time when her own body is still maturing. The mother-to-be would need to increase her own already high nutritive allowances by the amounts of nutrients needed for pregnancy. (See Chap. 12.)

FOOD SELECTION AND HABITS

As an age group, more teen-agers have poor food habits than any group in the life cycle. The diets of boys and girls most frequently fail to meet recommended allowances for calcium, vitamin A, and ascorbic acid. In addition, girls often do not get enough iron.

Of the food groups, milk requires special emphasis because of the great calcium needs and the substantial amount of protein provided. The 10-to-12-year-old should drink 3 or more cups of milk daily, and from 12 years on the boy or girl should drink not less than 4 cups daily. If dark-green leafy and deep-yellow vegetables and citrus fruits were more adequately consumed, the vitamin A and ascorbic acid intakes would be substantially improved.

The impression is sometimes gained that all teen-agers are poorly nourished and always eat great quantities of empty-calorie snacks. In fact, many teen-agers have good food habits, are well nourished, and might serve as good examples for others in their age group who need to improve their food habits. Perhaps we have not sufficiently appealed to the teen-ager himself in terms of his needs for better nutrition. Girls express a particular need for a good figure, a healthy skin, and beautiful hair. They need to understand the patterns of normal maturing of the body so that they do not indulge in bizarre reducing diets. Although a good diet is essential to a healthy skin, they also need to understand that skin problems may arise when rapid changes in hormone production are taking place.

Boys are more likely to be interested in tall stature, muscular development, and athletic vigor and stamina. They too have skin problems about which they are concerned. The large appetite of boys helps to ensure an increased intake of needed nutrients along with the foods that are supplying calories.

Among the particular problems during adolescence are these:

1. *Skipped meals.* Many high-school students keep late hours, get up too late in the morning to eat breakfast, eat a hurried lunch at school, and never quite make up during the rest of the day for their nutritional requirements.

2. *Overweight.* The pattern of overweight is often set in earlier childhood through a continuing excessive food intake. Active participation in sports rather than watching others engage in sports is important. Weight control should begin in childhood and during adolescence and not be delayed to middle age.

3. *Snacks.* Boys and girls, as a rule, need some snacks, but their selection should be substantially from the Four Food Groups. A correlation has been established between the excessive intake of soft drinks and sweets and the amount of tooth decay. This is not to say that any foods are altogether forbidden. Rather, if there is an adequate intake of foods from the Four Food Groups the amounts of empty-calorie foods to satisfy the appetite will be correspondingly reduced.

REVIEW QUESTIONS AND PROBLEMS

1. Visit a drug store or infant department in a department store to see the kinds of equipment available for formula preparation. Develop a list of minimum equipment a mother would need, keeping cost as low as possible.

2. Why is terminal sterilization of the formula preferable to the aseptic technique?

3. Write a schedule for a day for a seven-month-old infant, indicating the kinds and approximate amounts of foods to include at this time.

4. A baby eats one third of the contents of a can of strained fruit. What would you do with the rest of it?

5. Why is egg white not given until toward the end of the first year?

6. What is meant by a Type A lunch? Why is the school lunch program of such importance for the child? Plan a packed lunch for a 12-year-old boy who attends a school where there is no lunch program.

7. Develop suggestions for helping teen-agers to improve their food habits.

8. What nutrients require special emphasis during adolescence? What foods will meet these needs?

9. Write a menu for one day for adults. Modify this menu so that it is suitable for a three-year-old, an eight-year-old, and a 15-year-old boy. Include plans for snacks.

REFERENCES

Children's Bureau, U.S. Department of Health, Education and Welfare, Washington, D.C. *The Adolescent in Your Family*, 1964. *Infant Care*, 1966. *Your Baby's First Year*, 1962. *Your Child from One to Three*, 1964. *Your Child from One to Six*, 1963. *Your Child from Six to Twelve*, 1966.

Gregg, W. N. A *Boy and His Physique*. Chicago: National Dairy Council, 1963.

Leverton, R. M. A *Girl and Her Figure*. Chicago: National Dairy Council, 1962.

Lubchenko, L. O. "Formulas and Nutrition," *Amer. J. Nurs.*, **61**:73, May 1961.

Rasmussen, S. *Foundations of Practical and Vocational Nursing*. New York: The Macmillan Company, 1967, Chaps. 43, 44, 45, 46.

Richardson, F. H. "Breast or Bottle Feeding," *Today's Health*, **40**:62, May 1962.

Robinson, C. H. *Proudfit-Robinson's Normal and Therapeutic Nutrition*, 13th ed. New York: The Macmillan Company, 1967, Chaps. 23 and 24.

Smith, B. B. "Weaning the Breast-Fed Baby," *Today's Health*, **40**:26, July 1962.

Spindler, E. B. "Better Diets for Teenagers," *Nurs. Outlook*, **12**:32, February 1964.

U.S. Department of Agriculture, Washington, D.C.: *Food for Families with School Children*, 1963. *Improving Teen-Age Nutrition*, 1963.

TOWARD BETTER FOOD HABITS

Hunger is the urge to eat and is accompanied by a number of unpleasant sensations. It follows a period when one has been deprived of food, and is generally associated with contraction of the stomach. The individual begins to feel irritable, uneasy, and tired. If a blood sample is taken at this time, the blood sugar level is somewhat low. When food is taken, the individual begins to feel better almost immediately.

Appetite is the anticipation of and the desire to eat palatable food.

People eat not only to satisfy hunger. People also eat because food has many meanings for them. Good or bad food habits may result because of the interaction of social, emotional, and cultural factors. In order to help improve your own food habits and to help other people improve theirs, you need to appreciate and understand the variations people have in their likes and dislikes and their attitudes toward food.

Some people have good food habits because they have been fortunate in their early home and school environment. Other people through education have seen the need for change and have been willing to work to modify their habits. Are you one of these?

Many people remain indifferent and ignorant concerning nutrition. They are willing to believe only that which pleases them, and they often use childhood experiences as excuses for being finicky.

Factors Affecting Acceptance of Food

PHYSIOLOGIC VARIATIONS

Young children have many more taste buds on the tongue and in the cheek, and therefore they have a keener sense of taste than older individuals. Babies and young children prefer bland foods, whereas teenagers begin to like foods that are more spicy and highly flavored. The number of taste buds diminishes later in life, and old people often lose a sense of taste for certain foods.

The sense of taste varies widely from one individual to another. Some people notice slight differences in taste, and others do not. Some persons like much salt, others only a little; some like very sweet foods, others do not; some like spicy foods, and others prefer bland foods. From day to day, the senses of taste and smell also vary. Smelling food too long at a time, or having a steady diet of certain foods, may reduce the response of the sense organs.

The feel of foods is also important. A baby learns about food by feeling it as well as tasting it. We all react favorably to velvety ice cream, crisp rolls, fluffy mashed potatoes, but we are likely to object to sugary fudge, greasy meat, lumpy mashed potatoes, and stringy string beans. Young children don't like very hot or cold foods, but adults usually demand that their foods be piping hot or well chilled.

REGIONAL PATTERNS IN THE UNITED STATES

Food habits result from the foods that have been available in the various parts of the world. People everywhere tend to like the foods with which they are familiar. Even before tasting a food they will look with suspicion and dislike on something that is unfamiliar. The ease with which people travel from one part of the world to another is doing much to widen our food experiences and to make us more appreciative of other cultures.

Some regional differences still exist in the United States, but for the most part, these are exceptions rather than major departures from the diet. One is likely to associate New England with clam chowder, codfish cakes, Boston baked beans, and lobster; Pennsylvania Dutch, with seven sweets and sours, scrapple, German-type sausage, and shoofly pie; the South, with corn bread, hominy, fried chicken, hot biscuits, turnip and other greens, and sweet potatoes; Louisiana, with French and Creole cookery; the Southwest, with Mexican dishes; the Midwest, with its abundance of dairy products, eggs, and meat and the traditions of Scandinavian, Polish, and Germany cookery; the Far West, with its luscious fruits and vegetables, salmon, and the influences of the Orient.

NATIONAL FOOD PATTERNS

Although people of the United States come from nationality back-grounds from all over the world, the differences in their diets are evident primarily on holidays and family celebrations. Those who adhere more closely to national patterns can readily adapt to the varied supplies of foods in our markets when taught how to do so. A few of the more outstanding examples of some dietary patterns are described briefly below.

Puerto Rican. Many Puerto Ricans have come recently to the large cities of the eastern United States. They are frequently poor, lack employment skills, and live in crowded, often unsanitary, quarters. Because of difficulty in speaking and understanding English, they are likely to patronize small food stores that are owned by Spanish-speaking people. They usually pay much more for the foods they purchase than they would in a supermarket. These and other factors account for a high level of malnutrition, especially among children.

Their staple foods include rice, chick peas, kidneys beans, and other legumes, and a variety of *viandas* or starchy vegetables, such as plantain, green bananas, white sweet potato, and others. Dried codfish is often used. Although milk, chicken, and pork are well liked, they are infrequently used because of cost. Fruits and vegetables have always been available to them in abundance, but they have made limited use of them.

Rice (*arroz*) is eaten once or twice a day and may be combined with a little codfish, legumes, and occasionally chicken (*arroz con pollo*) or pork. The legumes are usually cooked and dressed with a highly seasoned tomato sauce (*sofrito*). The starchy vegetables are boiled and served with oil, oil and vinegar, or some dried codfish.

Mexican. The staple foods of Mexicans include corn, pinto or calico beans, and chili peppers; wheat is now replacing some of the corn. Milk is seldom used, and meat and eggs appear on the menu only two or three times a week. Mexican dishes are seasoned liberally with red chili powder, garlic, onion, and spices.

Dried corn is heated and soaked in lime water, washed, and pounded to a putty-like dough called *masa*. Thin cakes rolled from the masa and baked on a hot griddle are known as *tortillas*. Cheese and ground meat with onion and lettuce may be used to fill tortillas in preparations known as *enchiladas*. Tamales consist of highly seasoned ground meat and masa wrapped in corn husks, steamed, and served with chili sauce. (See Fig. 14-1.)

Italian. Pastas such as spaghetti, macaroni, and noodles in many sizes and shapes are characteristic of the Italian diet. Crusty Italian bread is widely used. Chicken, lamb, pork, and veal and a variety of cold cuts are popular but eaten less frequently than in typical American diets. Milk is

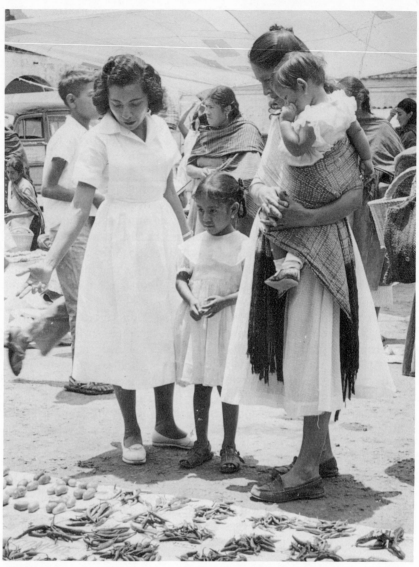

FIGURE 14–1 A community nurse in Mexico points out the importance of selecting fruits and vegetables for the family's meals. *(Courtesy, UNICEF.)*

not used much, but many varieties of Italian cheeses are favored. Vegetables boiled and dressed with oil or oil and vinegar are well liked. Salads and fruits are important parts of the day's meals.

Noodle doughs may be filled with meat, cheese, and vegetable mixtures for such dishes as *lasagne, ravioli,* and *pizza.* Chick peas, split peas, kidney beans, and lentils may be used in such substantial soups as *minestrone. Polenta* is a thick cornmeal mush often served plain or with tomato sauce and cheese.

Near East. Round, flat loaves of bread are the staff of life at every meal. Cracked parboiled whole wheat (bulgur) and rice are staple foods eaten as such or with vegetables and meat. Fermented milk (yogurt) is preferred to plain milk. Fresh fruits are widely used. Eggplant, zucchini, onions, peppers, okra, cabbage, and cauliflower are favorite vegetables.

Lamb and mutton are preferred, although other meats and poultry are also eaten. Meat is often ground or cut and cooked with wheat, rice, or vegetables. For example, ground meat may be baked in cabbage leaves, and pieces of cut lamb may be placed on skewers with tomato and onion slices for *shashlik*.

Oriental. Rice, wheat, and millet are staple cereals providing most of the calories and protein for people of the Orient. The Chinese use soybeans and soybean sprouts in many dishes. Finely sliced vegetables are cooked by the Chinese for a short time in a little oil and retain their color and crispness. Chicken, pork, eggs, fish, and shellfish serve as the foundation for many delicious dishes, such as shrimp egg rolls, sweet and sour pork, and chow mein, an American adaptation. Milk, cheese, and beef are not widely used. Sesame oil, peanut oil, and lard are much used. Soy sauce at almost every meal contributes to a high salt intake. Almonds, sesame seeds, and ginger are popular seasonings.

RELIGION AND DIETARY PATTERNS

Various foods have symbolic meanings in religion. Likewise, most religions place certain restrictions upon the use of food. The regulations for fasting placed upon Roman Catholics have been liberalized, but many Catholics still abstain from meat on fast days; to them fish and cheese may be associated with denial and penitence. Islamites abstain from eating pork, whereas Buddhists are vegetarians and will not eat the flesh of any animal. Seventh Day Adventists are lacto-ovo-vegetarians; that is, they do not eat meat but they use eggs, milk, nuts, and legumes as sources of protein.

Orthodox Jews adhere to dietary laws based upon tradition and the Bible. Animals and poultry are slaughtered according to ritual, and the meat is soaked in water, salted to remove the blood, and washed. This is known as *koshering*. Pork and shellfish are prohibited.

Milk, sour cream, cottage cheese, and cream cheese are widely used, but no dairy foods are served at a meal with meat. Usually two meals each day are dairy meals, and one meal is a meat meal. Separate utensils are used for the cookery of meat and dairy products. Fish, eggs, vegetables, fruits, cereals, and bread may be used at all meals; however, no milk or butter may be used with these foods if they are included in the meat meal.

No food preparation takes place on the Sabbath, and an Orthodox Jew may refuse to eat food that has been freshly cooked on the Sabbath. Religious festivals are celebrated with special dishes, and much symbolism is attached to food. For example, only unleavened bread is eaten during the Passover. Separate sets of dishes are used during the Passover week. On Yom Kippur (Day of Atonement), the most solemn day of the religious year, no food or drink is taken for 24 hours.

Among the widely used foods by Jewish people are *borsch* (a soup), *gefullte fish*, *blintzes* (thin rolled pancakes filled with cottage cheese or ground beef), *knishes* (pastry with ground meat), *challah* (a braided white bread), *bagel* (doughnut-shaped hard yeast roll), *kuchen* (coffee cake), *leckach* (honey cake served especially at Rosh Hashana, the New Year), and *strudel* (fruit-filled pastry).

FAMILY CUSTOMS AND SOCIAL PATTERNS

The family environment has much influence on food habits. Food is more likely to be well accepted when the entire family is together for meals in a happy, relaxed atmosphere. If the homemaker prepares only a few well-liked dishes over and over again, the family members will encounter some difficulty in adapting to other situations. Within the family some allowances may be made for individual likes and dislikes without preparing many separate dishes. If the homemaker selects a variety of foods and prepares them in different ways from time to time, the individual's food experiences are enriched.

Negative attitudes to food may be developed in the home. Children are quick to imitate their parents, who may not be eating certain foods. They rapidly note signs of worry, dislike, or anger on the part of the parents and may develop antagonisms toward particular foods. They dawdle when they learn it is a way to gain attention. Parents sometimes punish by refusing to give dessert to a child who hasn't finished his meal or bribe and reward with a favorite food like candy if a meal is finished.

Foods are often classed as being for babies, young children, or adults. Milk, cut-up food, peanut-butter-and-jelly sandwiches are looked upon as children's foods; hamburgers, pizza, and large sandwiches are teen-age fare; tea and coffee are for adults.

Meat, potatoes, and pie are considered to be typical of masculine meals, whereas soufflés, salads, and light desserts are more characteristic of feminine foods.

Some foods have more prestige value than others, and we may use them as company foods to honor or impress our friends. They cost more, are hard to get, take a lot of time to prepare, or are unusual. Examples of such status foods are filet mignon, wild rice, baked Alaska, and a fine imported wine. Other foods are sometimes considered to be only for those with low incomes; ground meat, margarine, dry skim milk, dry beans, and fish, for example. Yet any of the latter foods are just as nutritious and can be prepared in as many delicious ways as more expensive foods.

FOOD AND THE EMOTIONS

Did you ever go to a soda fountain for a fancy sundae after taking an examination? Or have you sometimes rewarded yourself for finishing a difficult job with an especially good meal in a restaurant? Do you recall with pleasure certain meals at birthday parties or holidays? Food is often used in one way or another to express or to cover up our feelings of happiness, love, security, worry, grief, loneliness, and so on.

The baby who is held when he is fed associates his food with warmth and security. But a child who is scolded for being messy may associate certain foods with unhappiness. The teen-ager may overeat to compensate for a poor record in school or unpopularity with his classmates. Elderly persons living alone often eat far too little, because they are lonely and unhappy. People who are grieving or who can't face the problems that beset them are known to gain excessive weight in some instances, because they find relief in eating excessive quantities of food.

Establishment of Good Food Habits

TECHNIQUES FOR CHANGING FOOD HABITS

Good food habits are easily acquired in youth, and it is more difficult to change the habits of people later in life. Perhaps you have found some of your food habits should be improved, or maybe you can help someone in your family or a friend to improve his. The following suggestions may be helpful.

1. A change in food habits is indicated only if the present habits lead to poor nutrition. Remember that persons who have good food habits need not like every nutritious food. Also, it is not necessary to omit all foods that are poor sources of the nutrients.

2. Find out what reasons are most likely to appeal to the individual. Boys are often motivated on the basis of growth in stature, physical vigor, and ability in sports. The teen-age girl, on the other hand, may be looking for a slim figure to be in the latest fashion, or for a clear skin and glossy hair. Neither boys nor girls are likely to be interested in the promise of health or of a good old age, but they might like to impress their friends with their cosmopolitan tastes in food. Older people, on the other hand, are interested in weight control from the standpoint of health or may be motivated by diet control of some disease problems.

3. Look at the whole diet pattern—not just at one meal pattern or the

snacks. List the good points of the diet as well as the weaknesses. Start with the good points for building a better pattern.

4. Be realistic in what can be accomplished. Expect only small changes at the time. Make allowances for strong likes and dislikes. Don't suggest foods that are too expensive, hard to get, or contrary to one's beliefs.

5. Encourage the individual to become adventurous in trying new foods at home or when eating out.

6. Provide practical suggestions for preparing foods in attractive ways.

Specific suggestions given below for infants and young children also apply in principle toward the improvement of food habits later in life.

FOOD HABITS FOR THE INFANT

Good food habits in infancy and childhood will lead in later life to a liking for a wide variety of foods and the willingness to accept change. Parents have a wonderful opportunity as well as a tremendous responsibility for the development of good food habits in the young infant. (See Fig. 14–2.)

1. Hold the young baby while he receives his formula to provide the feelings of satisfaction, security, and warmth.

2. Regulate the feeding schedule to the baby, not to the clock.

3. Introduce only one new food at a time.

4. Give new foods at the beginning of the meal when the baby is hungry.

5. Serve only small portions of a new food; a taste is enough.

6. Don't show your dislike of a food by the expression on your face or by refusing to eat the food yourself.

7. Babies, like adults, are more hungry at some times than others. Don't expect them to finish every bottle or everything at every meal.

8. Expect that the baby will feel his food and be messy. Don't scold him for spilling accidents.

9. Use a cup that does not tip easily, a deep bowl with rounded edges, and a spoon that can be managed by the baby. Provide safe and comfortable seating.

PRESCHOOL AND SCHOOL CHILDREN

1. Serve meals in a pleasant place and a calm unhurried atmosphere.

2. Provide meals that are colorful, varied in texture and flavor, and attractively served.

3. Don't serve the same food over and over again even if it is a favorite. Even well-liked foods can become tiresome.

4. Provide eating utensils and dishes that are easy for the child to hold and to use. Many vegetables, fruits, meats, and bread may be served as finger foods.

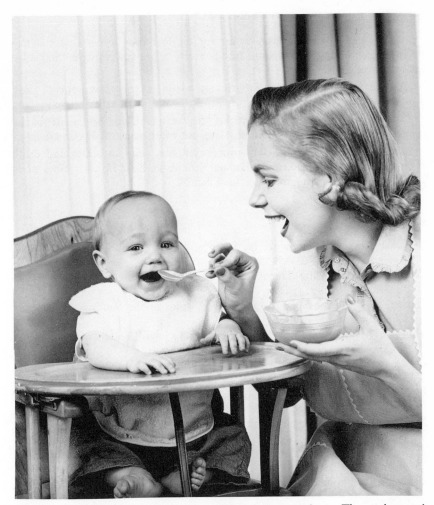

FIGURE 14-2 Good food habits are established during infancy. The environment should be pleasant, secure, and relaxed. (*Courtesy, Gerber Products Company.*)

5. Allow sufficient time for meals; breakfast need not be hurried if children are awakened early enough.

6. Don't let the child become too tired before meals. Plan for adequate rest and early bedtime.

7. Plan for snacks as carefully as the meal. Snacks can provide good nutrition. They should not be eaten so close to meals that the appetite is spoiled for the meal.

8. Remember that appetite decreases as the rate of growth slows down during the second, third, and fourth years of life. The toddler may refuse certain foods at this time in trying to assert his independence; don't make too much of this.

REVIEW QUESTIONS AND PROBLEMS

1. A young man away from home for the first time writes that the food he is getting is not to his liking. List as many reasons as you can that affect his food acceptance.

2. What nationality food patterns are found in your community? Write a menu for one day that would be well liked by one nationality group.

3. If possible, visit a food market that caters to particular nationality groups. What foods do you find that are not often seen in supermarkets?

4. A 14-year-old girl is 15 lb overweight. She skips breakfast and drinks little milk, eats no bread, and does not like vegetables. In what ways could you approach her to improve her food habits?

REFERENCES

Berkowitz, P., and Berkowitz, N. S. "The Jewish Patient in the Hospital," *Amer. J. Nurs.*, 67:2335, 1967.

Cantoni, M. "Adapting Therapeutic Diets to the Eating Patterns of Italian-Americans," *Amer. J. Clin. Nutr.*, 6:548, 1958.

Hacker, D. B., and Miller, E. D. "Food Patterns of the Southwest," *Amer. J. Clin. Nutr.*, 7:224, 1959.

Kaufman, M. L. "Adapting Therapeutic Diets to Jewish Food Customs," *Amer. J. Clin. Nutr.*, 5:676, 1957.

Longman, D. P. "Working with Pueblo Indians in New Mexico," *J. Amer. Diet. Ass.*, 47:470, 1965.

MacGregor, F. C. "Uncooperative Patients: Some Cultural Interpretations," *Amer. J. Nurs.*, 67:88, 1967.

Mayer, J. "The Nutritional Status of American Negroes," *Nutr. Rev.*, 23:161, 1965.

Torres, R. M. "Dietary Patterns of the Puerto Rican People," *Amer. J. Clin. Nutr.*, 7:349, 1959.

Valassi, K. V. "Food Habits of Greek-Americans," *Amer. J. Clin. Nutr.*, 11:240, 1962.

Wauneka, A. D. "Helping a People to Understand," *Amer. J. Nurs.*, 62:88, July 1962.

15

CAUSES OF FOOD SPOILAGE · **Illness from Food** | BACTERIAL INFECTIONS AND INTOXICATIONS | PARASITE INFESTATIONS | CHEMICAL POISONING · **Preservation of Foods** | OBJECTIVES FOR FOOD PRESERVATION | DEHYDRATION | COLD TEMPERATURES | HEAT PRESERVATION | CHEMICAL PRESERVATION | ANTIBIOTICS | RADIATION PRESERVATION · **Additives** · **Food Protection Through Legislation** | FEDERAL LAWS | STATE AND LOCAL LEGISLATION

THE FOOD SUPPLY AND PUBLIC HEALTH

Present-day public health standards provide an excellent safeguard for water and milk so that illness occurs infrequently from these sources. The food supply in the United States is more wholesome than at any time in history, and disease from food, in terms of the total population, is amazingly low. Nevertheless, illness from eating contaminated food still occurs more often than it should, and constant vigilance on the part of the government, the food industry, and the consumer must be taken to safeguard the food supply.

CAUSES OF FOOD SPOILAGE

Bacteria and parasites in food may lead to illness; yeasts produce fermentation, as in cider and fruit juices; molds attack wet berries, citrus fruits, bread, jellies and jams, and other foods. Chemical and physical changes also occur in food; enzyme activity leads to softening of the food, development of off flavors, and loss of some nutrients; in a few hours sunlight destroys much of the riboflavin in milk and changes the flavor; exposure to air leads to darkening of peeled fruit and to rancidity of fats.

Foods are contaminated by any of the following ways:

1. Preparation by persons whose hands have not been washed after each use of the handkerchief, toilet, or contact with other source of dirt and filth.

2. Exposure to dust, flies, insects, and nasal sprays of persons who cough or sneeze.

155

3. Use of equipment and dishes that are poorly cleaned and rinsed.

4. Failure to refrigerate fresh or cooked food promptly, thus speeding up the action of bacteria, molds, yeasts, and enzymes.

Illness from Food

BACTERIAL INFECTIONS AND INTOXICATIONS

Diphtheria, tuberculosis, streptococcic sore throat, typhoid fever, hepatitis, tularemia, undulant fever, dysentery, and gastrointestinal upsets including vomiting and diarrhea are examples of food-borne diseases. The illness occurs after the organism has been incubated in the human body for the usual period of time. In some instances the illness results from the toxin produced by the bacteria in food.

Staphylococcic food poisoning is caused by the toxin produced by the bacteria. Staphylococci may be present in the nose and throat of food handlers. Skin cuts, boils, and pimples are a frequent source of food contamination. The bacteria are not destroyed in foods cooked at low temperatures, including creamed dishes, puddings, cream-filled pies and pastries, and poultry stuffing. They also grow very rapidly in ground meats, and egg, meat, poultry, fish, and potato salads mixed with mayonnaise. The toxin produced by the bacteria is not destroyed by boiling for as long as 20 minutes or more. Foods that are kept at room temperature for three or four hours may look, smell, and taste all right but may contain enough of the toxin to produce severe cramps, vomiting, and diarrhea one to six hours after the food is eaten.

Salmonella infection is frequent, and results from eating contaminated eggs, custard-filled bakery products, poultry, and prepared meat products. The use of raw eggs in beverages and other dishes is now generally discouraged. *Salmonella* infections cause gastrointestinal upsets within 6 to 24 hours after the contaminated food is eaten.

Clostridium perfringens. This organism, also known as the gas gangrene organism, causes numerous gastrointestinal outbreaks every year. The bacteria are readily killed by heat, but the spores produced by the bacteria are destroyed only with very long heating. Thus, the spores will germinate and produce high numbers of bacteria if the food is kept at room temperature for one or more hours before serving.

Botulism is a rare but deadly poisoning that results from the toxin produced by *Clostridium botulinum.* The bacteria are present in soils and thus infect vegetables. The bacteria produce spores that are heat-resistant, and that germinate in the absence of oxygen as in canned foods. The growing bacteria produce botulin, a toxin that causes fatalities in about 65 per cent of all cases. Most instances of poisoning have occurred from eating inadequately sterilized home-canned meats, poultry, and nonacid vegetables, such as corn, beets, peas, beans, and asparagus. The high temperature attained with a pressure cooker for a sufficient length of time is the only way to be certain that the spores have been destroyed. Home-canned vegetables and meats should always be boiled for six to ten minutes before even tasting, because boiling destroys the toxin if it is present.

PARASITE INFESTATIONS

Foods may be contaminated by tapeworms, pinworms, and *Endamoeba histolytica*, which causes amebic dysentery. With increased world travel, the incidence of parasitic diseases may be expected to increase in the United States. Parasite infestations seriously affect the nutritional status, especially in young children.

Trichinella spiralis is a worm that becomes embedded in the muscle tissue of pork and leads to trichinosis in humans who eat raw or incompletely cooked pork. *Trichinella* is destroyed when pork is cooked to the well-done state, or when pork is kept frozen at $0°F$.

CHEMICAL POISONING

Some varieties of wild mushrooms and toadstools are deadly poisonous. Oxalic acid in rhubarb leaves, solanine in the green part of potatoes, and an alkaloid in Pacific coast mussels at certain times of the year are likely to cause severe illness.

Chemical compounds sometimes contaminate the food supply. A continuing problem of public health is that of the use of sprays for insects and other pests. The effect of a continuous ingestion of such sprays from unwashed fruits and vegetables is not known. The amount of such products that may be used in the growing of food is now defined by law.

Chemical poisoning sometimes results when an insecticide or cleaning agent is kept in an unlabeled container and is mistaken for a food product. Such chemicals should be clearly labeled, always stored in an area away from food, and kept out of the reach of children.

Preservation of Foods

OBJECTIVES FOR FOOD PRESERVATION

Food preservation aims (1) to destroy microorganisms as by heat, or (2) to retard their growth by removal of moisture or the use of cold temperatures. Chemical changes are minimized by avoiding exposure to air and light, by reducing the environmental temperature, and by destroying enzymes. Some losses in nutritive value, especially ascorbic acid and thiamine, are unavoidable. However, commercial techniques now ensure processed foods with a greater proportion of all nutrients still present.

DEHYDRATION

Drying is one of the oldest methods of food preservation. Modern techniques have made many of these foods attractive in terms of their ease of preparation, the variety they lend to the diet, and the fact that they can be stored at room temperature. Instant dry milk, instant potatoes, mixes for breads, cakes, cookies, and puddings, instant coffee, beverage powders, and mixes for soups, as well as dried fruit, are among the products we now take for granted.

COLD TEMPERATURES

Refrigeration. Perishable foods are now transported from coast to coast under refrigeration, are kept cold in the market until sold, and remain high in quality for several days to a week in the home refrigerator.

Freezing of food has been employed for centuries in cold regions of the world, but the advent of quick freezing of food in the 1930's has revolutionized the food industry. Foods are rapidly frozen at $-35°F$ and may be stored in the home freezer at $0°F$ for several weeks or months (depending upon the product) with minimum changes in texture, color, flavor, or nutritive value. Bacteria and enzymes are not destroyed at freezing temperatures, but they are inactive. Once food is thawed, however, spoilage occurs more rapidly because the cell walls have been broken by the tiny ice crystals. Thawed food should be used promptly and not refrozen.

Freeze-drying consists in quickly freezing the food product, drying it in a vacuum, and finally packaging it in the presence of an inert gas such as nitrogen. The food retains its original shape, and can be readily rehydrated with water. It is light in weight and requires no refrigeration. The method is not extensively used for products for home use at the present time.

HEAT PRESERVATION

Cookery. The boiling of food leads to destruction of microorganisms and of enzymes. Lower temperatures, such as those attained in a double boiler, are not sufficient to destroy certain organisms, such as *Salmonella* in eggs. *Trichinella* in pork is destroyed only when the meat is cooked so that no tinge of pink color remains. Some spores of bacteria and some toxins are not destroyed by the heat used in ordinary cooking methods.

Pasteurization is the application of heat to destroy pathogenic organisms, but it does not sterilize the product. In the high-temperature, short-time process now widely used, milk is held at 160°F for at least 15 seconds. Undoubtedly, the pasteurization of milk is the major reason why disease now rarely results from the drinking of milk. Milk and cream for the manufacture of cheese, ice cream, and butter are usually pasteurized.

Canning is still the primary means used to preserve foods for long periods of time. Commercial canning is done by steam under pressure; thus at 15 lb pressure the temperature is 250°F. Home canning is far less frequent than at one time. Meat, poultry, and nonacid vegetables, such as corn, peas, and green beans, should be canned only with a pressure cooker to ensure destruction of the spores of *Cl. botulinum*.

CHEMICAL PRESERVATION

Sugar has a preservative effect when used in high concentrations for jams, jellies, and preserves. Molds will grow on the surfaces of such products, however, unless they are protected from the air. Brine is used for pickles, sauerkraut, and pickled fish. Sodium benzoate may be used in a limited number of products, including margarine. Sulfur dioxide prevents the darkening of apples and apricots during dehydration. The growth of molds is retarded in bread with the use of calcium propionate and in cheese by using wrappings to which sorbic acid has been added.

ANTIBIOTICS

Antibiotics retard the growth of microorganisms and may be used under controlled conditions to extend the shelf life of dressed poultry and fish. Chlortetracycline (Aureomycin) and oxytetracycline (Terramycin) are diluted in water to rinse dressed poultry or in the ice slush to pack fish. No harm results to humans if the fish or poultry is cooked because the antibiotics are destroyed by heat.

RADIATION PRESERVATION

Small doses of irradiation will destroy the insects in grains and *Trichinella* in pork, delay the ripening of fruit, and prevent the sprouting of potatoes and onions. The complete destruction of bacteria and enzymes requires such high levels of irradiation that marked changes occur in color, flavor, and nutritive value. Much testing remains to be done on irradiation before it is used for commercial food processing.

Additives

Numerous compounds are used in agriculture, by the food processor, and by the homemaker for the growing, manufacture, and preparation of food. These compounds, now in excess of 1000, are known as *additives.* Even salt, baking powder, and baking soda are chemical additives.

Intentional additives. Many chemicals improve the flavor, texture, appearance, nutritive value, and keeping properties of some foods. Nutrients added to food include iron, thiamine, riboflavin, and niacin to flours, breads, and cereals; vitamin D to milk; vitamin A to margarine; and iodine to salt. Certified food colors, flavorings, and spices improve the appearance and flavor of many foods. Calcium propionate is added to bread and rolls to inhibit the growth of molds. Emulsifiers and stabilizers are used to keep the oil from separating out in peanut butter or French dressing and to maintain smoothness in ice cream. Carbon dioxide is present in pressurized cans of whipped cream. Antioxidants are added to fats to retard rancidity, and ascorbic acid retards the darkening of peeled fruit.

Incidental additives. Some chemicals enter into food accidentally rather than intentionally; for example, insecticides from unwashed fruits and vegetables and substances present in the package but not ordinarily in the food itself. Constant control is needed of the levels of insecticides used for spraying crops. The washing of fruits and vegetables before eating needs to be emphasized over and over again.

Radioactive fallout. Nuclear testing has increased the amount of strontium 90 and iodine 131 in the atmosphere and consequently in the soil. Cattle may transmit strontium 90 from the grasses they eat to their milk, and plants grown on such soils may also contain radioactive elements. The absorption of large quantities of iodine 131 by the body increases the possibility of thyroid cancer. About four fifths of the strontium 90 is excreted in the urine, but some is deposited in the bones and gonads. A liberal intake of calcium appears to be protective against excessive deposit of strontium 90. The Atomic Energy Commission and the United States Public Health Service measure the amounts of radioactive fallout in food supplies from time to time. Presently, the amounts are well below any danger levels.

Food Protection Through Legislation

FEDERAL LAWS

The first federal food and drug law was passed in 1906 and was replaced in 1938 by a more comprehensive Federal Food, Drug, and Cosmetic Act—also known as the "Pure Food and Drug Law." This law pertains to food, other than meat and poultry products, sold in interstate commerce and imported and exported foods. It requires that foods be pure, wholesome, and honestly labeled.

Amendments. Several amendments to the law have been enacted. The Miller Pesticide Amendment of 1954 enables the establishment of safe tolerances of pesticides that may remain in foods after they have been harvested. The Additives Amendment of 1958 provides that an additive may be used in a food product only if it can be shown to improve the nutritive quality, appearance, or keeping properties of a food and not to cover up the use of an inferior food. The amendment requires the manufacturer to submit evidence from experimental work on animals that an additive is safe before it may be included in a food product for sale. The Food and Drug Administration examines the evidence, seeks further proof if necessary, and then issues or refuses a permit for the use of the additive, depending upon its findings. The Color Additive Amendment of 1960 provides for the establishment of safe tolerance levels for all colors used in foods.

Special dietary foods and supplements must be labeled to give information on the composition of the product in terms of the intended use for modified diets. New regulations proposed by the Food and Drug Administration have not been finally adopted at this time.

Enforcement. The food and drug law, together with its amendments, is enforced by the Food and Drug Administration of the Department of Health, Education, and Welfare. Under the law, factories and warehouses may be inspected to ascertain that the raw materials together with processing, packaging, and storage facilities are sanitary. Adulterated and misbranded products may be seized by inspectors and destroyed or relabeled, depending upon the nature of the offense. Flagrant violations may result in the imposition of fines or imprisonment by the courts.

Interpretation of the law. A food is *adulterated* if it contains dirt, filth, or decomposed material or any substance harmful to health; if it is prepared, packaged, or stored under unsanitary conditions; if it is made from diseased animals; if it contains additives that conceal the poor quality of the food; if it contains unsafe additives, uncertified food colors, or pesticide residues in excess of tolerances; if the packaging material contains substances harmful to health.

Misbranded food is that which has a false, misleading label; a package that fails to specify the weight, measure, or count of the food; a package that is of misleading size, so that the consumer thinks he is getting more than he actually is; a label that does not clearly state the use of imitations, including artificial color, flavorings, and preservatives; a label that fails to list the name of the manufacturer, packer, or distributor; a label that does not list the amounts of nutrients in special dietary products. (See Fig. 15–1.)

The Food and Drug Administration also establishes what a product actually is by setting standards of *identity*, *quality*, and *fill*. Foods for which an official standard has been set must contain amounts of ingre-

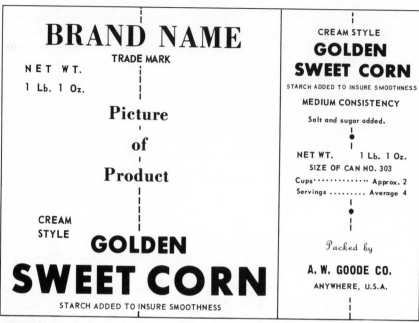

FIGURE 15–1 Sample food label. The label must bear (1) the name and place of business of the manufacturer, packer, or distributor; (2) an accurate statement of the quantity of the contents in terms of weight, measure, or count; (3) statement of any artificial coloring, artificial flavoring, or chemical preservative that may have been used. (*Courtesy, Food and Drug Administration.*)

dients not below the prescribed minimum nor above the legal maximum. This regulation applies also to the addition of required amounts of nutrients for enrichment and fortification. For nonstandardized products the ingredients are listed in order from the greatest amount to the least. Standards of quality for canned vegetables, fruits, and meats, and other products pertain to the color, flavor, and freedom from defects. Standards of fill specify how full a container must be.

Meat and poultry inspection. The Meat Inspection Act of 1906 and its amendments of 1967 and the Poultry Inspection Act of 1957 accomplish the objectives of the pure food law for meat and poultry. These acts provide for the inspection of premises for processing of animals and poultry, the live animals, and the carcasses. Meat that has been inspected and is fit for consumption is labeled "U.S. Inspected and Passed," and that which is unfit for human consumption is marked "Condemned." (See Fig. 15–2.) The Act also applies to manufactured meat products and provides for the proper use of additives, the correct labeling of the product, and the maintenance of standards of identity.

The **Federal Trade Commission** regulates advertising for products involved in interstate commerce. In recent years some of the food supple-

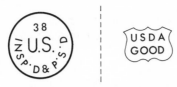

FIGURE 15–2 The round inspection stamp on meat indicates that the meat is wholesome. This stamp must appear on all meat shipped in interstate commerce. The shield indicates the grade of meat; this is not required by law. (*Courtesy, U.S. Department of Agriculture.*)

ments, such as vitamins and so-called health foods, were seized because false claims were made for nutritive values or for cures of disease.

STATE AND LOCAL LEGISLATION

Because federal legislation applies only to foods sold in interstate commerce, the individual states have passed laws that are similar to the federal laws. The state and local ordinances for the protection and pasteurization of milk, and the regulations for public eating establishments, have usually been patterned after the codes set up by the United States Public Health Service.

The United States Department of Agriculture maintains a voluntary grading service for the quality of livestock, poultry, dairy products, fruits, and vegetables. Many state departments of agriculture cooperate with the federal government in the training of state inspectors and in setting up comparable standards for intrastate products. (See Fig. 15–2.)

REVIEW QUESTIONS AND PROBLEMS

1. Visit a local market or restaurant to observe the practices in the handling of food. List the good practices and any that require improvement.

2. Who determines the regulations for the control of sanitation of food in your city? In your state?

3. What would you do if you opened a can of food that appeared to be spoiled?

4. Following a picnic many people became ill from eating chicken salad. What organism probably caused the illness? How did it probably gain entrance to the food? Give several rules for avoiding such illness.

5. What is meant by botulism? Trichinosis? How can they be avoided?

6. Read the labels on the following packaged foods and list the additives contained in them: hydrogenated fat, breakfast cereal, bread, gelatin dessert powder, cake mix, process cheese, and canned soup. What reasons can you give for the use of each additive?

7. What protection of our food supply is provided under national laws?

REFERENCES

Earl, H. G. "Food Poisoning: The Sneaky Attacker," *Today's Health*, **43**:64, October 1965.

Hasler, D., and Hasler, N. B. *Personal, Home, and Community Health*. New York: The Macmillan Company, 1967, Chaps. 10, 11, 14.

Martin, R. "What You Don't See Can Hurt You," *Today's Health*, **43**:42, November 1965.

Oser, B. L. "How Safe Are the Chemicals in Our Food?" *Today's Health*, **44**:61, March 1966.

Patterson, M. I., and Marble, B. "Dietetic Foods," *Amer. J. Clin. Nutr.*, **16**:440, 1965.

Setter, L. R. "Radioactive Contamination of Food," *J. Amer. Diet. Ass.*, **39**:561, 1961.

Strong, F. N. "Deleterious Compounds in Foods," *Amer. J. Clin. Nutr.*, **11**:500, 1962.

U.S. Department of Agriculture. *Protecting Our Food. The Yearbook of Agriculture 1966*. Washington, D.C.: Government Printing Office.

U.S. Department of Health, Education, and Welfare, Food and Drug Administration. *Food and Drug Administration—What It Is and Does*, 1965. *Read the Label on Foods, Drugs, Devices, Cosmetics*, Pub. 3, 1963. *What the Consumer Should Know About Food Additives*, 1964. *What the Consumer Should Know About Food Standards*, 1964.

U.S. Public Health Service. *You Can Prevent Foodborne Illness*, 1967.

Werrin, M., and Kronick, D. "Salmonella Control in Hospitals," *Amer. J. Nurs.*, **65**:528, 1965.

Woodburn, M. "Safe Food versus Foodborne Illness," *J. Home Econ.*, **59**:448, 1967.

16

Food Selection and Economy | IMPORTANCE OF WISE PURCHASING |
FOOD PLANS | GENERAL RULES FOR ECONOMY | MILK GROUP |
MEAT GROUP | VEGETABLE-FRUIT GROUP | BREAD-CEREAL GROUP |
FATS | SWEETS AND CONDIMENTS · Storage of Food in the
Home | FACTORS TO CONSIDER | DIRECTIONS FOR FOOD STORAGE ·
Emergency Food Supply | GENERAL RECOMMENDATIONS |
EMERGENCY FOOD SHELF

SELECTION AND CARE OF FOOD

Food Selection and Economy

IMPORTANCE OF WISE PURCHASING

At no time have homemakers faced as great a challenge in marketing
for food as today. The nurse who must help her patient plan for nutritious
meals at low cost will find much satisfaction in being able to give practical suggestions for wise use of the food money. (See Fig. 16–1.)

Literally thousands of food items are stocked in any supermarket.
Which is the best buy in meat, cheese, eggs, fruits, vegetables, milk,
breads, cereals? Should one buy fresh, canned, dehydrated, or frozen
products? Is a mix cheaper than a homemade product? Is the larger package a better buy? Which brand is best? Which grade is suitable? What
does the label state? What is the cost per pound, or ounce, of brand A as
compared with brand B?

More money is spent for food by many persons than for any other item.
Likewise, the dietary service in a hospital requires an important part of
the total budget. A severe shortage of money, of course, means that people
cannot buy sufficient food to meet their requirements. City, state, and
federal governments furnish much help in terms of welfare assistance
and direct food supplies. But a shortage of know-how in the wise purchase
of food is also a frequent problem. People who spend money wisely for
food can have more interesting meals and better nutrition at lower cost.

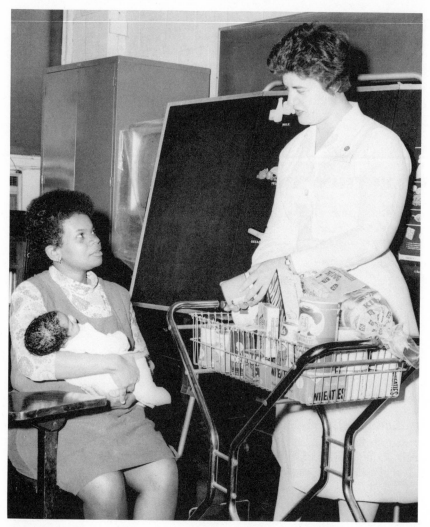

FIGURE 16–1 A market basket is used to illustrate the nutritive and economic values of foods. *(Courtesy, Thomas Jefferson University Hospital.)*

(See Fig. 16–2.) Such people find that there is also more money to buy some of the other things they want. Those people who have the lowest incomes probably require the greatest skill in food selection to get the most for their money; unfortunately, persons in this group have the least education in the planning of meals and the purchase and preparation of food. A nurse can be of particular assistance to such underprivileged people.

FOOD PLANS

Although the Four Food Groups provide a guide for menu planning, they are not adequate for the budgeting and purchase of food supplies. Other foods are also needed. The Consumer and Food Economics Research Division of the United States Department of Agriculture has developed five plans at varying cost levels. These plans specify the amounts of foods needed in a week by each member of the family in order to meet the Recommended Dietary Allowances. The Four Food Groups have been subdivided into 11 food groups. (See moderate-cost plan in Table 16-1.)

To use this plan follow these steps:

1. From the food plan, list the amounts of foods needed by each member of the family for each food group. Total the amounts for each food group. The weekly total represents the amount of food to be purchased. This total is used from week to week in planning menus.

2. Plan the menus for the week, keeping in mind the suggestions for economy discussed in the pages to follow.

3. Prepare the market order according to the menus.

Several bulletins have been published by the United States Department of Agriculture to assist in using these food plans. They contain examples of a week's menus, market lists, and hints on purchasing.

GENERAL RULES FOR ECONOMY

1. Read food columns in newspapers to learn which foods are plentiful and lower in cost. Take advantage of advertised specials in newspapers.

2. Plan menus in advance and prepare a market order. Be prepared to modify your plans if you find that some foods are too expensive when you get to the market or are not available.

3. Avoid buying foods on impulse.

4. Read labels and compare prices, weights, and grades of different brands.

5. Buy fresh foods in season. Fresh foods out of season are usually more costly than canned or frozen foods.

6. Compare cost of convenience and home-prepared foods. Many canned and dried products and some frozen products are about as low in cost as home-prepared foods and save considerable time for the homemaker. Highly perishable convenience foods, such as salad mixes of fruits or vegetables and bakery foods, are likely to be much more expensive.

7. Consider the nutritive value of the snack foods—popcorn, candy, pretzels, soft drinks, and others. Is too much of your food budget spent for these?

8. Purchase only the amounts that are likely to be used by the family. Use leftovers promptly.

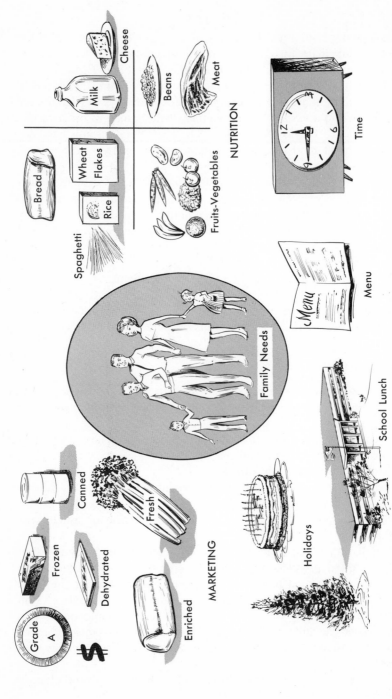

FIGURE 16-2 Good meal management includes consideration of nutrition, family needs, economics, time, attractive meals served in pleasant surroundings.

TABLE 16–1 MODERATE-COST FAMILY FOOD PLAN—REVISED 1964 *

Weekly Quantities of Food† for Each Member of Family

Sex-Age Group†	Milk, Cheese, Ice Cream§ (Qt)	Meat, Poultry, Fish‖ (Lb)	(Oz)	Eggs (No)	Dry Beans Peas, Nuts (Lb)	(Oz)	Flour, Cereals, Baked Goods# (Lb)	(Oz)	Citrus Fruit, Tomatoes (Lb)	(Oz)	Dark-green and Deep-yellow Vegetables (Lb)	(Oz)	Potatoes (Lb)	(Oz)	Other Vegetables and Fruits (Lb)	(Oz)	Fats, Oils (Lb)	(Oz)	Sugars, Sweets (Lb)	(Oz)
Children																				
7 months to 1 year	5	1	8	6	0	0	0	14	1	8	0	4	0	8	1	8	0	1	0	2
1 to 3 years	5	2	4	6	0	1	1	4	1	8	0	4	0	12	2	12	0	4	0	4
3 to 6 years	5	2	12	6	0	1	1	12	2	0	0	4	1	0	4	8	0	6	0	8
6 to 9 years	5	3	4	7	0	2	2	8	2	4	0	8	1	12	4	12	0	10	0	14
Girls																				
9 to 12 years	5½	4	4	7	0	4	2	8	2	8	0	12	2	0	5	8	0	8	0	12
12 to 15 years	7	4	8	7	0	4	2	8	2	8	1	0	2	4	5	12	0	12	0	14
15 to 20 years	7	4	8	7	0	4	2	4	2	8	1	4	2	0	5	8	0	8	0	12
Boys																				
9 to 12 years	5½	4	4	7	0	4	2	12	2	4	0	12	2	4	5	8	0	10	0	14
12 to 15 years	7	4	12	7	0	4	4	0	2	4	0	12	3	0	6	0	0	14	1	0
15 to 20 years	7	5	4	7	0	6	4	8	2	8	0	12	4	0	6	8	1	2	1	2
Women																				
20 to 35 years	3½	4	12	8	0	4	2	4	2	4	1	8	1	8	5	12	0	8	0	14
35 to 55 years	3½	4	12	8	0	4	2	4	2	4	1	8	1	4	5	0	0	6	0	8
55 to 75 years	3½	4	4	6	0	2	1	8	2	4	0	12	1	4	4	4	0	6	0	8
75 years and over	3½	3	8	8	0	2	1	4	2	4	0	12	1	0	3	12	0	4	0	8
Pregnant **	5½	5	8	8	0	4	2	12	3	4	2	0	1	8	5	12	0	6	0	8
Lactating **	8	5	8	8	0	4	3	12	3	8	1	8	2	12	6	4	0	12	0	12
Men																				
20 to 35 years	3½	5	0	7	0	4	4	0	2	4	0	12	3	0	6	8	1	0	1	4
35 to 55 years	3½	4	12	7	0	4	3	8	2	4	0	12	2	8	5	12	0	14	1	0
55 to 75 years	3½	4	8	7	0	2	2	8	2	4	0	12	2	4	5	8	0	12	0	14
75 years and over	3½	4	8	7	0	2	2	4	2	8	0	12	2	0	5	4	0	8	0	12

* Family Food Plans 1964. Consumer and Food Economics Research Division, U.S. Department of Agriculture, Hyattsville, Maryland, 1964.
† Age groups include the persons of the first age listed up to but not including those of the second age listed.
‡ Food as purchased or brought into the kitchen from garden or farm.
§ Fluid whole milk, or its calcium equivalent in cheese, evaporated milk, dry milk, or ice cream.
‖ Bacon and salt pork should not exceed ⅓ lb for each 5 lb of meat group.
Weight in terms of flour and cereal. Count 1½ lb bread as 1 lb flour.
** Three additional quarts of milk are suggested for pregnant and lactating teen-agers.

MILK GROUP

Of fluid milks, fresh milk costs most, and skim milk made from nonfat dry milk costs least. Fresh milk is available in many variations, all of which are pasteurized: whole; homogenized; 2 per cent milk; fortified with vitamin D; multivitamin fortified; chocolate; skim; and buttermilk. Homogenized milk is fresh pasteurized milk in which the fat has been so finely divided that it remains mixed throughout rather than rising as cream; it is usually fortified with vitamin D. Fresh milk purchased in a supermarket is less expensive than having it delivered to the home. Half-gallon and gallon containers are economical for families who require large amounts of milk.

Evaporated milk and nonfat dry milk are much less expensive than fresh milk. Evaporated milk is double-strength whole milk and is fortified with vitamin D. It has the same nutritive value as fresh milk when an equal amount of water is mixed with it. It may be used in any cooked dishes that require milk. For a recipe that calls for 1 cup milk, use ½ cup evaporated milk plus ½ cup water. Evaporated milk may be whipped for desserts and may be used on cereals and as cream in coffee.

Nonfat dry milk has the same nutritive value as the fresh skim milk from which it was made. People who must drink skim milk because of special dietary needs find the milk from nonfat dry milk to be just as acceptable as the fresh skim milk. It should be prepared several hours before serving and chilled thoroughly. It may be mixed half and half with whole milk for a very palatable beverage. Nonfat dry milk may be used in any recipe that requires milk. The directions on any package state the proportions to use.

Cream, yogurt, cream cheese, and ice cream are more expensive dairy products and should be used infrequently when the budget is limited. Half-and-half contains about 12 per cent fat, coffee and cultured sour cream about 18 per cent fat, and whipping cream 30 to 40 per cent fat.

Cottage cheese, American cheddar and Swiss cheese, and process cheeses are inexpensive sources of protein, and provide good occasional substitutes for a meat meal. Imported cheeses, such as Roquefort, Gouda, Camembert, Edam, Gorgonzola, and many others are more expensive.

MEAT GROUP

Meat, poultry, fish. It is difficult to provide firm rules for the purchase of meats, because the relative cost of one variety as compared with another depends upon the market supply. Beef, for example, may be more or less expensive than lamb. Lean beef, lamb, pork, veal, poultry, and fish are similar in nutritive value. Therefore a selection of the meat that is least expensive per pound of lean will save money.

Meat that bears the round purple stamp of the Meat Inspection Board is safe and wholesome, but this stamp is no indication of quality. The cost of meat depends upon the grade, with U.S. Choice, Good, Standard, and Commercial grades being most common. Prime grade is seldom seen on the retail market. Choice grades of meat come from the younger animals and are more tender than the cuts from older animals. The lean meat of choice grade is well marbled with streaks of fat. Such meat will give the most tender steaks, chops, and oven roasts.

Rib and loin cuts of meat, such as steaks, chops, and rib roasts, are tender and usually more expensive than cuts from the more exercised parts of the animal, such as the flank, the shoulder used for pot roasts, Swiss steak, and meat loaf. Less tender cuts are very flavorful if properly cooked. Liver, kidney, heart, and tongue are good buys. Beef, lamb, and pork liver are much less expensive than calves' liver and just as nutritious.

When comparing the costs of meat, one should note the amount of fat, bone, and gristle in relation to the lean. Some cheap cuts of meat are sometimes more expensive because there is so little lean. One pound of lean meat, such as ground beef or round steak, will serve three to four persons. Steak and chops, because of the amount of bone and fat, will usually require 1 lb for two persons. Meat with much fat and bone, such as brisket and short ribs, will serve only one to two persons per pound.

Chicken and turkey have been good buys in recent times. The relative proportion of bone and skin to lean meat is somewhat higher than in the meat of larger animals.

Fish, whether fresh, canned, or frozen, is likely to be less expensive than meat. Shellfish, such as oysters, lobsters, shrimp, and crabs, are luxury items except where locally available.

Eggs. Eggs are priced according to quality and size. Top-quality eggs, grade AA and A, have a strong, clean, unbroken shell and a tiny air cell (less than ⅛ in.) when the egg is exposed to light in the candling process. When the egg is broken, the white is thick and gelatinous, and the yolk is round, high, and does not break easily. Such eggs are good for poaching, cooking in the shell, and frying. Grade B and C eggs will show a somewhat larger air cell on candling and will have thinner whites and flatter yolks when broken. Such eggs are suitable for cooking and baking. They have a somewhat less delicate flavor for table use.

Eggs are sorted according to size, based on weight per dozen: extra large, 27 oz; large, 24 oz; medium, 21 oz; and small, 18 oz. Medium and small eggs are usually a good buy in the fall, whereas large eggs may be a good buy in the spring. Medium eggs are a better buy than large eggs if their cost is at least one eighth less per dozen. White and brown eggs are equally good. Always buy refrigerated eggs.

Legumes. Legumes are a good protein source when the budget is limited, and they lend themselves to a variety of uses. Split peas, navy beans, Lima beans, kidney beans, lentils, soybeans, chick peas, and peanuts are among the varieties available. Peanut butter is a good buy. Dry legumes require soaking and a longer cooking time.

VEGETABLE-FRUIT GROUP

Fresh, frozen, dehydrated, and canned fruits and vegetables may be purchased. Fresh fruits and vegetables, especially those locally grown, are often less expensive in season. Canned or frozen fruits and vegetables are likely to be better buys at other times of the year. Frozen orange juice is less expensive than freshly squeezed juice, but usually costs a little more than canned juice. Frozen vegetables prepared with butter or cream sauces are appreciably higher in cost than plain vegetables that would be seasoned at the time of cooking.

Fruits should be ripe, firm, free from decay spots, and not soft or with mold spots. Vegetables should be firm, crisp, and clean—not wilted or bruised. Overripe fruits or too mature vegetables are not good economy even though the price may be somewhat lower.

A canned product should be selected for its use; for example, whole fruit may be desired when it is to be served as a dessert, but fruit pieces are just as good for a mixed salad or for pastries. Likewise, grade A peas may be preferred for buttered peas, but grade B peas would be suitable for a casserole dish.

BREAD-CEREAL GROUP

Enriched or whole-grain breads, cereals, pastas, and flours should be purchased. Enriched white bread is the least expensive way to purchase bread. Day-old bread, when available, is somewhat reduced in price. Many specialty breads that contain butter, stone-ground flour, honey, or other flavor ingredients and sweet breads and rolls are considerably more expensive. Many homemakers today find much satisfaction in baking their own breads and rolls.

Cooked breakfast cereals are usually less expensive than dry breakfast cereals. For variety, some of each should be used. Sugar-coated cereals and those containing dried fruit are more expensive than their plain counterparts. Precooked rice is more expensive than uncooked rice. To compare the cost of cereals, divide the total number of ounces stated on the package into the cost of the package.

FATS

Butter and margarine are of equal nutritive value and are comparable in flavor. Margarine is much less costly, but there are considerable differences in price from brand to brand. Lard and hydrogenated fats are inexpensive cooking fats. With the current emphasis on vegetable oils, corn, cottonseed, and soybean oils will be found to be just as satisfactory as the more expensive oils sometimes advertised.

SWEETS AND CONDIMENTS

Cane and beet sugars are inexpensive, whereas brown and confectioners' sugars are somewhat higher in cost. Molasses is a good buy, because it contains iron as well as carbohydrates. It can be used for many dishes, such as baked beans, gingerbread, cookies, puddings, and sometimes in a glass of milk for children. Honey, maple sugar and syrup, and candies represent expensive ways to buy sweets.

Spices, flavoring extracts, and herbs are important additions, because they enhance the flavors of food so much. Flavors are rapidly lost to the air, and only small containers of infrequently used seasonings should be purchased. Coffee, tea, catsup, meat sauces, pickles, and relishes add interest to meals. Depending upon the choices made, these food adjuncts may increase the food expenditure appreciably.

Storage of Food in the Home

FACTORS TO CONSIDER

The agents responsible for food spoilage have been discussed in Chapter 15. Bacteria, molds, yeast, and enzymes bring about food spoilage. Moist foods spoil rapidly, but changes take place more slowly in dry foods. Low temperatures retard food spoilage.

The quality of fresh fruits and vegetables is reduced when they are exposed to the air and become wilted. Foods also pick up undesirable flavors when they are in contact with each other; for example, milk and onions or cantaloupe. Fats may be oxidized and become rancid so that they are inedible.

DIRECTIONS FOR FOOD STORAGE

1. Follow directions on package labels for proper storage of foods.

2. Store dry cereals, flours, sugars, and mixes in the original container or another covered container in a dry cupboard. Use whole-grain cereals and flours promptly, especially in warm weather; they become rancid and may become infested with weevils if kept too long.

3. Canned foods may be kept in a cupboard indefinitely. Losses of vitamins are less if the cans are stored in a cool room. Discard any cans with bulging ends. Once canned food is opened, store any leftover food in the refrigerator and use in a day or two. The food may be kept in the

original container and covered, thereby reducing bacterial contamination.

4. Frozen foods may be kept for about a week in the freezing section of a refrigerator. If they are to be kept for longer periods of time, a freezer unit at 0°F is necessary. The directions on packages concerning storage, thawing, and preparation of frozen foods should be followed.

5. Store leftover foods in covered dishes in the refrigerator. Use in 24 hours.

6. Store fresh milk and cottage cheese in the original container in the coldest part of the refrigerator (under 40°F). Avoid exposure of milk to sunlight, because riboflavin is rapidly destroyed by light. Keep nonfat dry milk and evaporated milk at room temperature. When dry milk is mixed with water or evaporated milk is opened, refrigerate as for fresh milk.

7. Refrigerate all cheese. Use cottage cheese within four to five days and other soft cheese within two weeks. Wrap hard cheeses tightly in wax, plastic, or foil wrapper to reduce drying out. Mold that sometimes appears on hard cheese may be cut off and the rest of the cheese used.

8. Refrigerate eggs in the purchase carton. A high-grade egg rapidly loses its freshness if kept at room temperature. Do not wash eggs until they are to be used, because washing removes the protective covering.

9. Remove store wrappings from meat, poultry, and fish, and wrap loosely in wax paper. Store in the coldest part of the refrigerator. Use fresh fish, organ meats, and ground meat within 24 hours, poultry within two days, and roasts, steaks, ham, and chops within five to six days.

10. Sort fruit to remove injured pieces, and place the fruit in the hydrator of refrigerator. Unripe tomatoes, pineapple, melons, peaches, and pears should be kept at room temperature until ripened. Bananas are not refrigerated. Berries should not be washed until just before use.

11. Potatoes, rutabagas, sweet potatoes, onions, and hard-shell squash may be kept for about a week at room temperature with a good circulation of air, and somewhat longer at a dark cool temperature. Other vegetables should be washed and stored in the hydrator of the refrigerator. Cut off the tops of carrots, beets, radishes. Leave husks on corn; use fresh corn on the day of purchase, if possible. Leafy vegetables may be kept in plastic bags.

12. Butter and margarine should be kept in the purchase container or in covered dishes. Oils, mayonnaise, and salad dressings should be tightly capped and refrigerated once the container has been opened.

Emergency Food Supply

Following a flood or storm, normal facilities for obtaining and preparing foods may not be available. In the event of a nuclear bomb explosion, radioactive fallout would contaminate food and water supplies.

TABLE 16–2 SUGGESTED FOODS FOR EMERGENCY FOOD SHELF *

Food Class	Amount per Person Per Day	Kinds and Serving Portions
Milk	2 cups equivalent	Evaporated and nonfat dry milk
Meat, poultry, fish	2 servings	Canned meat, poultry, fish—2 to 3 oz
		Canned mixtures of meat, poultry, fish with vegetables, rice, macaroni, noodles, or cooked dry beans—8 oz
		Condensed soups with meat, poultry, fish, dry beans or dry peas—½ of 10½-oz can
Fruits and vegetables	3–4 servings	Canned juices—4 to 6 oz
		Canned fruits and vegetables—4 oz
		Dried fruit—1½ oz
Cereals and baked goods	3–4 servings	Ready-to-eat or dry cereals, crackers, cookies, flour mixes, flour—1 oz
		Canned bread, steamed puddings, cake—1 to 2 oz
		Macaroni, spaghetti, noodles, dry—¾ oz; cooked, canned—6 oz
Spreads for bread, crackers	According to family practice	Cheese spreads, peanut butter, marmalade, jam, jelly, preserves, syrup, honey, apple butter; relish, catsup, mustard
Fats and oils	Up to 1 lb	Kinds that do not require refrigeration
Sugars, sweets, nuts	1 to 2 lb	Sugar, hard candy, gum, nuts, instant puddings
Miscellaneous	Depending on family practices	Coffee, tea, instant cocoa; dry cream product; bouillon cubes; beverage powders; salt, pepper; flavoring extracts, vinegar; soda, baking powder

* Adapted from *Family Food Stockpile for Survival*. Home and Garden Bull. No. 77. Washington, D.C.: U.S. Department of Agriculture, 1964, pp. 4–5.

GENERAL RECOMMENDATIONS

Among the recommendations published by the United States Department of Agriculture * are these:

* Adapted from *Family Food Stockpile for Survival*, Home and Garden Bull. No. 77. Washington, D.C.: U.S. Department of Agriculture, 1964.

1. Keep a two-week supply of regular food in the home at all times, or assemble and maintain a special two-week stockpile of survival foods in the fallout shelter or home.

2. Select foods that will keep for months without refrigeration and can be eaten with little or no cooking.

3. Keep foods in cans, jars, or tightly sealed paper or plastic containers. Store paper boxes in tightly closed metal cans to protect against rodents and insects.

4. Rotate the food supply every 6 months so that the stock is always fresh.

5. Provide equipment for emergency cooking and serving: compact cooking unit such as used by campers; cooking pans; disposable knives, forks, spoons; paper plates, towels, cups and napkins; can and bottle openers; nursing bottles and nipples for a baby; measuring cup; medicine dropper for measuring water purifier; matches; pocket knife.

6. Store 7 gallons of water for each person for a two-week period. Another 7 gallons of water is recommended per person for dishwashing and personal care.

EMERGENCY FOOD SHELF

The foods stored should be those that the family likes and that require a minimum of facilities. Half the meals could be planned for use with no cooking facilities, and half with some facility to heat water or food but without extended cooking. Suggestions for an emergency food shelf are given in Table 16–2.

REVIEW QUESTIONS AND PROBLEMS

1. Examine the labeling on a package of each of the following foods: frozen green beans, frozen strawberries, ready-to-eat cereal, nonfat dry milk, process cheese, canned baked beans, canned mushroom soup. Prepare a table that shows the following: (1) weight; (2) grade, if listed; (3) list of ingredients; (4) directions for storage, if given; (5) directions for preparation for a meal.

2. Compare the cost per pound of round steak, short ribs, chuck roast, rib roast.

3. What would you do with leftover orange juice?

4. Using the moderate-cost food plan, write menus for a week for a family that includes father, mother, 16-year-old boy, 12-year-old girl, and seven-year-old girl. Make up a market list, keeping the totals for the market list as close to the totals from the food plan as possible.

5. What shopping guide would you provide for a woman who told you she had no refrigerator?

6. Plan menus for two days that would use only foods available from an emergency food shelf. Assume that no heating facilities are available for one of these days, and that a camper unit is available for one day.

REFERENCES

United States Department of Agriculture, Washington, D.C. *Family Food Budgeting for Good Meals and Good Nutrition*, HG 94, 1964. *Family Food Stockpile for Survival*, HG 77, 1964. *Food for Families with School Children*, HG 13, 1962. *Food for Families with Young Children*, HG 5, 1963. *Food Guide for Older Folks*, HG 17, 1963. *Food, the Yearbook of Agriculture* 1959. *Shopper's Guide to U.S. Grades of Food*, HG 58, 1966.

17 GOALS IN FOOD PREPARATION │ METHODS OF COOKERY │ EFFECTS OF COOKERY ON FOOD QUALITIES │ PROTEIN COOKERY │ VEGETABLE-FRUIT COOKERY │ CEREAL COOKERY │ GENERAL PROCEDURES FOR FOOD PREPARATION │ MAINTENANCE OF GOOD SANITATION

BASIC PRINCIPLES AND PROCEDURES FOR FOOD PREPARATION

GOALS IN FOOD PREPARATION

Good nutrition, attractive menus, economy, cultural patterns, individual preferences—all of these must be considered if one wishes to achieve meals that are tantalizing to the nose, attractive to the eye, and satisfying to the palate. Many a meal that is planned to be nutritionally and therapeutically correct is destined to fail if the patient at home, or those who cook for him, do not understand how to adapt daily meals to the requirements of a particular diet.

Most of the questions that patients ask about nutrition are concerned with the nutritive values of foods, the foods that may or may not be used on a modified diet, and the methods of preparation for specific foods. People also ask for suggestions on varying the diet, how to improve the quality of their family menus, and how to improve children's food habits. Every nurse who is able to give accurate, practical information of this kind is helping the patient to achieve realistic goals in managing his diet. (See also Chap. 18.) Although they are rarely called upon to prepare meals, nurses should be able to plan, prepare, and serve a simple meal for a patient in an emergency.

For her professional development and her personal satisfaction, it is hoped that the student will accept the challenge to broaden her horizons pertaining to food choice, to learn to judge when food is really good in quality, to be imaginative in menu planning, to develop skill in the kitchen based upon the fundamental principles of cookery, and to use artistry in

178

food arrangement and service. Such inclusive goals are not achieved overnight, nor is it the intention of this chapter to provide detailed guidance. Only the most basic principles of preparation for the Four Food Groups will be discussed.

METHODS OF COOKERY

Foods may be cooked by moist heat, dry heat, or frying. The moist-heat methods include boiling, simmering, stewing, braising, and steaming. Dry-heat methods include broiling, pan-broiling, baking, and roasting.

Boiling is cooking in water at 212°F. The bubbles break rapidly on the surface of the water.

Simmering is cooking in water just below the boiling point—about 200°F. Small bubbles rise slowly through the liquid to the surface.

Stewing is cooking foods such as less tender cuts of meat or poultry for a long time at about 200°F. The liquid is sometimes thickened at the end of the cooking period.

Braising is cooking with a small amount of water in a tightly covered pan at low temperature with direct heat or in an oven. Meats and vegetables are often braised.

Steaming is cooking by the heat of direct steam as in a steamer or in a double boiler. By increasing the pressure of steam, as in a pressure cooker, the temperature is raised and the cooking time is greatly shortened.

Broiling is cooking by direct heat from a gas flame, electric wires, or over live coals.

Pan-broiling is cooking in a hot metal pan on top of the range with just enough fat to prevent sticking. The fat is poured off as it accumulates.

Baking or *roasting* is cooking in an oven in open or covered pan. We generally refer to cakes as being *baked* and meats as being *roasted*.

Deep-fat frying is cooking by immersing the food in fat; French fried potatoes or doughnuts, for example.

Sautéeing is cooking in a small amount of fat in a frying pan; the food is turned often.

EFFECTS OF COOKERY ON FOOD QUALITIES

Color. Some of the changes in color with cookery increase the attractiveness of food; for example, the pink, gray, and brown colors of meat that was once bloody red, or the golden crust of baked rolls. But the green of vegetables can also become an unappetizing olive green if the vegetable is overcooked. An acid or alkaline reaction of the cooking water also affects color change. Red cabbage remains red if a trace of vinegar is used in cooking, but becomes blue if the water is alkaline. Green vegetables such as peas and green beans remain a bright green if a tiny pinch of baking soda is added to the cooking water, but this practice is not recommended because some of the vitamin C and thiamine are lost.

Texture. Cookery softens the connective-tissue fibers of meat and the cellulose fibers in fruits, vegetables, and cereals. Sometimes meats are tenderized by using a marinade of acid and oil, or an enzyme preparation to partially break down the fibers.

Microbial changes. Most bacteria and parasites are killed by heat, but cookery is not an absolute guarantee that food will be safe. See Chapter 15. Cookery should never be used as an excuse for poor practices in food handling.

Enzyme changes. You may have wondered why an apple, pear, or peach darkens so soon after it is cut; you have also noticed that this does not happen if the food is promptly cooked. As soon as foods are cut, the enzymes normally present in the food are activated. The oxidation by the enzymes not only changes the color, but also begins to soften the cell walls of the meat, fruit, or vegetables, and reduces the content of ascorbic acid and B-complex vitamins. The enzymes are inactivated at temperatures below freezing ($0°F$) but are rapidly reactivated at room temperatures; the warmer the room, the more rapid the action will be. Because enzymes are protein in nature, they are destroyed at high temperatures.

Digestibility. Many foods are more easily digested when cooked. The softening of connective tissue and cellulose fibers and the rupturing of the starch granules shortens the time required to digest meats, cereals, fruits, and vegetables. Moreover, the softer fibers are less likely to irritate the linings of the gastrointestinal tract.

Nutritive values. The mineral and vitamin content of foods is often reduced in cookery. Partly this comes about because some mineral salts and vitamins are soluble in water and are lost when the liquids are drained off. Also, ascorbic acid and thiamine are easily destroyed by heat. Thus, vegetables cooked for a short time in a little water may retain as much as 90 per cent of the original vitamin C, but if cooked in a large amount of water for a long time may have only 50 per cent of the initial amount of vitamin C. Meats that are stewed may retain as little as 25 per cent of the thiamine, but if the stewing liquid is also used an additional 25 per cent is conserved. Broiled and roasted meats retain 65 to 70 per cent of the thiamine. The losses of riboflavin and niacin are considerably lower than those for thiamine. Vitamin A values are not adversely affected by ordinary cooking temperatures.

PROTEIN COOKERY

Because foods of the milk and meat groups are protein in nature, the general rules for many dishes of these groups are the same. You know that a raw liquid egg mixture becomes solid when heated, and that you cannot reverse the solid back to the liquid state again. This change is known as *coagulation* and *protein denaturation*. You have also observed that cheese in a grilled sandwich sometimes becomes stringy, and that a well-done steak may be tough. To avoid the toughening of protein and the drying out of products, two general rules are observed in the cookery of milk and meat products:

1. Maintain low cooking temperatures. Thus, recipe directions may state: "Simmer," "Set in pan of hot water and bake in slow oven," "Cook in double boiler until thickened," "Cook over low heat, stirring constantly," and so on.

2. Cook only until tender. Meats that are cooked too long are dry and tough or stringy; overcooked fish is dry; overcooked custards tend to curdle.

Milk and cheese. Milk and cheese lend themselves to numerous uses in the diet. Many milk beverages, soups, and desserts form the basis for full-fluid diets and increase the protein for high-protein diets. Milk beverages should be thoroughly chilled before they are served. Cheese may be used in a variety of casserole dishes such as macaroni and cheese, escalloped vegetables, cheese soufflé; for sauces on vegetables or on toast; and in grilled sandwiches.

When milk is heated some of the protein sticks to the bottom and sides of the pan so that scorching occurs easily. A scum also forms over the top of the milk and it becomes difficult for steam to escape and the milk may boil over. The scum formation can be prevented by constant stirring, or by covering if a double boiler is used.

Eggs. Egg cookery is really quite simple and easy, but the results can be disastrous if one does not carefully observe the time-temperature directions. Soft- and hard-cooked or poached eggs are cooked in simmering, not boiling, water. Baked custard is set in a pan of hot water, and baked just until the tip of a knife inserted about one third from the edge of the baking dish comes out clean. Eggs serve many functions in the preparation of foods: as a binding agent in meat loaf; to hold crumb coatings on foods to be fried; as thickening agent in custards and puddings; for the leavening of sponge, angel food, and other cakes; for the emulsification of oils in the preparation of mayonnaise.

Meats. Tender cuts of meat have little connective tissues and are well marbled with fat. They are cooked by broiling, pan-broiling, or roasting. Tender beef roasts are roasted in an uncovered pan at 300° to 325°F to a rare, medium, or well-done stage as preferred. Pork must always be cooked until no tinge of pink remains in the meat. A meat thermometer inserted into the center of the thickest muscle of meat is the best guide for determining when the meat is cooked.

Steaks and chops are placed 2 to 3 in. from the source of heat when they are broiled. They are browned on one side, sprinkled with salt and pepper, and turned to cook on the other side. Broiling is not usually recommended for pork chops since they must be well done and they are likely to be dried out.

Broiling and frying chickens are also cooked with dry-heat cookery or by frying in fat or oil. Fish contains little connective tissue and requires only a short broiling or baking time before it flakes when gently touched with a fork. Low-fat white fish usually requires a light brushing with oil or butter if it is broiled.

Moist heat is used for less tender cuts of meat and poultry. A pot roast is an example of moist heat cookery; the meat is usually browned and then placed in a covered pan such as a Dutch oven and cooked at low heat on top of the range or in an oven at 300°F. Potatoes and other vegetables are often added when the meat is partially cooked. Swiss steak, braised short ribs, and stews are other examples of moist-heat cookery.

Meat is also made more tender by grinding it, as for hamburgers or meat loaf, or by treating it with a meat tenderizer. The tenderizers are enzyme products that soften the fibers, thus shortening the cooking time.

VEGETABLE-FRUIT COOKERY

Vegetables and fruits present the greatest challenge in cooking in order to preserve the maximum amounts of ascorbic acid and thiamine. Fresh raw fruits and vegetables may be served in many attractive ways: fruit cup, fruit and vegetable salads, relish assortments. Citrus fruit sections and juices and tomatoes and tomato juice retain ascorbic acid very well, even with overnight storage, because of their acid reaction.

Salads should be important parts of the meal. They should be colorful, crisp, and cold. The foods should be cut in attractive, bite-size pieces, and retain the identity of the food. The type of salad should complement the meal in nutritive composition, flavor, color, and texture. For example, a tomato aspic salad is not a good choice when all other foods are also soft; a sliced tomato salad would then be preferable. A salad containing some protein would be better than a tossed salad for a vegetable plate luncheon.

When fruits such as peaches, apples, and pears are cooked, the pieces will retain their shape if they are dropped into gently boiling syrup (cane sugar and water) and cooked until just tender. Dried fruits are cooked by adding water to cover and to allow for fruit to absorb water. They should be simmered until tender, and may be sweetened at the end of the cooking period if desired. Stewed dried fruits seem to be improved in flavor if kept in the refrigerator for a day or two before serving.

Properly cooked vegetables should be fork-tender yet slightly firm and crisp; they should not be mushy or soft, or tough and hard. Although some color change is bound to occur, the color remains attractive if the vegetables are not overcooked. Vegetables, depending upon choice, may be cooked by boiling, steaming, baking, deep-fat frying, broiling, or panning. They may be served with butter, margarine, or oil dressing and seasoned with salt, pepper, or herbs. Sauces such as cream sauce, cheese sauce, or hollandaise sauce are often used to dress vegetables.

Observance of the following rules will result in maximum retention of ascorbic acid and thiamine, and best eating qualities. Can you give the reasons why each rule is important?

1. Remove peelings as thin as possible.

2. Peel and cut vegetables just before cooking. Avoid soaking in water.

3. Use a small amount of water in cooking. With a tightly covered saucepan the water need not cover the vegetable.

4. Bring water to the boiling point and add salt. Plunge fresh or frozen vegetable into the boiling water, and bring again to the boiling point as rapidly as possible.

5. Cook fresh green vegetables uncovered for the first few minutes to give mild acids a chance to go off in steam and thereby minimize the color change. Then cover the vegetable to finish cooking. Frozen vegetables and spinach are covered from the beginning of the cooking period.

6. Adjust heat so that vegetables are kept just at boiling temperature.

7. Do not add baking soda.

8. Cook vegetables until just tender and still slightly crisp.

9. Serve vegetables promptly. Avoid cooking ahead of time and reheating.

10. Finely cut or mashed vegetables lose more ascorbic acid than those in larger pieces.

11. Cover any leftover vegetables and place in the refrigerator promptly. Use within 24 hours. Do not count on leftovers for ascorbic acid.

CEREAL COOKERY

The inexperienced cook soon learns that a cup of dry rice or macaroni will serve several people when cooked. Starch granules absorb water and swell when cooked, thus increasing the volume and thickening the mixture. The dry cereal is added gradually to rapidly boiling, salted water and kept boiling until just done. The proportion of cereal to water is important for breakfast cereals. Macaroni, noodles, and spaghetti are cooked in a large volume of water. Rice is preferably cooked in just enough water to be completely absorbed by the grains. Too long cooking of rice, macaroni, noodles, and other pastas gives a sticky, gummy product.

The losses of thiamine are not appreciable in cooked breakfast cereals, because the water in which they are cooked is consumed. The baking of bread results in a 10- to 20-per-cent loss of thiamine that is unavoidable.

Where rice is an important part of the diet, the washing of rice and the use of large amounts of water may significantly reduce the thiamine content of cooked rice.

GENERAL PROCEDURES FOR FOOD PREPARATION

Numerous cookbooks are available, food manufacturers distribute free booklets concerning their products, and magazines and newspapers abound in recipes. In addition, cookbooks and leaflets for many modified diets are available. The nurse should become familiar with these sources for ideas in menu planning and for specific directions in food preparation.

Not to be ignored are the many packaged mixes and frozen and canned foods now available in supermarkets. With a little imagination attractive meals can be prepared within a few minutes' time, using ready-to-heat and partially combined foods: soups; plain meats, poultry, fish, or combinations in a variety of dishes; bread, biscuit, muffin, roll mixes, or brown-and-serve breads and rolls; frozen vegetables already mixed with their sauces; salad combinations; dessert mixes or desserts that require only thawing; and so on. At no time are convenience foods more appreciated than during illness in the home. Time saved from food preparation means additional time for the patient. Not all convenience foods, however, may be used for modified diets. Only careful reading of labels and general understanding of food preparation will ensure correct choice for therapeutic diets.

The preparation of good food requires management of time, equipment, and food supplies. These general directions should be followed.

1. If you are inexperienced select recipes that are simple and easily prepared. Consider the amount of time you can spend on food preparation. A simple meal well prepared will succeed; a complicated menu for which you have insufficient time and skill has little chance of success.

2. Read the recipe carefully to be sure you understand the directions in every detail. Check whether all ingredients and the necessary equipment are on hand.

3. Follow directions exactly: preparation of cooking pans; heating of oven; measurement of ingredients; order of mixing; amount of mixing; temperatures of cooking or baking; length of baking time; procedures for cooling; method of serving; and so on.

4. Use level measurements. Use standard measuring equipment: ¼, ½, and 1 teaspoon; 1 tablespoon; nest of cups for dry measure: ¼, ⅓, ½, and 1 cup; glass cup for liquid, with divisions for parts of a cup.

5. To measure dry ingredients, spoon sugar, dry milk, stirred no-sift flour, or cereals lightly into the cup until heaped up. Level off with the back of a knife. Brown sugar is measured by packing it tightly into the cup or spoon.

6. To measure liquids (water, milk, oil, juices): use glass measuring

cup, and fill to the correct mark. Be sure to keep the mark on the cup at eye level.

7. To measure soft fat: spoon fat into cups used for dry measure; press fat down firmly; level off with the back of a knife.

8. To measure hard fat: cut off correct amount indicated on sticks of butter or margarine. Or use the water-displacement method. Suppose you need to measure ⅔ cup fat: put ⅓ cup cold water into a glass measuring cup; add fat until the water comes to the 1-cup line; pour off the water; ⅔ cup of fat remains in the cup.

MAINTENANCE OF GOOD SANITATION

Anyone who prepares food should observe the following rules for food handling to help ensure the safety of the food supply, as discussed in Chapters 15 and 16.

1. Clothing should be clean and hair should be well groomed; if necessary, hair spray or a hairnet may be used to keep hair from blowing about.

2. Avoid touching the face or hair while preparing food.

3. Cover the mouth and nose if you must cough or sneeze.

4. Wash the hands with soap and water before beginning food preparation. Wash hands after using the toilet or the handkerchief.

5. Pick up foods with forks, tongs, and so forth, when practical.

6. Use a separate spoon for tasting; never return it to the food mixture.

7. Wash dishes and utensils in warm, soapy water, and rinse with hot water.

8. Refrigerate cooked foods promptly if they are not to be served immediately.

REVIEW QUESTIONS AND PROBLEMS

1. Define each of these terms: simmering, broiling, dry heat, moist heat, marinating, braising, sautéeing.

2. Look up in a cookbook a method recommended for cooking each of these cuts of meat: lamb chop, veal roast, beef chuck roast, pork chop, fish steak, hamburger, round steak, porterhouse steak, slice of ham. Which use moist heat? What conclusions can you make about the tenderness of meat?

3. Why are soft custards cooked in a double boiler? Why do they sometimes curdle?

4. List five ways for using eggs in the diet.

5. Write out the rules you would suggest for the preparation of this meal: baked chicken legs with mushroom sauce, mashed potatoes, buttered green beans, tossed green salad.

6. Plan a luncheon menu based upon convenience foods available in your markets.

REFERENCES

General Mills. *Betty Crocker's New Picture Cook Book.* New York: McGraw-Hill Book Company, Inc., 1961.

Heseltine, M., and Dow, U. M. *The Basic Cookbook,* 5th ed. Boston: Houghton Mifflin Company, 1967.

McWilliams, M. *Food Fundamentals.* New York: John Wiley & Sons, Inc., 1966.

Rombauer, I. S., and Becker, M. R. *Joy of Cooking.* New York: The Bobbs Merrill Company, Inc., 1962.

U.S. Department of Agriculture. *Conserving the Nutritive Values in Foods,* G 90, 1965. *Eggs in Family Meals,* HG 103, 1965. *Family Fare: Food Management and Recipes.* HG 1, 1960. *Food, the Yearbook of Agriculture, 1959,* pp. 495–554. *Green Vegetables for Good Eating,* HG 41, 1964. *Meat for Thrifty Meals,* HG 27. *Money-Saving Main Dishes,* HG 43, 1962. *Milk in Family Meals,* HG 127, 1967. *Vegetables in Family Meals,* HG 105, 1965.

DIET THERAPY

18

ILLNESS AND NUTRITION | ILLNESS AND FOOD ACCEPTANCE | DIET
THERAPY | NORMAL DIET AND ITS MODIFICATIONS |
NOMENCLATURE | THE NURSE'S ROLE IN NUTRITIONAL CARE |
GOOD TRAY SERVICE | THE PATIENT AND HIS MEALS | FEEDING THE
HELPLESS PATIENT | A SURVEY OF MODIFIED DIETS

NUTRITION AND DIET FOR
THE PATIENT

ILLNESS AND NUTRITION

Illness has many effects on the body's ability to use nutrients and upon
the specific requirements. Lack of appetite, vomiting, and pain often
prevent the intake of a sufficient amount of food. In severe diarrhea the
absorption of all nutrients is poor, so that loss of weight, dehydration, and
signs of malnutrition may be found. A fever increases the rate of metabolism, thus increasing the need for calories, protein, and vitamins. In
metabolic diseases nutrients are not utilized fully; for example, the untreated diabetic patient will not make adequate use of carbohydrate. The
patient who must remain in bed or in a wheel chair for a long time usually
loses increased amounts of nitrogen and calcium from his body. As the
student continues her study of diet therapy and becomes more experienced
in the care of patients, she will undoubtedly find numerous examples of
the effects of illness upon nutrition. (See also Table 18–1.)

ILLNESS AND FOOD ACCEPTANCE

The many physiologic, cultural, economic, and emotional factors affect-
ing food acceptance have been discussed in Chapter 14. The person who
is ill must face added problems related to his meals. Diet is related to both
the comfort and the treatment of the patient, but sometimes it is necessary to take therapeutic measures that may distress rather than provide
immediate comfort. The nurse plays an essential role in helping to bridge
this gap. (See Fig. 18–1.)

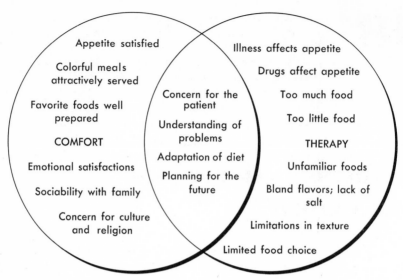

FIGURE 18–1 Patients seek comfort through food. Modified diets may present many problems. The nurse must help the patient solve these problems.

Illness itself may reduce interest in food because of anorexia, gastro-intestinal distention, or discomfort following meals. Inactivity and some drugs also reduce the desire for food.

The patient in a hospital may be away from home for the first time. He probably misses his family and the sociability of family meals. He finds that the food pattern in the hospital and the time for meals differ, more or less, from his usual pattern. He finds it difficult to manage a tray in bed. His food intake may be affected by his worries about mounting hospital bills, about return to work, or about the extent of his return to full health.

If the diet is modified, the patient may be getting less or more food than he normally eats. The change in flavor or texture of some diets may not be appealing. He may be unwilling to accept any change, he may be worried about how he will get the new foods for his diet at home, or he may be bothered about the inconvenience of sticking to a diet that is different from that of his family or friends. His modified diet may make him feel that he is deprived and punished.

In his illness the patient often becomes more self-centered, and he may react by being irritable or even angry. He may complain incessantly about his food in order to get more attention, or he may be quite indifferent to his diet, eat poorly, and ignore the suggestions made by doctors, nurses, or dietitians.

DIET THERAPY

An appropriate diet is essential in the total-care plan developed for every patient. Usually it supplements medical and surgical care; sometimes it is the specific treatment for disease. Diet therapy accomplishes one or more of these aims: (1) maintains normal nutrition; (2) corrects nutritional deficiency, for example, high-protein diet; (3) changes body weight, as with low- or high-calorie diets; (4) adjusts to the body's ability to use one or more nutrients, for example, diabetic diet; (5) permits maximum rest to the body or an organ, as with a soft, low-calorie diet in six feedings.

NORMAL DIET AND ITS MODIFICATIONS

The normal, regular, general, or house diet is the most frequently used of all diets. A normal diet, like a modified diet, is of great importance in a therapeutic sense. With satisfactory food intake the body's tissues are continuously maintained, and there is opportunity for repair from the effects of illness. On the other hand, the patient's failure to eat a normal diet could lead to loss of body tissue and a prolonged convalescence.

The normal diet in hospital usage follows the principles outlined in the preceding units, and is planned to provide the Recommended Dietary Allowances. The Four Food Groups offer a convenient basis for menu planning, and diets in this section will be arranged according to these groups. The normal diet in the hospital requires no restrictions upon food choice. Strong flavored vegetables, fried foods, cakes, pies, pastries, spicy foods, and relishes all have a place on the menu, but they should be used with discretion.

The normal diet may be modified for (1) consistency and texture; (2) flavor; (3) energy value; (4) nutrient levels such as fat, protein, carbohydrate, sodium, and others; or (5) food categories such as types of fats or elimination diets for allergies.

Often a combination of modifications is required; for example, 500-mg sodium, 1200-calorie, soft diet. In planning modified diets the normal diet should always be used as the frame of reference. The aim should always be to keep as many characteristics of the normal diet as possible.

NOMENCLATURE

Diets that are changed from the normal are referred to as *modified* or *therapeutic*; the term "special diet" has little meaning, and should be avoided. Diets should be described exactly in terms of the change made in consistency, flavor, and the level of nutrients. The words "high" and "low" have meaning only when they are used with reference to the normal diet or when a given diet manual specifies the nutritive level. For example, a low-calorie diet might mean 800 calories to one individual, 1200 calories to another, and 1800 calories to a man whose normal calorie requirement is 2800 per day. Diets should not be named for persons or for diseases; the latter practice is likely to be a continual reminder to the patient of his condition.

THE NURSE'S ROLE IN NUTRITIONAL CARE

All people responsible for care should consider each patient as a person and should recognize his physical, psychologic, cultural, and emotional needs. Thinking only in terms of treating a specific disease is inexcusable, for it denies to each patient the right to be an individual. A correct, nutritious, attractive, and well-prepared meal for the patient requires the teamwork of the medical, nursing, and dietary services. The physician always prescribes the diet. In the hospital the dietitian translates the diet prescription into a menu and supervises the food preparation and service to the patient. The nurse has the most continual direct contact with the patient and makes certain that he receives and consumes his meals under the best circumstances.

If a selective menu is used, the nurse may help the patient to select his meals according to his diet prescription. As a nurse you would expect to prepare the patient for his meals and to see that his tray is served as soon as it arrives. Perhaps you may need to feed him. Helping the patient to accept his diet by giving encouragement and praise is a decided contribution. This also means that you avoid criticism if he is not eating well, or pity because the diet is one you would not like very much.

Observing, listening, and reporting are three important functions performed by the nurse in nutritional care. How well the patient eats his food, what kinds and amounts of food are refused, and the patient's attitude toward his food are readily determined. You are more likely than anyone else to observe problems such as these: poorly fitting dentures and inability to chew; a sore mouth and pain when acid juices are taken; arthritic fingers that make it difficult to cut up food; portions that are too large for some elderly persons or too small for teen-agers; difficulty in breathing so that eating a large meal at one time is not possible; between-meal feedings interfering with the appetite for the meals; fatigue and poor appetite at the end of the day; and many others.

By listening you show your general interest in and your understanding of the patient, and help him to express his feelings and perhaps to "blow off steam." You begin to learn that some foods are favorites, others are thoroughly disliked, and still others cannot be eaten because of religious beliefs. You become aware of what food means to the patient, and what concerns the patient may have about the diet he will have when at home.

Acting upon your information is essential to the best care of the patient. Sometimes it is direct action on your part. More often it involves reporting to the nursing supervisor, dietitian, or physician depending upon the circumstances.

As a nurse you have opportunity for some informal teaching. Patients often ask questions about their diets. Some of these you will be able to answer, but if you are not certain of the correct reply you should consult with your nursing supervisor or the dietitian. When the patient has been given instructions for the diet to be used at home, you may be able to reinforce this by helping the patient to review his diet. For example, the lists of foods for a diet might seem very confusing at first. As you help the patient to see that foods on his tray correspond to these lists, you help him to become familiar with planning for the diet when he goes home. Patients often ask about food fads, meal planning, the kinds of foods needed for good health, tips for buying and preparing foods, and so on. Such questions give you an opportunity to emphasize the essentials of food nutrition.

GOOD TRAY SERVICE

Meals are often the high point of the day for patients. An attractive tray of well-prepared food presented cheerfully to a patient who has been gotten ready for his meal goes a long way toward ensuring acceptance. (See Fig. 18–2.) The essentials of good tray service are:

1. A tray of sufficient size for uncrowded arrangement of dishes.

2. An immaculately clean, unwrinkled tray cover and napkin of linen or good quality paper.

3. An attractive pattern of spotless china without chips or cracks; sparkling glassware; and shining silverware.

4. Convenient orderly arrangement of all items on the tray so that the patient can easily reach everything.

5. Portions of food suitable for the patient's appetite.

6. Food attractively arranged with appropriate garnishes.

7. Meals served on time.

8. Hot foods served on warm plates and kept warm with a food cover; cold foods served on chilled dishes.

9. Trays promptly served to the patient so that food is at its best.

THE PATIENT AND HIS MEALS

A pleasant cheerful environment is essential to the greatest enjoyment of food. Before the tray is served the nurse should make every effort to

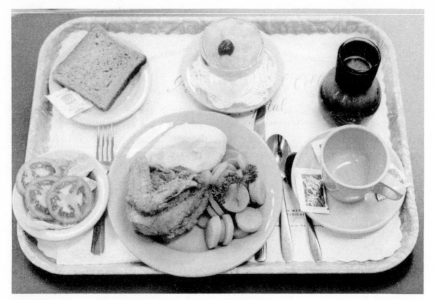

FIGURE 18–2   Color, texture, and flavor variations of foods that are attractively and conveniently arranged help to make mealtime enjoyable. (*Courtesy, Thomas Jefferson University Hospital.*)

provide surroundings that are clean, orderly, and well ventilated. Activities not associated with meal service should be avoided as far as possible while patients are eating. If an interruption in a meal is unavoidable because of a doctor's visit, or if there is a delay because of a laboratory test, arrangements should be made to keep food hot (or chilled, as the case may be) in a nearby kitchen.

Before the trays arrive the patient's hands should be washed, and if the patient is in bed, he should be positioned so that he is comfortable and able to feed himself. The tray should be checked as soon as it reaches the patient's room to be certain that everything needed is there and is convenient for the patient. Nurses or other persons responsible should cheerfully present trays to patients without delay. The nurse may butter the bread or cut the meat, if needed. The patient should be encouraged to eat, but should not be made to feel that he must hurry. Trays should be removed promptly when the patient has finished his meal.

FEEDING THE HELPLESS PATIENT

Acutely ill and elderly infirm patients often must be fed. Feeding a patient requires patience and understanding, especially if the patient eats slowly. If you can imagine how you would want someone fed who is very dear to you, you could probably set up a good guide. Here are some suggestions:

Before starting to feed the patient, make certain that you have everything you need. If the patient eats very slowly, it is a good idea to keep food hot by placing the plate over a hot-water container. Sit, rather than stand, so that you and the patient will be more comfortable and relaxed. If the patient is blind, give an attractive description of the food you are about to feed him. Offer small amounts of food at a time, and encourage the patient to chew his food well. Alternate one food with another, as the individual would normally do if he were feeding himself. Offer a beverage as seems indicated or as the patient requests it.

Focus upon the patient, rather than on the feeding process. Avoid giving the impression that the feeding is a bother to you and that you must hurry. Talk to the patient about pleasant things, and also give him a chance to talk. Listen thoughtfully and with interest to what he has to say. Explain the reasons for any change in his diet, and give encouragement when he makes progress.

A SURVEY OF MODIFIED DIETS

The chapters that follow will give full details of the most widely used therapeutic diets and the conditions for which they are usually prescribed. Many symptoms and laboratory findings are common to a wide variety of diseases. Some of these are listed in Table 18–1 together with the probable dietary considerations when they are present. Frequently occurring diseases and the typical dietary modifications for each are listed in Table 18–2.

It must never be assumed, however, that a dietary prescription is inflexibly and arbitrarily made for a given disease state. On the other hand, dietary adjustments must always be individualized for each patient according to his nutritional needs and the associated clinical findings. In some instances, priority must be given to one aspect of diet and other requirements may have to be deferred for a later time. For example, very low-residue diets are likely to be lacking in some vitamins, but the diet may be the only useful one in certain gastrointestinal disorders. The vitamin lack for a few days would not be serious; if it is prolonged, supplementation would be essential.

Symptom or Laboratory Finding	Typical Dietary Modifications
Anemia	Type must be determined. *Iron-deficiency:* Iron salts usually prescribed; normal diet. May increase protein and ascorbic acid intake. *Pernicious:* Vitamin B_{12} by injection; normal diet. Restrict fat and use bland diet, if intolerance to food
Anorexia	Do not force food; encourage eating prescribed diet. Attractive environment, appetizing food (18)
Constipation	
Atonic	High-fiber diet (19). Liberal fluid intake
Spastic	Soft high-fiber *or* bland diet (19). Liberal fluids
Dehydration	Force fluids. May need parenteral fluids. Adjust electrolyte balance
Diarrhea	No food by mouth → clear-fluid diet → full-fluid *or* low-residue *or* soft diet (19). When prolonged, high-protein, high-calorie; vitamin-mineral supplements
Edema	Sodium-restricted diet, usually 500–1000 mg (25)
Fever	Food and fluids as tolerated. Clear-fluid → full-fluid *or* soft → regular diet (19)
Short time	
High, prolonged	Liberal fluids; high-protein (23), high-calorie (21); low-residue, or soft if gastrointestinal tract is involved
Moderate, prolonged	Protein, 80–100 gm (23), 2500–3000 calories (21); 4 to 6 meals. Additional calcium and vitamin supplements for tuberculosis
Hypertension	Moderate sodium restriction (25). Severe sodium restriction or rice-fruit (Kempner) diet now seldom used. Fat-controlled (24) low-calorie (21) diets sometimes ordered
Hypoproteinemia	High-protein diet (23); adequate calories
Indigestion (heartburn)	Bland diet (19); small meals, pleasant environment (18)
Malabsorption	Must determine cause for appropriate dietary modification. Replacement of protein, calories, minerals, vitamins usually required
Obesity	800–1500-calorie diet (21)
Oliguria	Protein restriction, 20–40 gm (23); sodium restriction (25); usually fluid restriction
Steatorrhea	Must determine cause. Fat-restricted diet (24); if sprue, gluten-free diet (23)
Vomiting	No food by mouth → clear-fluid diet → full-fluid *or* low-residue *or* soft (19). If severe, replace fluids and essential nutrients parenterally
Weight loss	High-calorie diet (21); increased protein (23)

Disease Condition	Usual Dietary Considerations and Progression
Diseases of the gastrointestinal tract	
Esophageal obstruction	Tube feeding (19)
Gastritis, acute	Clear-fluid → full-fluid *or* low-residue → bland diet (19)
Gastritis, chronic	Low-residue *or* bland diet (19); 4 to 6 small meals
Peptic ulcer	Progressive bland diet with frequent meals (19)
Cancer, nonoperable	Diet as tolerated; full-fluid, soft. Cater to preferences
Hiatus hernia	Bland diet (19); 4 to 6 small meals
Regional ileitis	Low-residue diet (19); correct malnutrition with high-protein (23); high-calorie diet (21); iron and vitamin supplements
Diverticulitis	Nothing by mouth → clear-fluid → low-residue (19)
Ulcerative colitis	Bland diet (19); 100–150 gm protein (23); 3000–4000 calories (21); vitamin and mineral supplements. Possible allergies must be considered
Sprue, celiac disease	Gluten-free diet (23); vitamin-mineral supplements
Diseases of the liver, gallbladder, pancreas	
Infectious hepatitis	100–150 gm protein (23); high-calorie (21); full-fluid → soft → regular (19)
Cirrhosis	100–150 gm protein, if no liver failure (23); high-calorie, moderate fat. Vitamin and iron supplements. If ascites, 250–500 mg sodium (25). If esophageal varices, very low-fiber (19)
Hepatic coma	Protein-free to low-protein, 20 to 40 gm (23); high carbohydrate
Gallbladder disease	Fat-restricted (24), bland (19)
Pancreatic disease	Very low-fat (24); bland (19); 6 small meals
Cardiovascular and renal systems	
Coronary occlusion	Nothing by mouth → bland, 6 small meals. Usu-
Congestive heart failure	ally sodium-restricted (25); low-calorie (21); may be fat-controlled (24)
Atherosclerosis	Fat-controlled diet (24)
Acute nephritis	20–60 gm protein (23); 500–1000 mg sodium (25); bland (19); clear-fluid → full-fluid or soft
Chronic nephritis	Sodium-restricted, if edema (25); protein to replace urinary losses (23)
Renal failure	Protein-free to low-protein (23); sodium and potassium restriction (25)

TABLE 18–2 (*Continued*)

Disease Condition	Usual Dietary Considerations and Progression
Kidney stones	Fluids forced. Emphasize acid-producing *or* alkali-producing foods, depending upon type of stone (9)
Metabolic disorders	
Diabetes mellitus	Diet calculated for carbohydrate, protein, fat according to individual needs (22)
Functional hyperinsulinism	Calculated diet; high-protein, high-fat, marked restriction of carbohydrate (22)
Addison's disease	High-carbohydrate diet (22); 6 meals; bland to regular
ACTH therapy	1000 mg or mild sodium restriction (25)
Hyperthyroidism	If severe weight loss, high-protein (23) high-calorie (21)
Gout	Moderately low-purine diet (23)
Some surgical conditions	
Burns	High-protein, 150 gm (23); high-calorie (21); may require tube feeding (19)
Tonsillectomy	Sips of water, cold liquids, soft foods as tolerated. No tart fruit juices
Laryngectomy	Tube feeding (19)
Gastrectomy	Sips of water, parenteral feedings; small, frequent feedings of bland diet
Dumping syndrome	115–150 gm protein (23); 170–225 gm fat, 0–100 gm carbohydrate; 6 small meals; no fluids at meals
Peritonitis	Nothing by mouth; parenteral fluids; low-residue diet (19) when peristalsis returns
Ileostomy, colostomy	Nothing by mouth; intravenous fluids; low-residue diet (19)
Other abdominal operations	Clear fluids → full-fluid *or* low-residue *or* soft → regular diet (19). Parenteral fluids initially, if required

REVIEW QUESTIONS AND PROBLEMS

1. List some changes that occur in illness and that affect the nutrition of the patient.

2. Keep a record for a few days of the things that annoy you about food service. Also list the comments about food made by your friends and by patients. What reasons can you assign for these complaints? How would you as a nurse help the patient to better acceptance of his diet?

3. Become familiar with the arrangement of trays in your hospital. Arrange a tray for meals so that it is attractive and convenient.

4. What is meant by *diet therapy*? What purposes can be served by diet therapy?

5. Why are the following names for diet undesirable: cardiac diet, Meulengracht diet, ulcer discharge diet, low-salt diet?

6. Prepare a detailed list of ways in which you, as a nurse, can assist the patient with his nutrition.

7. Observe the meals served to patients for whom a house diet has been prescribed. How do they differ from normal diets with which you are familiar? Explain any differences you have noted.

REFERENCES

Babcock, C. G. "Attitudes and the Use of Food," *J. Amer. Diet. Ass.*, 38:546, 1961.

Buckley, B. R. "Feeding the Aged Person," *Amer. J. Nurs.*, 59:1591, 1959.

Dawson, M. J. "New Patients Dine with the Nurse," *Amer. J. Nurs.*, 66:287, 1966.

MacGregor, F. C. "Uncooperative Patients: Some Cultural Interpretations," *Amer. J. Nurs.*, 67:88, January 1967.

Morris, E. "How Does a Nurse Teach Nutrition to Patients?" *Amer. J. Nurs.*, 60:67, January 1960.

Rasmussen, S. *Foundations of Practical and Vocational Nursing*. New York: The Macmillan Company, 1967, Chap. 10.

Robinson, C. H. *Proudfit-Robinson's Normal and Therapeutic Nutrition*, 13th Ed. New York: The Macmillan Company, 1967, Chaps. 27 and 28.

Tarnower, W. "Psychological Needs of the Hospitalized Patient," *Nurs. Outlook*, 13:28, July 1965.

Young, C. M. "Teaching the Patient Means Reaching the Patient," *J. Amer. Diet. Ass.*, 33:52, 1957.

19

FIBER | FLAVOR | FLAVOR AND DIGESTION | OTHER FACTORS IN
FOOD TOLERANCE · Liquid Diets | CLEAR-FLUID DIET |
FULL-FLUID DIET | TUBE FEEDINGS · Modifications in Fiber
and Flavor | NOMENCLATURE AND INDICATIONS | MECHANICAL
SOFT DIET | SOFT, BLAND, AND VERY LOW-RESIDUE DIETS | BLAND
DIET FOR PEPTIC ULCER | HIGH-FIBER DIET

MODIFICATIONS OF DIET FOR CONSISTENCY AND FLAVOR

FIBER

The terms "fiber" and "residue" are not clearly differentiated. Fiber consists of the indigestible parts of foods. It includes cellulose, hemicellulose, lignins, gums, and related substances of plants, and the tough connective tissue from meats. Residue refers to the bulk remaining in the lower part of the gastrointestinal tract. It is derived from the indigestible fibers of the food, but may also be modified by the effect of the food on the growth of intestinal bacteria and their residues. For example, milk that contains no fiber may increase the residue in the feces.

Some foods contain much more fiber than others. Contrast the fibrous nature of cabbage, celery, and pineapple with the finer texture of spinach, lettuce, and banana; or the toughness of mature peas and Lima beans with the tenderness of the young seeds. The structural parts of the plant, skins, and seeds are indigestible. They lend bulk to the normal diet and encourage normal elimination.

The fiber content of the diet may be reduced in the following ways:

1. Selecting only young tender vegetables.

2. Omitting those foods that have seeds, tough skins, or much structural fiber; for example, berries, celery, corn, cabbage, stalks of asparagus, mature beans, and peas.

3. Peeling fruits and vegetables, such as apples, pears, potatoes, stalks of broccoli.

4. Cooking foods to soften the fiber.

200

5. Pressing foods through a sieve (puréeing or straining).

6. Using refined cereals and white breads in place of whole-grain cereals and breads.

7. Omitting fruits and vegetables entirely; using only strained juices.

Strained vegetables and fruits are extremely unpopular with patients. They have lost appeal in appearance, texture, and in flavor, and are looked upon as baby foods. Undoubtedly, these foods are necessary when a very smooth diet is required, as for a patient with bleeding esophageal varices; they are also useful in the construction of tube feedings. However, physicians have questioned the need for these foods in many diets for gastrointestinal disorders. Thus the soft and bland diets to be described in this chapter are much more liberal than they were a number of years ago.

Meats on low-fiber diets must be tender. Steaks, chops, and roasts with little connective tissue may be broiled and roasted. The less tender cuts of meat become tender when cooked with moist heat at low temperature; for example, stews that are simmered rather than boiled and pot roasts cooked at low heat. Tender cuts of meat need not be ground except when the patient should not exert the effort to chew or when the patient has no teeth.

FLAVOR

The flavors that are conveyed by foods are a composite of the taste qualities and the odors. Characteristic flavors are given to foods by various oils and water-soluble compounds. Fruits may taste sweet or sour, depending upon the amounts of sugar or acid. Fruits also give off typical odors that add much to their enjoyment.

Vegetables are classed as strong- or mild-flavored, depending upon the amounts of sulfur compounds that are present. Such compounds enhance the flavor of properly cooked vegetables, but they may be objectionable when vegetables are overcooked.

Meat extractives (purines) are nonprotein, nitrogen-containing compounds that are responsible for the flavor of meat. They give rich flavor to a gravy or soup.

The flavor of a food is modified by cooking procedures. The volatile substances that escape into the air lead to some loss and change of flavor. Would you expect cabbage to be stronger in flavor if cooked in an open or covered saucepan? Overcooking may lead to much loss of flavor, because some of the flavor compounds are dissolved out into the cooking water. On the other hand, some vegetables like cabbage develop strong flavors if overcooked.

The flavor of foods is often enhanced by the addition of flavoring substances, including spices, herbs, salt, vinegar, sugar, and flavoring extracts.

The effect of their use depends upon the choice of the condiment and the amount that may be used. Good cooks know that they must use a light hand in the use of herbs, for a little goes a long way. Chili con carne is normally classed as a highly flavored dish; yet it could range in seasoning from relatively mild to decidedly hot.

FLAVOR AND DIGESTION

Certain categories of foods are considered by many to cause gastrointestinal discomfort. Included are strongly flavored vegetables—broccoli, Brussels sprouts, cabbage, cauliflower, cucumber, leeks, onions, radishes, turnips; melons; and dry beans and peas.

Other foods are thought to be chemically stimulating; that is, they presumably increase the flow of gastric juices. Among these are meat extractives—broth, gravies, all meat stock soups; certain spices and seasonings—catsup, chili, garlic, horseradish, meat sauces, mustard seed, pepper, pickles, excessive salt, tabasco sauce, vinegar, Worcestershire sauce; and coffee and tea.

Considerable difference of opinion exists concerning the effects of eating the foods just discussed. On the one hand, people of several cultures—Indians and Africans, for example—use highly seasoned foods all their lives and appear to suffer no ill effects. Contrariwise, you undoubtedly know someone who complains of indigestion with the merest suggestion of garlic, onion, cucumber, or other items in the diet.

Specialists in medicine and dietetics believe that bland diets need have fewer restrictions placed upon them. Many persons should be permitted the wider range of many food choices that so often appear on "avoid" lists. Omissions of food should be made without hesitation for those individuals who have a definite intolerance for them.

OTHER FACTORS IN FOOD TOLERANCE

Disorders of the gastrointestinal tract have often led to a state of malnutrition because of the patient's inability to eat, his fear of eating certain foods, or the poor absorption of nutrients from the small intestine. High-protein and high-calorie adaptations of the diets described on the following pages are frequently ordered.

Patients with gastrointestinal disturbances are often nervous, anxious, worried, and tense. Their emotions may influence the digestion of foods. They may have many dislikes and expressed intolerance to food. It is important to give every consideration to the planning of meals that are enjoyable to the patient. The patient must also see the need for including nutritionally important foods from all major food groups.

Rapid eating and failure to relax are frequently noted in these patients.

They need to take adequate time for meals and to learn to eat slowly. They need, moreover, to learn to rest before and after meals and to look for diversions that are relaxing.

Liquid Diets

CLEAR-FLUID DIET

This is an allowance of tea, coffee or coffee substitute, and fat-free broth. Ginger ale, fruit juices, gelatin, fruit ices, and water gruels are sometimes also given. Small amounts of fluid are offered every hour or two to the patient. The diet is used for 24 to 48 hours following acute vomiting, diarrhea, or surgery.

The primary purpose of this diet is to relieve thirst and to help maintain water balance. Broth provides some sodium, and broth and fruit juices contribute potassium. Carbonated beverages, sugar, and fruit juices, when used, furnish a small amount of carbohydrate.

FULL-FLUID DIET

This is a nutritionally adequate diet consisting of liquids and foods that liquefy at body temperature. It is used for acute infections and fever of short duration and for patients who are too ill to chew. It may be ordered as the first progression from the clear-fluid diet following surgery or in the treatment of acute gastrointestinal upsets.

The diet is offered in six feedings or more. Initially, amounts smaller than those represented by the plan below may be given. To increase the caloric intake, 1 pt light cream may be substituted for 1 pt milk. The protein level of the full-fluid diet may be increased approximately 30 gm by including 3 oz nonfat dry milk each day. This may be added to fresh milk, to cream soups, to cereal gruels, or to custards. Strained meats may be added to broth or to hot tomato juice. Raw eggs are sometimes a source of *Salmonella* infection. Therefore, only commercially pasteurized eggnogs or beverages prepared from pasteurized dried egg powder should be used.

FULL-FLUID DIET

Food Allowance for One Day

6 cups milk
2 eggs
1–2 oz strained meat
1 cup strained citrus juice
½ cup tomato juice

Sample Menu

Breakfast
Grapefruit juice
Strained oatmeal with butter, hot milk, and sugar

Food Allowance (Continued)
½ cup vegetable purée
½ cup strained cereal
2 servings dessert: soft custard,
    Junket, plain ice cream, sherbet,
    or plain gelatin
2 tablespoons sugar
1 tablespoon butter

Protein: 85 gm
Calories: 1950

Sample Menu (Continued)
Milk
Coffee with cream and sugar

Midmorning
Orange juice
Soft custard

Luncheon
Broth with strained beef
Tomato juice
Vanilla ice cream
Milk

Midafternoon
Milk

Dinner
Cream of asparagus soup
Eggnog, commercial, pasteurized
Strawberry gelatin with whipped
    cream
Tea with lemon and sugar

Bedtime
Chocolate malted milk

TUBE FEEDINGS

A tube feeding is a nutritionally adequate allowance of liquefied foods that can be administered through a tube in the stomach or duodenum. A tube feeding is used in paralysis or obstruction of the esophagus, following mouth or gastric surgery, in severe burns, for unconscious patients, or in any situation where the patient is unable to chew or swallow.

A wide choice of these types of tube feedings is available: (1) blenderized feedings; (2) milk-base formulas; and (3) commercial preparations. Blenderized feedings include foods from a normal diet that are liquefied in a blender at high speed. These are generally preferred because diarrhea is a less frequent complication. To prepare a blenderized feeding the foods of a normal diet are placed in a blender with sufficient milk and other liquid to allow them to be blended. Homogenized milk must be used because plain milk would be churned into butter. The liquid mixture is strained several times through a fine-mesh sieve to remove all fiber. These feedings are usually given with a food pump.

Of the many formulas in use, two examples are shown in Table 19–1. The blenderized feeding includes strained baby foods, thereby reducing the amount of fiber and the need for repeated straining.

TABLE 19–1 TWO FORMULAS FOR TUBE FEEDING

Blenderized Feeding*			Milk-Base Formula	
Strained liver	150	gm	Water (3 cups)	720 gm
Egg	50	gm	Nonfat dry milk	150 gm
Applesauce	50	gm	Pasteurized egg powder	30 gm
Carrots, strained	50	gm	Sugar (¼ cup)	50 gm
Orange juice, frozen,			Molasses (¼ cup)	60 gm
reconstituted	100	gm	Brewer's yeast	15 gm
Nonfat dry milk	175	gm		
Sugar	15	gm		
Brewer's yeast	2.5	gm	Total volume	1000 ml
Water to make	1000	ml	Add supplement of vitamin	
			A to one feeding daily	
			Give 8 oz strained orange	
			juice in separate feeding	
Protein	90	gm	Protein	72 gm
Calories	1000		Calories	1100

* Stumpf, G. L. *Diet Manual—University of Michigan Hospital*, Ann Arbor, Mich.: The George Wahr Publishing Company, 1963, p. 41.

The normal daily intake of the formulas is about 2000 ml. The protein level may be reduced by decreasing the amount of nonfat dry milk. The calorie level may be adjusted by using light cream for part of the fluid.

Initially tube feedings are given hourly in 1½- to 2-oz portions; then the feedings are given in larger amounts at two- to four-hour intervals. The feedings may be heated over hot water to body temperature, care being taken that the mixture does not curdle.

Modifications in Fiber and Flavor

NOMENCLATURE AND INDICATIONS

The Mechanical Soft Diet differs from the normal diet only in that it is limited to soft foods for those who have difficulty in chewing because of no teeth or poorly fitting dentures. No restriction is made upon the diet for seasonings or method of food preparation.

The Soft Diet is a nutritionally adequate diet that differs from the normal diet in being reduced in fiber content, soft in consistency, and bland in flavor. It is used intermediately between the Full-Fluid Diet and the regular diet following surgery, in acute infections and fevers, and in gastrointestinal disturbances.

The Bland Diet is a nutritionally adequate diet (except in some stages used in peptic ulcer) that includes foods that are bland in flavor, soft in consistency, and mechanically and chemically nonstimulating. Variations of it are used for gastritis, peptic ulcer, ulcerative colitis, diverticulitis, ileitis, and similar gastrointestinal disorders.

The Very Low-Residue Diet is one designed to leave a minimum of residue in the colon. It is sometimes the first diet ordered following abdominal surgery, and may progress to the soft or regular diet. Prior to and following surgery on the colon or rectum, the diet is used to delay bowel movement. The diet is also used initially for acute diarrhea, diverticulitis, ileitis, colitis, and may progress to the bland or soft diet.

The High-Fiber Diet is a normal diet with special emphasis upon foods that are important sources of indigestible fiber. It is indicated for atonic constipation (sluggish colon).

MECHANICAL SOFT DIET

The normal diet is modified in the following ways:

1. Meat and poultry are minced or ground; fish usually is sufficiently tender without further treatment.

2. Vegetables are cooked. They may be cooked a little longer than usual to be sure they are soft, and may be diced or chopped; for example, diced beets, chopped spinach, and so on.

3. Chopped raw tomatoes, chopped lettuce, and finely chopped cabbage may sometimes be used.

4. Soft raw fruits may be used: banana, citrus sections, diced soft pear, peach, apple, apricots, melons, berries. All canned and frozen fruits are suitable.

5. Soft rolls, bread, and biscuits are used instead of crisp rolls, crusty breads, and toast.

6. All desserts on a normal diet that are soft may be used, including pies with tender crusts, cakes, puddings. Nuts and dried fruits are used only if they are finely chopped.

SOFT, BLAND, AND VERY LOW-RESIDUE DIETS

The food allowances and samples menus in Tables 19–2 and 19–3 provide opportunity to compare the three types of diets. Note the following changes from the normal diet:

1. Tender, minced, or ground meats.

2. Elimination of sharp cheeses, most raw fruits and vegetables; fibrous foods; hot seasonings and spices; fried foods; rich pastries, pies, and desserts.

The Bland Diet differs from the Soft Diet in that meat extractives and meat soups are omitted, and coffee and tea are limited to one cup daily.

TABLE 19–2   FOOD ALLOWANCES FOR DIETS MODIFIED
IN FIBER AND FLAVOR

Soft Diet	Bland Diet	Very Low-Residue Diet
Beverages—coffee, tea, carbonated	Coffee with milk— 1 cup; weak tea	Coffee, tea, carbonated beverages
Bread—white, fine whole-wheat, rye without seeds; white crackers	Same	White enriched only
Cereal foods—dry, such as cornflakes, Puffed Rice, rice flakes; fine-cooked, such as corn meal, farina, hominy grits, macaroni, noodles, rice, spaghetti; strained coarse, such as oatmeal, Pettijohn's, whole-wheat	Same	Cornflakes, Puffed Rice, rice flakes; corn meal, farina, hominy grits; macaroni, noodles, rice, spaghetti
Cheese—mild, soft, such as cottage and cream; Cheddar; Swiss	Same	Same. Hard cheeses in sauces only
Desserts—plain cake, cookies; custards; plain gelatin or with allowed fruit; Junket; plain ice cream, ices, sherbets; plain puddings, such as bread, cornstarch, rice, tapioca	Same	Same. Milk desserts sometimes omitted
Eggs—all except fried	Same	Same
Fats—butter, cream, margarine, vegetable oils and fats in cooking	Same plus salad dressings	Butter, cream, margarine, oils and cooking fats
Fruits—raw: ripe avocado, banana, grapefruit or orange sections without membrane; canned or cooked: apples, apricots, fruit cocktail, peaches, pears, plums—all without skins; Royal Anne cherries; strained prunes and other fruits with skins; all juices	Same	Strained juices only; applesauce sometimes
Meat—very tender, minced, or ground; baked, broiled, creamed, roast, or stewed: beef, lamb, veal, poultry, fish, bacon, liver, sweetbreads	Same	Same
Milk—in any form	Same	None
Soups—broth, strained cream or vegetable	Cream; no broth or stock	Broth or stock; no cream
Sweets—all sugars, syrup, jelly, honey, plain sugar candy without fruit or nuts, molasses Use in moderation	Same	Same
Vegetables—white or sweet potato without skin, any way except fried; young and tender asparagus, beets, carrots, peas, pumpkin, squash without seeds; tender chopped greens; strained cooked vegetables if not tender; tomato juice	Same plus raw tomato, tender salad greens	White potato and vegetable juices only
Miscellaneous—salt, seasonings and spices in moderation, gravy, cream sauces	Same	Same

TABLE 19–3   SAMPLE MENUS FOR SOFT, BLAND, AND
VERY LOW-RESIDUE DIETS *

Soft Diet	Bland Diet	Very Low-Residue Diet
Breakfast		
Orange sections	Orange sections	Strained orange juice
Oatmeal	Oatmeal	Cream of wheat
Milk	Milk	Milk for cereal
Sugar	Sugar	Sugar
Soft-cooked egg	Soft-cooked egg	Soft-cooked egg
Whole-wheat toast	Fine whole-wheat toast	White toast
Butter or margarine	Butter or margarine	Butter or margarine
Coffee with cream, sugar	Coffee with half milk—1 cup	Coffee with cream, sugar
Luncheon		
Tomato bouillon	Cream of tomato soup	Tomato bouillon
Melba toast	Melba toast	Melba toast
Roast chicken	Roast chicken	Roast chicken
Buttered rice	Buttered rice	Buttered rice
Asparagus tips	Asparagus tips	No vegetable
Parkerhouse roll	Parkerhouse roll	Parkerhouse roll
Butter or margarine	Butter or margarine	Butter or margarine
Golden cake with fluffy white icing	Golden cake with icing	Golden cake with icing
Milk; tea, if desired	Milk	Tea with lemon and sugar
Dinner		
Grapefruit juice	Grapefruit juice	Grapefruit juice
Small club steak	Small club steak	Small club steak
Baked potato without skin, butter	Baked potato, no skin, with butter	Baked potato without skin, butter
Buttered julienne green beans	Buttered green beans	No vegetables
Dinner roll with butter	Roll with butter	Roll with butter
Apple crisp	Apple crisp	Whipped raspberry gelatin with cream
Milk	Milk	Sugar cookie
Tea or coffee, if desired		Tea with lemon and sugar

* NOTE: These menus may be given in six feedings by saving part of the food from the preceding meal:

Midmorning: cereal from breakfast
Midafternoon: milk and crackers or dessert from lunch
Bedtime: milk and crackers or dessert from dinner

A more restricted fiber content could be obtained if fruits and vegetables were puréed and if only refined breads and cereals were used.

The Very Low-Residue Diet differs from the soft diet in that (1) all fruits and vegetables are omitted, except for a limited amount of strained juice; (2) only refined cereals and white breads may be used; and (3) milk is frequently omitted. This diet is used for only a short time, because it will be inadequate in vitamin A, iron, and sometimes protein, calcium, and riboflavin.

BLAND DIET FOR PEPTIC ULCER

The dietary treatment for peptic ulcer illustrates the use of the Bland Diet. Particular emphasis is placed upon (1) nutritive adequacy, (2) ability of the diet to dilute, neutralize, or reduce the secretion of acid by the stomach, and (3) ability of the diet to avoid mechanical, chemical, or thermal irritation.

Nutritive adequacy is expected of any diet used for a long period of time. Unfortunately, many restricted diets used for patients with peptic ulcer do not provide sufficient protein, minerals, or vitamins, and poor nutrition results when they are used too long. Other diets may be adequate in terms of calculated nutritive content, but the ground meats and puréed foods are so poorly eaten that the patient is still malnourished. The trend today is toward more liberal diets that the patient can enjoy and that thus improve nutrition. Sufficient protein and ascorbic acid are especially important for healing of the ulcer.

The most important therapeutic quality of a diet for peptic ulcer is that it assist in diluting or neutralizing the stomach acid. This is accomplished by giving small, frequent feedings, so that the acid can mix with the food, thus giving the ulcer a better chance to heal. Foods rich in protein have somewhat greater ability to neutralize acid than low-protein foods; thus milk, eggs, mild cheese, and meat, poultry, and fish are effective.

Fat has some ability to inhibit the secretion of acid. It also delays the emptying of the stomach. The fats of milk, cream, butter, and eggs are easily digested and may be beneficial in this respect.

Meat extractives, caffeine and tannins in coffee, tea, and cola beverages, some spices, alcohol, and tobacco appear to stimulate the flow of acid. They are ordinarily omitted.

Numerous interpretations of the bland diet are to be found in diet manuals of various hospitals. Generally, these diets are based upon the principles of progression from marked restriction to a more liberal diet, as described by Sippy and others half a century ago. The *Meulengracht* diet is a more liberal adaptation of the Sippy diet, and includes two hourly feedings of all foods permitted on the full bland diet.

The following outline of the four stages of diet progression illustrates the regimen used in many hospitals. Note that these stages range from fiber-free diets to only mild restriction of fiber; that they are bland in flavor; and that the initial stages are nutritionally inadequate. A patient may be started on stages 1, 2, or 3; he progresses within a few days, as a rule, to stage 4 and remains on this indefinitely.

Stage 1: Two to three ounces of milk and cream given hourly to the patient. The mixture may be fortified with nonfat dry milk for extra protein. This stage is used for only a few days.

Stage 2: Six ounces milk and cream feedings at two-hourly intervals. In addition, 3 to 4 oz of any one of these foods are offered at the three mealtimes: strained cream soup, eggs, cottage cheese, white potato, white toast or crackers, refined cereals, custards, and plain puddings.

Stage 3: Six to eight ounces of milk are offered six times a day. In addition, at the three mealtimes approximately 6 oz of any food listed for stage 2 are allowed. The selection of food may also include one serving of puréed fruit or vegetable.

Stage 4: The bland diet as described on pages 206 to 209 is used. Mid-morning, midafternoon, and bedtime feedings are always used. These interval feedings include plain milk or a milk beverage plus crackers, plain cookies, plain cake, a sandwich, or simple dessert.

HIGH-FIBER DIET

Since this diet is indicated primarily for atonic constipation, it is well to remember that the condition occurs more frequently in elderly persons who have little exercise, who confine their food selection to low-fiber foods, who drink little liquid, who resort to the use of laxatives, and who have irregular habits of elimination. Obviously, these practices must be changed in attempting to correct the constipation. Unless the physician indicates otherwise, the patient should be encouraged to drink six to eight glasses of fluid daily, with at least a glass (hot or cold, plain or flavored with lemon) before breakfast; to exercise as his condition warrants; and to develop regular habits of elimination.

The normal diet is increased in fiber content by including two or more servings of raw fruit and vegetable daily. A salad may be given at the noon and evening meals. Raw fruit may be used in place of dessert. Whole-grain breads and cereals with some bran are substituted for refined breads and cereals. Prunes and prune juice have particular laxative properties.

REVIEW QUESTIONS AND PROBLEMS

1. What are the sources of fiber in the diet? What is meant by *residue*?

2. What foods are usually allowed on a clear-fluid diet? What nutrients are supplied by this diet? When is it used?

3. Keep a record of the normal diet served to a patient for one day. What changes would you make in this menu so that it would be suitable for a patient who has no teeth? What changes would be likely if the physician has ordered a soft diet for a patient following surgery?

4. List four situations when a soft diet might be used.

5. How does a very low-residue diet differ from a soft diet?

6. How does a bland diet differ from a soft diet?

7. What are the important factors to consider in a diet for a patient with peptic ulcer? What is meant by *progressive regimen?*

8. A patient with ulcerative colitis complains that he cannot take milk. What nutrients would be lacking if milk is omitted? How could you supply these? What steps can you take to include some milk?

REFERENCES

Davenport, R. R. "Tube Feeding for Long-Term Patients," *Amer. J. Nurs.,* **64**:121, January 1964.

Dericks, V. C. "Rehabilitation of Patients with Ileostomy," *Amer. J. Nurs.,* **61**:48, January 1961.

Friedrich, H. N. "Oral Feeding by Food Pump," *Amer. J. Nurs.,* **62**:62, February 1962.

Jay, A. N. "Is It Indigestion?" *Amer. J. Nurs.,* **58**:1552, 1958.

———. "Colitis," *Amer. J. Nurs.,* **59**:1133, 1959.

Joint Committee of the American Dietetic Association and the American Medical Association. "Diet as Related to Gastrointestinal Function," *J. Amer. Diet. Ass.,* **38**: 425, 1961.

Kramer, P., and Caso, E. K. "Is the Rationale for Gastrointestinal Diet Therapy Sound?" *J. Amer. Diet. Ass.,* **42**:505, 1963.

Larsen, R. B. "Dietary Needs of Patients Following General Surgery," *Hospitals,* **39**:133, July 16, 1965.

McKittrick, J. B., and Shotkin, J. M. "Ulcerative Colitis," *Amer. J. Nurs.,* **62**:60, August 1962.

Mason, M. A. *Basic Medical-Surgical Nursing,* 2nd ed. New York: The Macmillan Company, 1967, Chaps. 14 and 15.

Ratcliff, J. D. "America's Laxative Addicts," *Today's Health,* **40**:52, November 1962.

Robinson, C. H. *Proudfit-Robinson's Normal and Therapeutic Nutrition,* 13th ed. New York: The Macmillan Company, 1967, Chaps. 33, 34, 35, 36.

Secor, J. "The Patient with Emphysema," *Amer. J. Nurs.,* **65**:75, July 1965.

White, D. R. "I Have an Ileostomy," *Amer. J. Nurs.,* **61**:51, May 1961.

DIETARY CALCULATIONS WITH
FOOD EXCHANGE LIST

NEED FOR CALCULATED DIETS

A number of conditions require control of the quantities of one or more constituents of the diet: obesity, diabetes mellitus, hyperinsulinism, and others. A daily calculation for the specific foods of the menu would be extremely time-consuming and impractical. As a matter of fact, even the detailed calculation would give only an approximate value for the actual intake because no two samples of the same kind of food are completely identical in their composition. Furthermore, people vary considerably in their metabolism from day to day.

FOOD EXCHANGE LISTS

This chapter describes a practical, rapid method for planning diets by using average values for groups of foods. The Food Exchange Lists (Table A–2) were prepared some years ago by a joint committee of the American Dietetic Association, American Diabetes Association, and Diabetes Section of the United States Public Health Service. Initially intended for simplification of diabetic diets (Chap. 22), the lists soon found wide use in the planning of low-calorie diets (Chap. 21). More recently fat-controlled diets (Chap. 24) and sodium-restricted diets (Chap. 25) have been developed with the use of food lists.

An *exchange* list is a grouping of foods in which the carbohydrate, protein, and fat values are about equal for the items listed. For example, any fruit in List 3, in the amounts stated, will supply 10 gm carbohydrate: one small apple, or one-half grapefruit, or two prunes, or one-half small banana, and so on. From List 4, Bread Exchanges, ½ cup cooked rice, or one small potato, or ¾ cup cornflakes could be exchanged for one slice bread. The six exchange lists include milk, vegetables—groups A and B, fruit, bread, meat, and fat. A seventh list includes items of negligible food value such as lemon juice, bouillon, and dill pickles that may be used as desired. (See Figs. 20–1, 20–2, 20–3, and 20–4.)

METHOD FOR DIETARY CALCULATIONS

A physician prescribes the amounts of carbohydrate, protein, and fat that are to be used in measured diets. Using the values for the exchange lists, the dietitian or nurse calculates the number of exchanges to be furnished by the diet.

The steps in planning the measured diet are listed below. A sample calculation in Table 20–1 illustrates the procedure.

1. Become familiar with the patient's usual pattern of meals, the food likes and dislikes, and so on. Whether the patient eats at home, carries lunches, or eats in a restaurant will affect the planning. The amount of money that can be spent, the preparation facilities, and the cultural patterns must be considered.

2. Include basic foods to ensure adequate levels of minerals and vitamins: 2 cups milk (3 or more for children); 5 oz meat; two servings vegetables; two servings fruit; breads and cereals.

3. List the carbohydrate, protein, and fat values for the milk, vegetables, and fruit.

4. Subtract the carbohydrate value of these foods (61 in the example) from the carbohydrate level prescribed (150 gm). Divide the difference by 15 to determine the number of bread exchanges (6 in the example).

5. Total the protein values of the milk, vegetables, and bread exchanges (30 in the example). Subtract from the protein prescribed (70). Divide the difference by 7 to determine the number of meat exchanges (6 in the example).

6. Total the fat values for milk and meat (50 in the example) and subtract from the total fat prescribed (70). Divide the difference by 5 to determine the number of fat exchanges (4 in the example).

7. Check the calculations to be certain that they are correct. It is not a good idea to split the fruit, bread, and meat exchanges into half. The calculations for carbohydrate should be within 7 gm of the prescribed level, and those for protein within 3 gm of the prescribed level.

8. Divide the total exchanges for the day into meal patterns according to the physician's diet order and the patient's preference. A meal pattern and sample menu illustrate the diet calculated in Table 20–1.

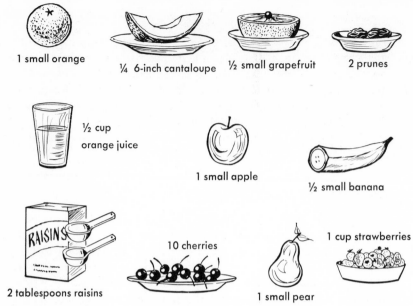

1 small orange

¼ 6-inch cantaloupe

½ small grapefruit

2 prunes

½ cup orange juice

1 small apple

½ small banana

2 tablespoons raisins

10 cherries

1 small pear

1 cup strawberries

FIGURE 20–1   Fruit exchanges. Each exchange supplies 10 gm carbohydrate and negligible protein and fat. See List 3 of Table A–2 for additional choices.

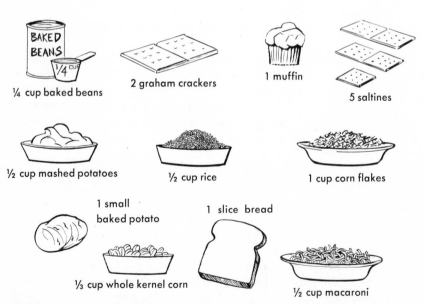

¼ cup baked beans

2 graham crackers

1 muffin

5 saltines

½ cup mashed potatoes

½ cup rice

1 cup corn flakes

1 small baked potato

⅓ cup whole kernel corn

1 slice bread

½ cup macaroni

FIGURE 20–2   Bread exchanges. Each food illustrated above yields approximately 15 gm carbohydrate and 2 gm protein. See List 4 in Table A–2 for additional choices.

214

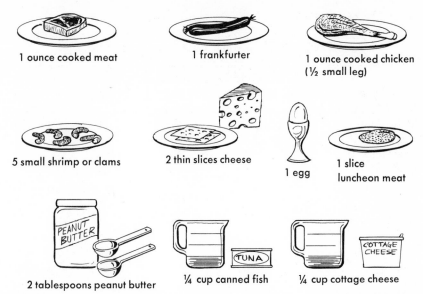

FIGURE 20–3 Meat exchanges. Each exchange provides 7 gm protein and 5 gm fat. About 3 meat exchanges are used for an average dinner serving of cooked meat; use 4 oz raw, lean meat to equal 3 oz cooked. See List 5 in Table A–2 for additional choices.

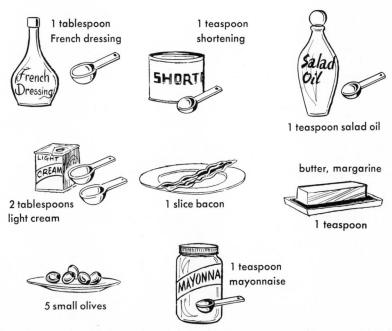

FIGURE 20–4 Fat exchanges. Each of the foods illustrated above provides approximately 5 gm fat. See List 6 in Table A–2 for additional choices.

TABLE 20–1 SAMPLE CALCULATION OF DIET

Exchange List	Number of Exchanges	Carbohydrate gm	Protein gm	Fat gm
Milk	2	24	16	20
Vegetables A	1–2	—	—	—
Vegetables B	1	7	2	—
Fruit	3	30	—	—
		(61)*		
Bread	6	90	12	—
			(30)†	
Meat	6	—	42	30
				(50)‡
Fat	4	—	—	20
Totals for the day		151	72	70

* 150 — 61 = 89 gm carbohydrate to be supplied from bread exchanges
  1 bread exchange = 15 gm carbohydrate
  89 ÷ 15 = 6 bread exchanges
† 70 — 30 = 40 gm protein to be supplied from meat exchanges
  1 exchange meat = 7 gm protein
  40 ÷ 7 = 6 meat exchanges
‡ 70 — 50 = 20 gm fat to be supplied from the fat exchanges
  1 fat exchange = 5 gm fat
  20 ÷ 5 = 4 fat exchanges

Meal Pattern	Sample Menu

Breakfast

Milk—1 exchange	Milk—1 cup
Fruit—1 exchange	Cantaloupe—¼ medium
Bread—2 exchanges	Wheat flakes—¾ cup
	Toast—1 slice
Meat—1 exchange	Egg—1
Fat—2 exchanges	Butter—1 teaspoon
	Cream, light—2 tablespoons

Luncheon

Milk—1 exchange	Milk—1 cup
Vegetable, group A	Radishes and celery sticks
Fruit—1 exchange	Apple—1 small
	Sandwich
Bread—2 exchanges	Bread—2 slices
Meat—2 exchanges	Roast beef—2 oz
Fat—1 exchange	Mayonnaise—1 teaspoon

Dinner

Vegetable, group A   Asparagus tips
Vegetable, group B—1 exchange   Baked acorn squash—½
Fruit—1 exchange   Pears, water-packed—2 halves
Bread—2 exchanges   Potato, baked—1 small
                                        Roll, dinner—1
Meat—3 exchanges   Roast pork, lean—3 oz
Fat—1 exchange   Butter on potato—1 teaspoon

REVIEW QUESTIONS AND PROBLEMS

1. List the foods in the vegetable group A that are especially rich in vitamin A; in ascorbic acid.

2. Which vegetables are included in the bread list?

3. Plan a breakfast that includes the following exchanges: milk, 1; fruit, 1; bread, 2; meat, 1; fat, 3.

4. Calculate the carbohydrate, protein, and fat value of the following day's allowance: milk, 2; vegetable, group A, 1; vegetable, group B, 1; fruit, 3; bread, 4; meat, 7; fats, 5.

5. Arrange the day's allowance from question 4 into three meals. Write a sample menu for the pattern you have set up.

LOW- AND HIGH-CALORIE DIETS

Problems of Weight Control

HAZARDS OF OVERWEIGHT AND UNDERWEIGHT

Obesity or excessive fatness of the body is a hazard to health. Imagine your reaction if you were told to carry a 25-lb package with you wherever you went! That is exactly what the overweight person must do—10, 25, 50 lb or whatever the excess may be. It goes with him whether he walks upstairs, or ties a shoelace, or tries to hurry for a train. The extra weight makes demands upon his heart, his blood circulation, his back, his feet, and so on. It is no surprise that obese people more often have heart disease; they also have gallbladder disease, diabetes, and other chronic diseases more frequently. They face an extra risk if they require surgery. The obese pregnant woman is more likely to have complications than the woman of normal weight.

Underweight, though less emphasized, also presents dangers to health. Underweight persons are more likely to have infections and disturbances of the gastrointestinal tract. Tuberculosis is most frequent among young, underweight people.

BALANCING ONE'S WEIGHT

The degree of obesity or undernutrition is most often judged by comparing what one weighs with a height-weight table (see Table A–3). If one weighs 10 to 19 per cent more than is desirable for his height and body frame, he is *overweight*; if he weighs 20 per cent or more over desirable weight, he is *obese*. People who are 15 per cent or more below normal weight are *underweight*. The degree of body fatness may also be determined by measuring the thickness of skin folds of the upper arm or abdomen with a caliper.

Gaining or losing weight is simply a question of balancing food calories with the body's need for calories. One pound of fat is equal to about 3500 calories. Thus, if you have 500 calories extra every day, you will gain about 1 lb a week. If you have 500 calories less every day than your body needs, you will lose about 1 lb in a week.

Suppose you need 2000 calories a day, but your diet adds up each day to 2100 calories. In 30 days this excess amounts to 3000 calories. You would gain about 0.9 lb in the month ($3000 \div 3500 = 0.9$). Perhaps this does not seem like much, but it amounts to about 11 lb in a year!

To keep in balance you would need to eliminate the surplus calories from your diet. You could also avoid gaining weight by increasing your activity. By walking a mile a day the average adult uses about 100 to 125 calories; so this increase in exercise would help to avoid weight gain.

CAUSES OF OVEREATING AND UNDEREATING

Too often we assume that obese people simply eat tremendous amounts of food. In fact, however, obesity more often results because of the little extras day by day; perhaps an extra pat of butter, a second roll, a snack, a second piece of candy, or a rich dessert each day rather than a low-calorie dessert.

Not all obese people eat more than normal-weight people. Several recent studies have shown that many obese boys and girls actually eat less than normal-weight boys and girls. However, they were found to be much less active. Failure to get enough exercise meant that their diets, which seemed quite normal, furnished too many calories for them. Likewise, many adults probably do not eat large amounts of food, but they may be so inactive that their intakes are excessive for them.

The following list presents some of the factors that might be responsible for failing to balance one's calories with body weight.

Some Reasons for Calorie Intake in Excess of Needs	*Some Reasons for Inadequate Calorie Intake*
1. Family patterns of rich, high-calorie foods; mother often has reputation of being a good cook	1. Family pattern places emphasis upon low-calorie foods; few rich desserts, for example
2. Good appetite; likes to eat; likes many rich foods; may dislike fruits and vegetables	2. Small appetite; has little interest in eating; may have many dislikes; unpalatable therapeutic diets

3. Ignorance of calorie value of foods

3. Ignorance of essentials of an adequate diet

4. Skips breakfast; is a frequent nibbler; coffee breaks with high-calorie snacks

4. Skips meals; seldom makes up for skipped meals; rarely nibbles

5. Pattern of living
   a. Sedentary occupation; idleness
   b. Riding to work or school
   c. Little exercise during leisure
   d. Often sleeps more as he becomes older

5. Pattern of living
   a. Often tense
   b. Overactive
   c. Not enough sleep and rest

6. Emotional outlet: eats to overcome worry, boredom, loneliness, grief

6. Emotional outlet: unhappy, worried, grieving, but refuses to eat

7. Many social events with rich foods; frequent eating in restaurants

7. Often lives alone; misses sociability; doesn't like to eat alone

8. Lower metabolism with increasing age, but failure to reduce intake

8. Illness and infection; fever, diarrhea; hyperthyroidism

9. Influenced by pressures of advertising for many high-calorie foods

9. Affected by claims for fad diets; may get inadequate diet

PREVENTION OF OBESITY

To avoid obesity one must first understand fully the reasons for excessive calorie intake as described in the preceding section. But there must also be the will to take prompt measures when the first few extra pounds appear. It is much easier to prevent obesity than to treat it. Prevention is most effective when patterns of diet and exercise are established early in life. Mothers need to know that the fat baby is not necessarily the healthiest baby, and that they should not force the infant to eat every last bit of food. Preschool children should not be bribed or rewarded with food; they should have a variety of activities so that they do not depend too much upon food for pleasure.

In families where one or both parents are obese, children are very likely to become obese and remain so throughout life. This can be prevented by changing the eating patterns so that fewer calorie-rich foods are eaten. Use fruits for desserts often and cakes, pies, or pastries seldom; broil, stew, or roast meats instead of frying; put less butter and cream on vegetables and learn to use other flavorings.

Children should be urged to get more exercise and should be expected to perform some chores requiring daily physical activity. Family recreation needs to include more participation in physical activity and somewhat less of the quiet pastimes such as watching television and riding about in automobiles.

Diets for Obesity

PLANNING FOR WEIGHT LOSS

Any program of weight loss of more than a few pounds should be directed by a physician. If a weight-losing program is to be successful, the individual must be convinced of the rewards that will come: better health, a slimmer figure, more pep, and perhaps a longer life. Although a low-calorie diet is used only so long as weight needs to be lost, each obese person must be convinced that he needs to modify his lifetime eating habits. If he fails to do this, he will gain back all the pounds he has lost.

It is important to set a reasonable goal. A weekly weight loss of one or two pounds is better than a crash program that leaves one tired and unwilling to continue. If one needs to lose 50 lb, six to nine months is not an unreasonable time allowance.

Keeping a weekly weight chart is a good idea. The person should weigh at the same time every week on the same scale and with the same amount of clothing. He needs to know that the scales might not show any weight loss for the first week or two because, in some instances, water is temporarily held in the tissues when people are placed on reducing diets. After a while this water will be released from the tissues, and the weight loss will show up.

Exercise has its place in a weight-reduction program. Walking is one of the best exercises. People can walk a few extra blocks to work or make it a practice to see a little more of the outdoors on foot rather than from an automobile window. Moderate exercise does not increase the appetite as some claim. For very obese persons, or those who have been ill, the recommendation for exercise by the physician should be followed closely. It is never a good idea for a person who has been sedentary to suddenly engage in violent exercise.

THE LOW-CALORIE DIET

Women usually lose satisfactorily on diets restricted to 1000 to 1500 calories, whereas men lose satisfactorily on diets furnishing 1200 to 1800 calories. Bed patients, such as those with heart disease, are often placed on diets restricted to 800 to 1000 calories, and sometimes less.

The daily food allowances for the 1000-, 1200-, and 1500-calorie diets are somewhat higher in protein than normal. (See Table 21–1.) This is desirable, because it provides most people with a feeling of satisfaction. Also, it helps to correct the greater losses of muscle tissue that occur during reducing. The extra protein is provided from the meat group, with some restriction of the bread-cereal group.

The food exchange lists are used for planning the daily food choices

TABLE 21-1 LOW-CALORIE DIETS BASED ON FOOD EXCHANGE LISTS *

		1000 Calories	1200 Calories	1500 Calories
Milk, skim	Cups	2	2	3
Vegetables, group A		As desired	As desired	As desired
group B	Cups	½	½	½
Fruit	Exchanges	3	3	3
Bread	Exchanges	2	2	4
Meat	Exchanges	8	9	9
Fat	Exchanges	0	2	4
	Protein, gm	78	85	97
	Fat, gm	40	55	65
	Carbohydrate, gm	91	91	133
	Calories	1036	1199	1505

* Food choices are listed in Table A–2.

for the low-calorie diets. The patient with a little practice becomes familiar with the kinds of foods included, the correct size of portions, and the methods of food preparation. For example, if he is allowed one exchange fruit for breakfast, he may have two prunes, not five or six; or one-half banana, not a whole banana. If his diet permits four meat exchanges for dinner, he may have 4 oz of steak, not 8 oz as many men prefer. Since the 1000-calorie diet allows no fat exchanges, he would eat his roll or bread without butter, and substitute lemon juice or herbs for the flavoring of vegetables.

Usually the food allowances are divided into three approximately equal meals. Skipping breakfast is not a good idea. Some people prefer to have a midafternoon or bedtime snack, and these may be included by saving some milk or fruit from the meal. Of course, tea or coffee without cream or sugar, and bouillon may also be used.

Meals on a low-calorie diet should be attractive and palatable. Herbs and spices may be used to lend variety to vegetables and meat preparation. Meats, fish, and poultry should be lean, and prepared by broiling, roasting, or stewing. Fresh fruits or canned unsweetened fruits are used. Group A vegetables may be used in salads for variety in texture and flavor, and add bulk to the diet. Low-calorie salad dressings are available commercially or may be prepared at home.

Low-calorie diets would not include alcoholic beverages, sweetened carbonated beverages, cakes, candy, cookies, cream, fried foods, sweetened fruits, pastries, pies, potato chips, pretzels, puddings and so on. One needs to be especially conscious of the little extras not included in the diet such as a teaspoon of butter, a tablespoon of cream, or a little gravy. Of course, even occasionally eating a piece of pie or cake will wreck the efforts that may have been made toward dieting all day!

A sample menu for a 1200-calorie diet is shown in Table 21–2.

FAD DIETS

People who are overweight do not always remember that they did not become so in just a few days, and yet they often expect to return to normal weight in a short time. They are frequently misled by advertising as well as articles in magazines or newspapers that promise spectacular losses in a few days; for example, "Lose 9 pounds in 9 days." Some fad diets do not supply the protein, minerals, and vitamins needed by the person who is reducing. As a result, such diets lead to weakness and ill health if they are used for a long time. Other fad diets are based upon bizarre food combinations or unusual proportions of carbohydrate, fat, and protein. No specific food or combination of foods has any special ability to increase the rate of weight loss, nor does the proportion of carbohydrate to fat or protein make any difference. Among the fad diets that come and go and that are not recommended are the nine-day diet; drinking man's diet; "Air Force" diet (the U.S. Air Force did *not* recommend this diet); the egg diet (also known as the "Mayo diet" although the Mayo Clinic did *not* subscribe to it); banana–skim milk diet; grapefruit diet; grape juice diet; meat and fat diet.

Formula diets are widely used, and people often ask about their value. Unlike most fad diets the formulas include all the nutritional essentials; they are convenient to use; and they take away the problems of dietary planning. An important disadvantage is that they do not retrain the individual to a new pattern of eating once the weight has been lost. If used exclusively, the formula diets provide little bulk, and constipation may be a problem. Formula diets are probably most useful for individuals who substitute them for one or two meals a day and who need to lose only a few pounds.

Reducing candies and pills of various kinds have no place in the reducing program. They are a waste of money and may be dangerous. Some pills cause diarrhea and increased excretion of water by the kidney—a temporary weight loss that is soon replaced; it is fat, not water, that one should lose. Other pills lead to overactivity of the thyroid, increase in metabolism, and increase in heart rate; the results could be disastrous. Obesity is rarely caused by endocrine disturbances.

TABLE 21–2 SAMPLE MENUS FOR LOW- AND HIGH-CALORIE DIETS

1200-Calorie Diet	High-Calorie Diet (3000–3200 calories)
Breakfast	
Half grapefruit	Half grapefruit
Soft cooked egg—1	Dry cereal—1 cup
Toast—1 slice	Milk, whole—1 cup
Butter—1 teaspoon	Soft cooked egg—1
Coffee—no cream or sugar	Toast—1 slice
	Butter—2 teaspoons
	Sugar for cereal and coffee—2 teaspoons
	Cream for coffee—2 tablespoons
	Coffee
Luncheon	
Salad plate:	Cream of mushroom soup—1 cup
Whole tomato stuffed with	Saltines—2
Tuna fish—2 oz	Salad plate:
Diced celery	Whole tomato stuffed with
French dressing—1 tablespoon	Tuna fish—2 oz
Lettuce	Diced celery
Sliced hard-cooked egg	French dressing—1 tablespoon
Muffin, plain—1	Lettuce
Milk, skim—1 cup	Sliced hard-cooked egg
Plums, unsweetened—2	Muffin, plain—1
	Butter—2 teaspoons
	Jelly—1 tablespoon
	Milk, whole—1 cup
	Plums in syrup—3
	Sugar cookie—1
Dinner	
Roast leg of lamb, lean—4 oz	Roast leg of lamb, lean—4 oz
Broccoli with lemon	Mashed potato—⅔ cup
Carrots	Broccoli, buttered
Milk, skim—1 cup	Dinner roll—1
Tea with lemon	Butter, on vegetables and for roll—2 pats
	Milk, whole—1 cup
	Cherry pie
Bedtime	
Apple—1 small	Milk, whole—1 cup
Cheese—1 oz	Chicken sandwich:
	Bread—2 slices
	Mayonnaise—1 teaspoon
	Butter—1 pat
	Chicken—1½ oz

Diet for Underweight

INDICATIONS FOR HIGH-CALORIE DIET

Long illness not infrequently leads to much weight loss because of nausea, lack of appetite, and inability to eat. In some individuals vomiting and diarrhea may lead to failure to absorb all nutrients, so that weight loss and undernutrition become severe. Moreover, the individual with an upset gastrointestinal tract is often so uncomfortable that he is reluctant to eat.

Other patients with a high fever lose much weight, because each degree Fahrenheit rise in body temperature increases the rate of metabolism by about 7 per cent. Thus a temperature of 102° or 103° would considerably increase the calorie needs. Occasionally, an individual has a very high metabolic rate because of an overactive thyroid. Although hyperthyroidism is usually treated by drugs or surgery, many individuals have lost much weight before they sought medical advice.

THE HIGH-CALORIE DIET

About 500 calories daily above the normal caloric requirements are needed in order to gain 1 lb per week. Ordinarily, a 3000- to 3500-calorie diet is considered to be high in calories for the adult. In some cases of marked weight loss and greatly increased metabolism, 4000 to 4500 calories are indicated. A sample menu for a high-calorie diet is shown in Table 21–2. Note that the menu items used in the low- and high-calorie diets were, for the most part, the same. The increase in calories was brought about by substituting a high-calorie dessert and adding butter, sugar, jelly, bread, soup, and so on.

Weight loss is often accompanied by loss of protein tissue as well as fat tissue. Therefore it is necessary to provide a liberal protein allowance— usually 100 gm per day. When the undernutrition is severe, the physician may prescribe mineral and vitamin supplements.

Weight gain for some people is just as difficult as weight loss is for others. Usually the person who requires a 3000-calorie diet will be found to be consuming only half as many calories. To suddenly place before him a tray loaded with food can only result in further loss of appetite and reluctance to eat. The high-calorie diet, then, must begin with the patient's present intake. Perhaps some changes are first made to a menu selection that is somewhat higher in calories but that does not contain much extra bulk. The increase in the amount of food is usually achieved gradually.

All the following foods rapidly increase the calorie content of the diet:

light or coffee cream on fruit or on cereal, sour cream for baked potato or in salad dressings, whipping cream, half milk and half cream, ice cream; butter, margarine, mayonnaise, and other salad dressings; jelly, jam, marmalade, honey, sugar, candy; cake, cookies, puddings, pie, and pastry.

Many persons find an excess of fats or sugars to be nauseating, so it is important that the above foods be used with care. On the other hand, one should avoid filling up the patient on too many bulky low-calorie foods, such as vegetables and fruits.

Three meals a day plus a bedtime snack are, as a rule, preferable to three meals plus midmorning and midafternoon feedings. Often the between-meal feedings take the edge off the appetite, so that the meals are less well eaten. However, such quickly digested and absorbed foods as fruit juice with crackers and cookies may increase the calorie intake without interfering with the appetite. Three examples of calorie-rich bedtime snacks are:

Chicken salad sandwich	Chocolate milk shake	Strawberry ice cream
Milk	Plain sugar cookies	Angel food cake

The high-calorie diet may need to be modified in consistency. For example, some postoperative patients might require a high-calorie fluid or soft diet. Usually patients who have a chronic diarrhea, as in ulcerative colitis, require a high-calorie soft diet. (See Chap. 19.)

REVIEW QUESTIONS AND PROBLEMS

1. What are the effects of obesity on health?

2. A patient is 25 lb overweight. If he needs 1800 calories a day but eats a diet that provides 1200 calories a day, how long would it take him to lose this weight?

3. List eight factors in the American way of life that make it easy to gain weight.

4. Plan menus for three days for a man on a 1500-calorie diet, using the food allowances in Table 21–1.

5. Visit a supermarket and make a list of five types of products that are claimed to be low in calories. Read the label information. What conclusions do you reach?

6. If a person eats all his meals in a restaurant, what are some suggestions you could give him so that he does not gain weight?

7. Plan five bedtime snacks for a person who is trying to gain weight. Be certain that these snacks also provide a good supply of nutrients.

8. Discuss ways by which you might improve the food intake of a patient who has a very poor appetite and for whom a high-calorie diet has been ordered.

REFERENCES

Choose Your Calories by the Company They Keep. Chicago: National Dairy Council, 1966.

Leverton, R. M. *Food Becomes You,* 3rd ed. Ames, Iowa: Iowa State University Press, 1965, Chaps. 6 and 7.

Mayer, J. "Obesity Control," *Amer. J. Nurs.,* **65**:112, June 1965.

Obesity and Health. U.S. Public Health Service, Pub. No. 1485, Washington, D.C.: Department of Health, Education and Welfare, 1966.

Page, L., and Fincher, L. J. *Food and Your Weight.* Home and Garden Bull. 74. Washington, D.C.: U.S. Department of Agriculture, 1964.

Rosenberg, B. A., *et al.* "Three Views of the Treatment and Hazards of Obesity," *J. Amer. Med. Ass.,* **186**:45, 1963.

Step Lively and Control Weight. Leaflet. Chicago: The American Dietetic Association.

Trulson, M. F., and Stare, F. J. "The Great Balancing Act: Eating vs. Activity," *Today's Health,* **41**:35, June 1963.

Young, C. M. "Planning the Low Caloric Diet," *Amer. J. Clin. Nutr.,* **8**:896, 1960.

MODIFICATIONS FOR CARBOHYDRATE, PROTEIN, AND FAT: THE DIABETIC DIET

Diabetes Mellitus

NATURE

Diabetes mellitus is a metabolic disease that affects the endocrine system of the body and the use of carbohydrate and fat. Specifically, there is not enough insulin available for the body's needs. In some patients the islands of Langerhans of the pancreas are unable to produce enough insulin; in others the pancreas requires some stimulation to manufacture enough insulin; and in still others the insulin that is produced cannot, for some reason, be used by the tissues.

Because glucose cannot be used, the level in the blood rises (hyperglycemia) until finally some of it is excreted in the urine (glycosuria). To excrete sugar, water is taken from the tissues. Thus the patient complains of frequent urination (polyuria) and increased thirst (polydipsia). The appetite is often increased (polyphagia), because the patient is not fully using the food he normally eats. He may also lose weight.

When the body is unable to use carbohydrate, it oxidizes more and more fat to supply energy. The liver breaks down the fatty acids to ketones (acetone, beta-hydroxy-butyric acid, acetoacetic acid). Normally, the ketones are further broken down to yield energy and the end products carbon dioxide and water. However, in diabetes the breakdown of fatty acids is more rapid than the body can care for. The ketones are acid products. When they accumulate in the blood the pH of the blood is lowered; the patient then has symptoms of acidosis or diabetic coma.

Two types of diabetes are recognized. *Juvenile* diabetes occurs at any age from birth through adolescence. It is severe, requires insulin for treatment, and is difficult to manage. Some adults who have so-called *brittle* diabetes are also hard to control; they fluctuate widely between diabetic acidosis and insulin shock.

Adult-type diabetes occurs primarily in obese people who first become diabetic in middle age. The disease is usually mild, stable, and well regulated by diet alone or by diet and oral compounds.

INCIDENCE

Between 4 and 5 million persons in the United States have diabetes, although almost half are unaware that they are diabetic. People should be urged to have tests made at the annual detection campaigns conducted by the American Diabetes Association. Diabetes occurs at all ages, but it is most common in middle age. More women than men are affected.

Persons who have a family history of diabetes and who are overweight are more likely to have diabetes. Weight control throughout life can do much to delay the onset of diabetes and to keep it in a mild form when it does appear.

LABORATORY TESTS

After a night's fast the blood sugar of a diabetic patient is quite a bit above the normal level of 70 to 90 mg per 100 ml. Some or all of the urine samples give a positive test for sugar, depending upon how high the blood sugar level is. A *glucose tolerance test* is sometimes used to measure how well a patient uses a standard amount of sugar. The procedure is about as follows: (1) a blood sample is taken after a night's fast; (2) a weighed amount of glucose—usually about 50 to 100 gm, depending on body weight—is given in water to the patient; (3) samples of blood and urine are collected at one half, one, two and three hours after drinking the glucose solution; (4) the glucose is determined in each of the blood samples and compared with the response of a normal individual; and (5) each urine sample is tested for sugar. From Figure 22–1 it is seen that the sugar curve for the diabetic patient begins at a higher level and stays higher than the curve for a normal person. The curve comes down slowly for the diabetic person, but sharply for the normal person. The diabetic patient shows some glycosuria; the normal individual does not.

DIET

Each diabetic patient must learn to regulate these aspects of his daily life: (1) diet, (2) activity, (3) insulin or oral compounds, if he needs them, and (4) body hygiene.

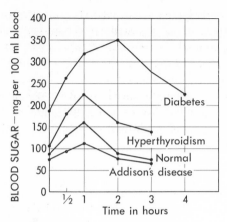

FIGURE 22-1 **The glucose tolerance test shows differences in various disorders of carbohydrate metabolism.**

The amount of diet control required depends upon the severity of the disease and whether the physician recommends strict control or moderate control. Some physicians require that all foods be weighed on a gram scale. At the other extreme is the so-called "free diet," which means that the food is not measured, but the patient learns about the essentials for good nutrition and is told to avoid concentrated sweets.

Most patients are expected to use a measured diet, using the food exchange lists described in Chapter 20. The prescription planned by the physician is based upon the age, sex, weight, body build, activity, severity of diabetes, and the need for insulin or oral compounds. The patient's economic status, time and place for meals, food preparation facilities, and cultural and religious preferences must be considered.

The diet is essentially a normal one, except that the amounts of food and their distribution in meals are controlled from day to day. Some diet control will be necessary for the rest of the patient's life.

Energy. Overweight diabetics are initially placed on low-calorie diets, because weight loss results in better tolerance to carbohydrate. Individuals of normal weight are given sufficient calories to maintain weight:

In bed	11–12 calories per pound
Sedentary	13–14 calories per pound
Moderately active	15–16 calories per pound

Protein. About 1 to 1½ gm protein per kilogram body weight (½ to ⅔ gm per pound) is usually allowed. The higher level is more typical for patients who show a preference for protein-rich foods, as many Americans do.

Carbohydrate and fat. After subtracting the calories provided by protein, the remainder of the calories for the day are usually divided about equally between carbohydrate and fat. The number of grams of fat is ordinarily about the same as the number of grams of protein; the amount of carbohydrate is roughly twice the number of grams of protein.

Carbohydrate distribution. In diabetic diets the physician indicates how the carbohydrate is to be divided between the meals and snacks, if any. The division depends upon whether the patient is taking insulin, the type of insulin used, and the urine sugar tests. For example, the 150 gm of carbohydrate in the calculation of Table 20–1 might be divided as follows:

Breakfast	Lunch	Dinner	Bedtime	
50	50	50		No insulin
25	50	50	25	Small breakfast; long-acting insulin like protamine zinc insulin
41	42	42	25	Long-acting insulin, such as NPH, lente

Diet plans. The American Dietetic Association has developed nine plans for diabetic diets that provide varying levels of calories, carbohydrate, protein, and fat. (See Tables 22–1, 22–2.) These plans are easily adapted to the individual needs of most patients. Plans are available from the Association for diabetic patients who also require bland or sodium-restricted diets.

FOOD PREPARATION AND SERVICE

All foods for the diet are measured according to the amounts in the food exchange lists. Level measures with standard measuring cups and

TABLE 22–1   CALORIC LEVELS OF SAMPLE MEALS FOR DIABETICS *

Meal Plan	Carbohydrate gm	Protein gm	Fat gm	Energy Calories
1	125	60	50	1,200
2	150	70	70	1,500
3	180	80	80	1,800
4	220	90	100	2,200
5 †	180	80	80	1,800
6 †	250	100	130	2,600
7 †	370	140	165	3,500
8	250	115	130	2,600
9	300	120	145	3,000

* Turner, Dorothea: *Handbook of Diet Therapy*, 4th ed. © 1946, 1952, 1959, and 1965 by The University of Chicago.
† Planned particularly for children.

TABLE 22–2 SAMPLE MEAL PLANS FOR DIABETICS *

Diet	Milk	Veg. A	Veg. B	Fruit Exchanges	Bread Exchanges	Meat Exchanges	Fat Exchanges
1	1 pt	As desired	1	3	4	5	1
2	1 pt	As desired	1	3	6	6	4
3	1 pt	As desired	1	3	8	7	5
4	1 pt	As desired	1	4	10	8	8
5 †	1 qt	As desired	1	3	6	5	3
6 †	1 qt	As desired	1	4	10	7	11
7 †	1 qt	As desired	1	6	17	10	15
8	1 pt	As desired	1	4	12	10	12
9	1 pt	As desired	1	4	15	10	15

* Turner, Dorothea: *Handbook of Diety Therapy*, 4th ed. © 1946, 1952, 1959, and 1965 by The University of Chicago.

† These diets contain more milk and are especially suitable for children.

spoons are used. When purchasing meat, for 3 oz of cooked meat allow:

4 oz raw lean meat or fish, if there is no waste;

5 oz raw meat, fish, or poultry, if there is a small amount of bone or fat to be trimmed off;

6 oz raw meat, fish, or poultry, if there is much waste.

Foods are prepared using only those allowed on the meal pattern. No extra flour, bread crumbs, butter, or other foods may be used. Many recipes are available from diabetic cookbooks and can be adapted to the patient's prescription.

Meats may be broiled, baked, roasted, or stewed. If they are fried, some of the fat allowance must be used.

Water-packed fruits (canned without sugar) are available in most food markets and may be used according to the exchange lists. Frozen or canned fruits packed with sugar must be avoided. It is important to read labels carefully. (See Fig. 22–2.)

Special dietetic foods usually have some food value even though they are low in carbohydrate. They seldom need to be used, and they are usually expensive. The patient should consult the physician or dietitian before using such foods, so that any protein or fat in them can be calculated in the diet.

Concentrated sweets and desserts are avoided: sugar, candy, jelly, jam, marmalade, syrup, honey, molasses, soft drinks, cake, cookies, pie, pastry, sweet rolls.

Snacks are permitted only if they are calculated in the diet plan. They are necessary with the long-acting insulins. The patient may have coffee, tea, fat-free broth, unsweetened gelatin, and vegetables from the 2A group at any time, without calculating them.

Each patient's tray is a teaching aid. The patient should be instructed

Dietetic Peaches

Packed in water without added sugar

PROXIMATE ANALYSIS
(including liquid in this can)

Protein	0.6%	Milligrams sodium per	
Fat	0.03%	100 grams	6
Crude fiber	0.4%	Milligrams sodium per	
Ash	0.3%	4 ounce serving	7
Moisture	92%	Calories per 100 grams	31
Available carbohydrate	6.7%	Calories per ounce	9

FIGURE 22–2 Foods intended for therapeutic diets must be labeled with the information concerning their nutritive values.

to become visually accustomed to the size of portions. He should learn to relate the specific foods on his tray to the exchange lists. (See Fig. 22–3.)

As a nurse you should consistently check the patient's tray after each

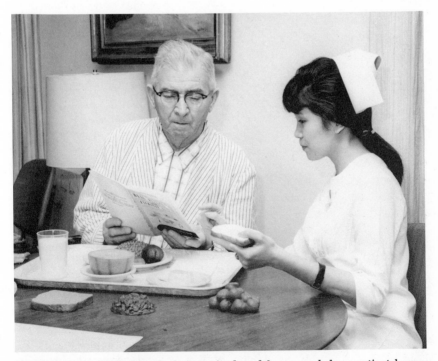

FIGURE 22–3 With the aid of plastic food models a nurse helps a patient become familiar with the Food Exchange Lists in his instruction booklet. (*Courtesy, Thomas Jefferson University Hospital.*)

meal to know how well he is eating. If he is taking insulin and refuses food, an arrangement is made for a substitution so that he will not go into insulin shock.

A typical pattern and sample menu for Diet 3 of the ADA plans is shown in Table 22–3. Note that this pattern provides three meals of approximately equal carbohydrate value plus a bedtime meal.

TABLE 22–3 A TYPICAL MEAL PATTERN AND SAMPLE MENU
FOR DIET No. 3 (C, 180; P, 80; F, 80)

Meal Pattern	Exchanges	Carbohydrate gm	Sample Menu
Breakfast			
Fruit	1	10	Orange, sliced—1 small
Bread	2	30	Dry cereal—¾ cup
			Toast—1 slice
Milk	1	12	Milk—1 cup
Meat	1		Egg, poached—1
Fat	1		Butter—1 teaspoon
		—	Coffee or tea as desired; no
		52	sugar
Luncheon			Packed Lunch
Meat	2		Sandwiches—1½
Bread	3	45	Bread—3 slices
Fat	2		Cheese—1 oz
			Boiled ham—1 oz
			Mayonnaise—1 teaspoon
			Butter—1 teaspoon
			Lettuce
Vegetable A			Whole tomato
Fruit	1	10	Apple—1 small
		—	Coffee or tea, if desired
		55	
Dinner			
Meat	4		Roast beef—4 oz
Vegetable A	1		Tossed green salad
Vegetable B	1	7	Peas—½ cup
Bread	2	30	Potato, baked—1 small
			Roll—1 small
Fat	2		French dressing—1 table-
			spoon
			Butter—1 teaspoon
Fruit	1	10	Strawberries—1 cup fresh
		—	
		47	

Meal Pattern	Exchanges	Carbohydrate gm	Sample Menu
Bedtime			
Milk	1	12	Milk—1 cup
Bread	1	15	Graham crackers—2
		27	

INSULIN AND ORAL COMPOUNDS

Insulin must be given by injection, because it would be digested and made inactive if given by mouth. The amount and kind of insulin are determined by the physician. Most insulins now used are long-acting, which means that one injection a day is usually needed. For some insulins, the action is delayed so that a small breakfast is preferred. There is some danger of insulin reaction during the night. To prevent this, the patient is given a bedtime snack of carbohydrate food, also including some protein. This feeding is calculated as part of the diet. (See Table 22–3.)

Oral agents may be used by adult patients with mild diabetes who cannot be regulated by diet alone. These compounds are not insulin. The sulfonylurea compounds, including tolbutamide (Orinase), chlorpropamide (Diabinese), and acetohexamide (Dymelor), stimulate the pancreas to produce insulin. Another type of preparation, phenformin (DBI), increases the peripheral utilization of glucose in the muscle.

INSULIN SHOCK

Insulin shock is the effect of too much insulin. It may occur because the patient has failed to eat some of his food; he may have increased his activity; or he may have a gastrointestinal upset so that the nutrients are not being normally absorbed.

The symptoms of insulin shock result from the marked lowering of the blood glucose. The patient becomes weak, nervous, pale, and hungry. He trembles, perspires, complains of headache, and may become irrational in behavior as if intoxicated. If he is not given carbohydrate promptly he becomes drowsy, disoriented, and eventually unconscious. Prolonged hypoglycemia is damaging to the brain cells because glucose is the only form of energy used by nervous tissue.

Patients who take insulin should always carry some lump sugar or hard candy in case they feel the signs of a reaction. Orange juice or other fruit juice or tea with sugar may be given to the patient who has signs of insulin shock. When the patient is unconscious glucose is given intravenously.

DIABETIC COMA (DIABETIC ACIDOSIS)

Diabetic coma is caused by inadequate insulin to meet body needs. The patient may have failed to follow his diet, or to take the prescribed insulin, or may have an infection.

When the insulin supply to the body is inadequate, the blood sugar rises and glycosuria occurs. A rapid increase of incompletely metabolized fatty acids in the blood leads to a low blood pH. The patient may complain of thirst, headache, frequent urination, fatigue, and drowsiness. His face becomes red, his skin is hot and dry, and his breath has a sweetish (acetone) odor. Nausea and vomiting sometimes occur. The respirations become rapid and the pulse is fast. Finally, the patient lapses into unconsciousness.

Immediate medical attention is required for the patient who goes into diabetic coma. Treatment includes insulin and fluid therapy.

Other Modifications of Carbohydrate

FUNCTIONAL HYPERINSULINISM

Certain individuals produce too much insulin and have typical symptoms of insulin shock. Eating additional carbohydrate aggravates the condition, because it stimulates the pancreas to produce still more insulin.

The diet is calculated by using the food exchange lists. Carbohydrate is restricted to 75 to 125 gm daily in order to reduce the stimulation of the pancreas. A high-protein intake, 120 gm or more, is prescribed. Fat furnishes the remaining calories. Fat and protein are slowly digested and are more gradually absorbed. Thus they reduce the stimulation of the pancreas.

In planning meals for the typical prescription, the bread exchanges are ordinarily omitted. Milk, vegetable, and fruit exchanges supply the prescribed carbohydrate. The number of meat and fat exchanges is considerably increased. The day's food allowance is divided into three meals of equal size.

ADDISON'S DISEASE

This is a serious disorder of the adrenal gland. The patient excretes excessive amounts of sodium and is unable to excrete potassium. The absorption of carbohydrate is not as good as normal, and the glycogen reserves in the liver are rapidly used up. The blood sugar drops to very low levels.

Today these patients are treated with synthetic adrenal hormone. Their diets must provide liberal carbohydrate, because the hormone does not correct the metabolism of carbohydrate. The diet is high in protein, high in carbohydrate, and high in calories. It is given in three meals, with between-meal feedings in order to avoid hypoglycemia.

REVIEW QUESTIONS AND PROBLEMS

1. What is the cause of diabetes mellitus?

2. What symptoms are seen in patients with diabetes?

3. What tests are used to determine whether an individual has diabetes?

4. A diabetic diet is essentially a normal diet. How does the diet differ from the normal pattern?

5. The menu for a family dinner is beef stew with potatoes, carrots, onions; tossed salad with Russian dressing; rolls and butter; lemon meringue pie; milk. Tell exactly how you would adapt this menu for a patient who is allowed the following exchanges: milk, 1; group B vegetables, 2; fruit, 1; meat, 3; fat, 2.

6. Why is a bedtime feeding ordinarily used for patients who are taking insulin?

7. List ten foods that diabetic patients usually should avoid.

8. Why must insulin be given by injection? What is meant by *oral compound*?

9. What symptoms would lead you to suspect that a patient is having an insulin shock? What would you do?

REFERENCES

Behrman, M. *A Cookbook for Diabetics.* New York: American Diabetes Association, Inc., 1959.

Caso, E. K. "Diabetic Meal Planning—A Good Guide Is Not Enough," *Amer. J. Nurs.*, **62**:76, November 1962.

Coultas, R. "Patients Use Props to Plan Diabetic Menus," *Amer. J. Nurs.*, **63**:104, August 1963.

Diabetes Mellitus—A Guide for Nurses. Public Health Service Publication No. 861. Washington, D.C.: U.S. Department of Health, Education, and Welfare, 1962.

Jay, A. N. "Hypoglycemia," *Amer. J. Nurs.*, **62**:77, January 1962.

Krysan, G. S. "How Do We Teach Four Million Diabetics?" *Amer. J. Nurs.*, **65**:105, November 1965.

Martin, M. M. "Diabetes Mellitus. Current Concepts," *Amer. J. Nurs.*, **66**:510, March 1966.

Martin, M. M. "Insulin Reactions," *Amer. J. Nurs.*, **67**:328, February 1967.

Mason, M. *Basic Medical-Surgical Nursing,* 2nd ed. New York: The Macmillan Company, 1967, Chap. 18.

Moore, M. L. "Diabetes in Children," *Amer. J. Nurs.*, **67**:104, December 1967.

Weller, C. "Oral Hypoglycemic Agents," *Amer. J. Nurs.*, **64**:90, March 1964.

NOMENCLATURE · **High-Protein Diet** | INDICATIONS | PLANNING THE DIET · **Low-Protein Diet** | INDICATIONS | PLANNING THE DIET · **Modification of Protein for Various Metabolic Disorders** | DUMPING SYNDROME | SPRUE | GOUT | PHENYLKETONURIA

PROTEIN MODIFICATION OF THE DIET

NOMENCLATURE

The protein content of the normal diet may be (1) increased to a *high-protein diet,* allowing 100 to 125 gm or more of protein daily; (2) decreased to a *low-protein diet* containing about 40 to 50 gm protein, a *very low-protein diet* providing about 20 gm protein, or a *protein-free diet;* or (3) modified in kinds of protein permitted: for example, *gluten-free diet, low-purine diet,* or *low-phenylalanine diet.*

High-Protein Diet

INDICATIONS

Poor protein nutrition results in loss of body weight, more frequent infections, a slow rate of recovery from illness, poor healing of wounds following injury or surgery, lowered blood serum proteins, and possibly nutritional edema.

A high-protein diet becomes necessary when any one, or a combination, of the following situations exist:

1. Inadequate intake of protein. Some persons fail to ingest enough protein because they do not understand the importance of protein in the diet. Their diets are often high in calories, but inadequate in protein as well as other nutrients. Elderly persons sometimes think they no longer

require protein. Illness may result in poor appetite and dislike for some protein foods, such as meat, eggs, or milk.

Alcoholics fail to get enough protein as well as other nutrients, because alcohol, which takes the place of food, is a source of energy only. Such persons may have cirrhosis of the liver. In this instance the disease is principally a problem of malnutrition. It may be successfully treated with a protein-rich diet.

2. Excessive metabolism of protein. A mild fever, such as found in tuberculosis, results in a slight increase in protein metabolism, whereas a high fever, as in infectious hepatitis (inflammation of the liver), typhoid fever, malaria, or undulant fever, results in a considerable destruction of body protein tissues. The hyperthyroid patient who is not treated with drugs also has a great increase in protein metabolism.

3. Loss of protein from the body. Patients with nephritis may lose small to rather large amounts of protein in the urine. Not infrequently the losses may be 10 to 20 gm daily. Patients with severe burns lose much protein through the oozing that occurs from the skin surfaces. Those who have had injuries or who are recovering from surgery lose protein through drainage from the wound. Any hemorrhage, whether small or large, represents loss of body protein. A slight but persistent hemorrhage into the bowel from an ulcer, colitis, or hemorrhoids, although undetected, may explain the anemia and loss of protein reserves in some patients.

4. Malabsorption of protein. Any disease in which diarrhea is present leads to problems of protein nutrition. Patients with ulcerative colitis and those with sprue are examples. Children with celiac disease, or cystic fibrosis of the pancreas, also have poor absorption of amino acids and all other nutrients.

5. Failure to synthesize proteins. This occurs in liver disease. The liver is responsible for the formation of the serum proteins. The lack of enough albumin is one of several factors leading to edema (ascites) in severe cirrhosis of the liver. The lower fibrinogen level increases the tendency to hemorrhage.

Hemoglobin is synthesized more rapidly when there is ample protein available in the diet. Patients with iron-deficiency anemia require liberal protein intakes as well as iron supplements.

PLANNING THE DIET

As in all therapeutic diets, the high-protein diet begins with the adaptation of the normal diet. In many instances requiring increased protein, the appetite is poor and has often been so for a long time. The patient's present intake should be gradually improved by giving emphasis at each meal to protein-rich foods. Portions given to patients should be such that the patient can eat all foods offered. A bedtime snack is a good way to increase protein and calorie intakes. A midafternoon feeding is possible if it doesn't interfere with the appetite for dinner.

Protein. The diet should be enriched with foods that are concentrated sources of protein. About two thirds of the protein should be provided from animal sources, because the quality is superior. The outline in Table 23–1 shows the food allowances for a diet containing about 125 gm protein. Compare this diet with the 60-gm protein level.

Additional milk is usually included. Nonfat dry milk is the least expensive way to increase the protein content. Depending upon the brand used, 4 to 5 tablespoons added to 8 oz milk will double the amount of protein. Nonfat dry milk may also be added to mashed potatoes, baked custard, cream sauces, cream soups, and other foods. When well liked, larger portions of meat may be used at luncheon or dinner. Perhaps two eggs at breakfast instead of one will be accepted; or egg may be added to milk for an eggnog, to a glass of orange juice, or used in baked custard or pudding. A meat, fish, poultry, cheese, or egg sandwich is a good way to incorporate additional protein. Two examples of protein-rich bedtime snacks are:

Sandwich
  2 slices bread
  2 teaspoons butter, mayonnaise
  1½ oz roast beef
  1 oz cheese
Milk, 1 cup

Protein, 29 gm; calories, 585

High-protein milk shake (tall glass)
  1 cup milk
  5 tablespoons nonfat dry milk
  2 tablespoons chocolate syrup

Protein, 16 gm; calories, 345

Energy. Whenever the protein allowance is increased, the caloric level of the diet must be sufficient to meet the body's energy needs. If the caloric intake is low, protein will be used to provide energy rather than for repairing and building body tissue. For bed patients without fever, 2000 to 2500 calories are sufficient. The diet will need to furnish 2500 to 4000 calories if there is a fever, marked loss of body protein, or poor absorption of food from the intestinal tract.

Minerals and vitamins. The foods added to the diet for protein also increase the intakes of calcium, iron, and the B-complex vitamins. Therefore supplements are required only for patients who have faulty absorption, especially of the fat-soluble vitamins.

Sodium. A 1000-mg sodium restriction is not uncommon in chronic nephritis or in toxemia of pregnancy. This presents no problem in providing sufficient protein. A diet containing as little as 250 mg sodium may be prescribed for patients with severe cirrhosis of the liver and who also have ascites. In order to achieve the liberal protein intake often required, 1 qt low-sodium milk must be used daily; no regular milk is permitted. Eggs would be restricted to one per day.

Texture and flavor. A high-protein diet may be given as a full-fluid, very low-residue, soft, or regular diet. See Chapter 19.

Some patients, such as those with cirrhosis of the liver, hepatitis, colitis, and pernicious anemia, may have a particular distaste and intolerance for fried and fatty foods, spices, hot seasonings, strongly flavored vegetables, and legumes.

TABLE 23–1   FOOD ALLOWANCES FOR DIETS AT LOW-, MODERATE-, AND HIGH-PROTEIN LEVELS *

	Daily Protein in Grams			
	20	40	60	125
Milk, cups	0	½	2	4
Cream, light, cups	½	½	0	0
Lean meat, poultry, fish, or cheese, ounces	0	1	2½	7–9
Eggs	0	1	1	1–3
Vegetables, one raw				
Potato or substitute, servings	2	2	2	1–2
Green leafy or deep-yellow, servings	1	1	1	1
Other, servings	1–2	1–2	1–2	1–2
Fruits				
Citrus, servings	1	1	1	1
Other, fresh, canned, or frozen, servings	2	2	2	1–2
Juice, cups	2	1	0	0
Cereals and breads, enriched or whole-grain, servings	4	5	5	6–7
Butter, margarine, salad dressings, tablespoons	3	3	3	6
Sugar, jelly, jam, tablespoons	7	4	4	4 or more
Daily calories	1990	2025	2020	2500

* Adapted from Robinson, C. H., *Proudfit-Robinson's Normal and Therapeutic Nutrition*, 13th ed. New York: The Macmillan Company, 1967, p. 646.

Low-Protein Diet

INDICATIONS

Protein restriction is essential when the kidney is unable to remove nitrogenous wastes from the blood. This may occur in the terminal stage of nephritis. A protein-free diet is a temporary expedient for a few days when the kidney is not functioning; this diet is followed by a very low-protein diet (20 to 40 gm) and then a moderately low-protein diet (40 to 50 gm) as the patient improves.

TABLE 23–2   TYPICAL MENUS FOR VERY LOW-PROTEIN
AND HIGH-PROTEIN DIETS

Very Low-Protein Diet (20 gm)	*High-Protein Diet (125 gm)*
Breakfast	*Breakfast*
Stewed prunes	Stewed prunes
Cooked rice *with*	Scrambled eggs, 2
Cream, ½ cup	Wheat flakes *with*
Brown sugar	Milk, 1 cup
Toast, enriched, 1 slice	Sugar
Butter	Toast, enriched, 1 slice
Jelly	Butter
Coffee with cream, sugar	Jelly
	Coffee with cream, sugar
Midmorning	
Grape juice with ginger ale, 1 cup	
Luncheon	*Luncheon*
Baked potato with butter	Cold sliced ham, bologna, cheese,
Zucchini squash	3 oz
Lettuce with sliced tomato	Potato salad
Mayonnaise	Lettuce, sliced tomato
Roll	Mayonnaise
Butter, jelly	Roll
Fresh peaches	Butter
Tea with sugar	Fresh peach ice cream
	Cookie
	Milk, 1 cup
	Tea, if desired
Midafternoon	
Orangeade, 1 cup	
Dinner	*Dinner*
Parsley buttered noodles	Swiss steak, 4 oz
French green beans	Parsley buttered noodles
Grapefruit avocado salad on water	French green beans with slivered
cress	almonds
French dressing	Grapefruit avocado salad on water
Dinner roll with butter, jelly	cress
Raspberry ice	French dressing
Tea or coffee with sugar	Dinner roll with butter
	Floating Island
	Milk, 1 cup
	Tea or coffee, if desired
Bedtime	*Bedtime*
Grapefruit juice with glucose, 1 cup	Egg salad sandwich
	Milk, 1 cup

242

Hepatic coma is a condition in which there is too much ammonia in the blood circulation. The brain is especially affected, and the patient becomes tremulous, disoriented, confused, and lapses into coma. The condition sometimes occurs in patients with severe cirrhosis of the liver. In these patients the ammonia from the gastrointestinal tract bypasses the liver and enters the general circulation. The protein metabolism must be drastically reduced in order to correct the high ammonia levels of the blood. The protein-free, very low-protein, and moderately low-protein diets may be used in sequence.

Moderate protein restriction is usually ordered for patients with acute glomerulonephritis.

PLANNING THE DIET

The protein-free diet and very low-protein diets are temporary measures. Because the breakdown of body protein can also lead to undesirable levels of nitrogen constituents in the blood, it is absolutely essential that the caloric intake be as liberal as practical. Even 100 to 200 gm carbohydrate is useful in reducing the breakdown of body protein.

A protein-free diet may be given by using a commercial sugar-fat emulsion.* A butter-sugar "soup" may be prepared by cooking together 2 tablespoons flour, ¾ cup sugar, ¾ cup butter, and 2 cups water. The mixture is flavored with vanilla, chilled, and served as six equal feedings. It provides approximately 1800 calories.

The allowances of foods for the 20-, 40-, and 60-gm protein levels are listed in Table 23–1. A sample menu is given for the 20-gm protein diet in Table 23–2. The protein allowed in each of these diets should be divided as evenly as possible between the three meals so that the tissues will make maximum use of the assortment of amino acids.

Nitrogen balance is usually not maintained at protein levels below 30 gm daily. Protein losses will be minimal if the caloric intake can be kept adequate.

Modification of Protein for Various Metabolic Disorders

DUMPING SYNDROME

Certain patients who have had a gastrectomy complain of nausea, weakness, sweating, and dizziness shortly after meals. Vomiting, diarrhea, and weight loss are common.

The condition is caused by rapid entry of the food material directly

* Ediol (Schenley Laboratories, Inc., New York); Lipomul® (Upjohn Company, Kalamazoo, Mich.).

into the intestinal tract. The large amount of carbohydrate draws water from the blood circulation into the small intestine and thus reduces the circulating blood volume. The sugars are rapidly absorbed into the blood. This causes too much insulin to be produced, and in a short time the blood sugar drops to very low levels. Thus the patient has the symptoms of insulin shock and also the symptoms that accompany reduction of the circulating blood volume.

The diet used for this condition is summarized below.

1. Give small meals every two hours consisting of meat, fish, poultry, eggs, or cheese with butter, margarine, or bacon.

2. As improvement occurs, add one to two small servings of one of these: bread, crackers, cereals, vegetables, and finally unsweetened fruits. Gradually increase the amounts and variety of these foods until the diet approaches a normal pattern.

3. Omit fluids at mealtime; they may be taken after at least 45 minutes have elapsed.

4. Omit very cold foods.

5. Avoid sugar, jelly, jam, syrup, candy, soft drinks, sweetened fruit, gravies, sauces, cakes, cookies, pastries, ice cream, and other sweetened foods.

6. Relax and rest before and after meals.

TYPICAL MENU FOR INITIAL STAGE

Breakfast, Noon, or Evening	*Midmorning, Midafternoon, Bedtime*
2 beef patties, or roast meat, chicken, fish, steaks, chops, or 2 to 3 eggs	3 oz meat, fish, poultry
2 to 3 pats butter or margarine	2 to 3 pats butter or margarine

TYPICAL MENU FOR FIRST PROGRESSION

Breakfast	*Midmorning, Midafternoon, Bedtime*
2 scrambled eggs	2 oz meat, fish, poultry
2 strips bacon	2 pats butter
½ piece toast with butter	2 thin slices bread for sandwich

Luncheon or Dinner

4 oz meat, poultry, or fish
1 small serving green or yellow vegetable
½ slice bread with butter or margarine

SPRUE

Nontropical sprue is a diarrheal condition in which excessive fat is excreted in the stool (steatorrhea). Nitrogen, minerals, and vitamins are also excreted in considerable amounts, so that the individual becomes severely malnourished.

Apparently many of these patients have an intolerance for gluten, a protein found in wheat, rye, oats, and to a lesser extent in barley and buckwheat. They respond well when all foods containing these cereal grains are rigorously omitted from the diet.

The general characteristics of the diet are as follows.

1. A high-protein diet (100 gm or more) is usually necessary. Mineral and vitamin supplements are often prescribed.

2. Cereals and breads containing wheat, rye, or oats must be omitted. Thickened soups, cooked salad dressings, cold cuts, breaded meats, meat loaf, and mixes of all kinds must be avoided. Read labels carefully.

3. Substitute corn and rice cereals. Use breads especially prepared with rice, corn, potato, or soybean flour, or gluten-free wheat starch. Use tapioca, cornstarch, potato starch, or wheat starch (gluten-free) to thicken soups, gravies, puddings.

4. A low-fat, low-fiber diet may be better tolerated during initial stages.

TYPICAL MENU FOR GLUTEN-FREE DIET

Breakfast
Tomato juice
Rice Krispies with milk, sugar
Poached eggs—2
Corn sticks (cornmeal; no wheat flour)
Butter, jelly
Coffee with cream, sugar

Luncheon
Baked breast of chicken (egg-cornflake crust)
Savory rice
Buttered spinach
Celery and carrot sticks
Vanilla tapioca pudding with sliced orange sections
Milk

Dinner
Pot roast of beef *with*
Gravy (thickened with cornstarch)
Parsley potato
Mashed winter squash
Tossed green salad
French dressing
Coffee ice cream
Coffee or tea

Bedtime
Strawberry milk shake

GOUT

Gout is a condition of abnormal purine metabolism. Purines are nitrogen-containing compounds that are broken down in the body to uric acid. Normally uric acid is eliminated in the urine. In gout some of the uric acid is deposited as an insoluble salt in the joints and causes pain, especially in the great toe.

Medications have largely replaced the need for a modified diet in gout. Patients are usually advised to avoid foods that are high in purines: liver, kidney, brains, sweetbreads, heart, sardines, anchovies, broth, bouillon, meat soups, and meat gravies.

Some physicians recommend the omission of all foods moderate in purine content during the acute attacks of gout. Liberal amounts of milk, eggs, and cheese would supply adequate protein in place of the meat, fish, poultry, and legumes normally included. When the acute attacks have subsided, small servings (2 to 3 oz) of meat, fish, and poultry are added three to four times a week.

PHENYLKETONURIA

Phenylketonuria is a defect at birth in which the infant is unable to use the amino acid phenylalanine. Consequently, the phenylalanine level of the blood increases, and this is especially damaging to the brain. An untreated infant will be mentally retarded.

All proteins contain about 5 per cent phenylalanine, which is far too much for the affected infant. Commercial formulas that are low in phenylalanine (Lofenalac) contain the correct amounts of amino acids needed by the infant for growth.

As the patient improves with the low-phenylalanine formula, carefully measured amounts of fruits, fruit juices, cereals, and vegetables are gradually added. The diet is complex and requires rigorous education of the parents or others responsible for feeding the infant. Many printed materials are available for the parents' guidance.

REVIEW QUESTIONS AND PROBLEMS

1. List at least eight conditions for which a high-protein diet is used. Name three conditions that require a low-protein diet. See Table 18–2.

2. What foods could you use to add 25 gm protein to a normal diet?

3. Why is it important to use a liberal carbohydrate and fat intake with a high-protein diet? A low-protein diet?

4. Modify the menu on page 242 for a soft high-protein diet.

5. Modify the menu for a very low-protein diet on page 242 to provide 40 to 50 gm protein.

6. What foods are often omitted on diets for patients with liver disease? Why?

7. Why is an increase in protein required for some patients with kidney disease? Why is it restricted for others?

8. What is hepatic coma? Why is a low-protein diet used?

9. What is meant by a low-purine diet? When is it used? What protein foods are the basis for this diet? Why are others omitted?

10. List the foods in the menu on page 242 that must be omitted for a gluten-free diet. What foods could you substitute?

11. What is meant by the dumping syndrome? What changes are made in the diet?

REFERENCES

Fisher, J. A. "The Dumping Syndrome," *Amer. J. Nurs.*, **58**:1126, 1958.

Hamilton, A. "Good News About Gout," *Today's Health*, **45**:16, December 1967.

Herman, I. F., and Smith, R. T. "Gout and Gouty Arthritis," *Amer. J. Nurs.*, **64**:111, December 1964.

"How to Eat Well on a Gluten-Free Diet," *Today's Health*, **43**:38, October 1965.

Mason, M. A. *Basic Medical-Surgical Nursing*, 2nd ed. New York: The Macmillan Company, 1967, Chaps. 16 and 19.

Pittman, A. C., and Robinson, F. W. "Dietary Management of the 'Dumping' Syndrome," *J. Amer. Diet. Ass.*, **40**:108, 1962.

Robinson, C. H. *Proudfit-Robinson's Normal and Therapeutic Nutrition*, 13th ed. New York: The Macmillan Company, 1967, Chaps. 31, 34, 36, 37, 43.

Umbarger, B. J. "Phenylketonuria. Dietary Treatment," *Amer. J. Nurs.*, **64**:96, January 1964.

FAT-RESTRICTED AND FAT-CONTROLLED DIETS

NOMENCLATURE

Fat-restricted diets are those in which the amount of fat is reduced from approximately 40 per cent of the total calories to 25 per cent of the total calories or less. In a moderately low-fat diet about 25 per cent of the calories are furnished by fat; this is equivalent to 35 to 65 gm fat, depending upon the calorie level. A very low-fat diet furnishes 10 to 15 per cent of the total calories from fat, or about 20 to 25 gm fat.

Fat-controlled diets are those in which the amount and kind of fat are regulated. The amount of fat may vary from 40 gm at 1200 calories to 85 gm when calories are not restricted. On the average, about 35 per cent of the dietary calories are supplied by fat. The polyunsaturated fatty acids are emphasized in the fat-controlled diets and saturated fats are kept at the lowest practical level. In these diets the linoleic acid is at least twice as high as the saturated fatty acids.

Fat-Restricted Diets

INDICATIONS

Gallbladder disease. The gallbladder concentrates and stores the bile, which is manufactured in the liver. When fat is eaten, the gallbladder contracts to force the bile through the common duct into the small intestine, so that the fats can be emulsified and digested.

248

In some individuals the gallbladder may become inflamed because of infection or irritation owing to the accumulation of gallstones. Sometimes the duct to the small intestine becomes obstructed. When fat is eaten and the gallbladder contracts, pain will result.

A reduction in fat intake will reduce the contraction of the gallbladder and thus provide relief for the patient. In acute attacks the very low-fat diet may be necessary, but ordinarily the moderately low-fat diet is satisfactory.

Diseases of the liver. It is no longer believed necessary to restrict the amounts of fat in hepatitis and in cirrhosis of the liver, although discretion is usually exercised in the amounts of fried foods, for example, that might be used. See Chapter 23 for recommended high-protein diet.

Malabsorption. Steatorrhea is the excessive excretion of fat in the feces. Usually the absorption of protein, minerals, and vitamins is also poor. The patient is poorly nourished as a rule and requires a high-calorie, high-protein diet with supplementary vitamins. The specific dietary modifications with respect to fat depend upon the causes of the disease.

Nontropical sprue in adults and celiac disease in children are examples of malabsorption in which nutrition may be seriously impaired. Although the excretion of fat may be excessive, the fault usually lies in the intolerance to gluten rather than to fat. The gluten-free diet described in Chapter 23 is usually successful.

Children with cystic fibrosis of the pancreas excrete large amounts of fat because the enzyme that splits fat in digestion is missing. They are initially placed on diets that are extremely low in fat and high in protein. Patients with pancreatic disease have a marked distaste for fats and poor tolerance for many foods. Pancreatic enzymes are often prescribed to facilitate the digestion of fats when the enzymes are not produced in the body.

DIETARY PLANNING

Food choices. The following foods would be included on a fat-restricted diet:

2 cups skim milk or buttermilk; nonfat dry milk may be used in place of fresh skim milk

3 or more servings vegetables, including at least one deep-green or deep-yellow vegetable

3 or more servings fruit, including at least one serving citrus fruit or other good source of ascorbic acid

4 to 7 servings breads and cereals, depending upon calorie need

6 oz lean meat, poultry, or fish; 3 eggs per week may be substituted for meat (1 egg = 1 oz meat)

Sugars and sweets as desired, and according to calorie need; see Dessert List, Table 24–2

Fats: *very low-fat diet*, none
      moderately low-fat diet, 1 to 2 tablespoons

Foods restricted. For the moderately low-fat diet, as well as the very low-fat diet, the following foods would be omitted:

whole milk, cream, ice cream
whole milk cheeses, fatty meats, fish, and poultry
chocolate, fried foods, gravies, cooking fats, lard
most baked foods: cakes, cookies, doughnuts, pastries, pies, sweet rolls

In addition, the daily intakes of these foods would be limited according to the fat level permitted by the diet:

lean meat, poultry, fish
egg yolk
butter, margarine, salad dressings

Vitamins. The principal sources of vitamin A in fat-restricted diets are deep-yellow and dark-green leafy vegetables and some yellow fruits. Because of their high cholesterol level, organ meats are usually omitted and egg yolks are restricted to about three per week. The absorption of the carotene from vegetables is reduced when the fat intake is low and is especially affected when there is interference with the production or flow of bile. Hence, the physician often prescribes a vitamin A supplement if a very low-fat diet is used for a long time.

Food preparation. Meats require particular attention to keep their fat content as low as possible. The meat selected should be lean rather than marbled with fat. All visible fat must be trimmed off. If the meat is stewed, it may be cooked a day ahead, cooled, and the fat skimmed off the top of the liquid. Meats that are roasted or broiled should be placed on a rack so that the drippings will be removed. If the diet permits no fat, meats, fish, and poultry may be basted with tomato juice, lemon juice, wine, or bouillon.

Vegetables cannot be dressed with butter, margarine, or sauces. Lemon juice, vinegar, and herbs lend variety to cooked vegetables. See flavoring suggestions for vegetables in Chapter 25.

Some patients complain of intolerance to legumes, strongly flavored vegetables, and hot seasonings. It may be necessary to incorporate the modifications suggested for soft and bland diets (see Chap. 19).

Vegetable or fruit salads may be included, but only lemon juice, vinegar, or low-calorie fat-free dressings should be used. Honey, jelly, or preserves may be used on bread instead of butter.

A sample menu for a very low-fat diet is shown in Table 24–3.

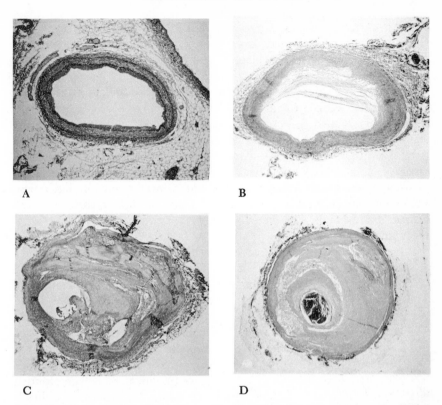

A B

C D

FIGURE 24–1 Gradual development of atherosclerosis in a coronary artery, leading to a heart attack. (A) Normal artery; (B) deposits formed in inner lining of artery; (C) deposits harden; and (D) normal channel is blocked by a blood clot. (*Courtesy, American Heart Association.*)

Fat-Controlled Diets

INDICATIONS

Atherosclerosis (hardening of the arteries) refers to the thickening of the inside walls of the blood vessels. (See Fig. 24–1.) It is caused by the accumulation of fatty materials including a high proportion of cholesterol, as well as other substances. The channel through which the blood flows becomes much narrower. In such a narrow channel a small blood clot can cause sufficient clogging so that no blood can flow through. The tissue that is supplied by such a blood vessel would be unable to receive its nutrients or dispose of its wastes and would die.

Atherosclerosis is the most common cause of heart attacks, also called coronary thrombosis, myocardial infarction, or just "coronary." If a major artery of the heart becomes clogged, death may be immediate. If a lesser artery is clogged, a small part of the heart tissue will be affected, scar tissue will form, and alternate circulation will be established. If an artery supplying the brain becomes clogged, the individual has a stroke or apoplexy.

Those who are most susceptible to atherosclerosis and to heart disease are (1) males between the ages of 45 and 64 years of age; (2) overweight persons; (3) diabetics; (4) those with high blood pressure; (5) those consuming a diet high in saturated fat; (6) those with high blood cholesterol levels; (7) those with a family history of heart and blood vessel disease; (8) sedentary individuals; (9) those who have much tension, frustration, emotional stress, and who must meet many deadlines; and (10) heavy smokers. It is apparent that many of these factors are interrelated; for example, the individual may be overweight because he is sedentary, and so on.

One of the widely held theories concerning diet is that a high intake of saturated fat leads to an increase in the blood of certain types of *lipoproteins* (large molecules containing fat and protein) and cholesterol. The increased blood levels are believed to lead to deposits in the blood vessel walls.

On the other hand, an intake of polyunsaturated fats helps to reduce the blood levels of the undesirable lipoproteins and cholesterol. Thus the objectives of the diet are (1) to reduce the intake of saturated fatty acids to the barest minimum, and (2) to increase the intake of polyunsaturated fatty acids as high as is possible within the calorie limitations. The diet is mostly likely to benefit persons who have a family history of heart disease, who have had a heart attack, or who are overweight.

DIETARY PLANNING

A joint committee of the American Dietetic Association, the American Heart Association, and the United States Public Health Service has developed booklets describing fat-controlled diets at 1200, 1800, and unrestricted calorie levels. A summary of the daily food allowances appears in Table 24-1. The food choices are an adaptation of the Food Exchange Lists used for diabetic diets. Note these points especially as you study the lists in Table 24-2: (1) only skim milk and buttermilk are allowed; (2) all meats, poultry, and fish must be lean; (3) restrictions are placed upon the use of beef, lamb, and pork; and (4) the fat list includes oils high in polyunsaturated fatty acids, with specified amounts of special margarines being allowed. See sample menu for 1800 calories in Table 24-3.

Food preparation. The booklets *Planning Fat-Controlled Meals* published by the American Heart Association include practical suggestions for menu planning, purchase, and preparation of food and for eating in restaurants.

TABLE 24–1 FOOD ALLOWANCE FOR FAT-CONTROLLED DIETS *

Food List		1200 Calories	1800 Calories	2000–2200 Calories	2400–2600 Calories
Milk, skim	Cups	2	2	2	3
Vegetables, at least one green or yellow	Servings	3	3	As desired	As desired
Fruits, one citrus	Servings	3	3	As desired	As desired
Breads and cereals	Servings	4	7	As desired	As desired
Meat, fish, poultry	Ounces, cooked	6	6	6–8	6–8
Eggs		3 per week	3 per week	3 per week	3 per week
Fat	Teaspoons	5	9	9	12
Special margarine	Teaspoons	1	3	3 or more	3 or more
Sugars, sweets	Tablespoons	—	2	As desired	As desired

* *Planning Fat-Controlled Meals for 1200 and 1800 Calories,* Revised. *Planning Fat-Controlled Meals for Approximately 2000–2600 Calories, Revised.* New York: American Heart Association, 1967.

TABLE 24–2 FOOD LISTS FOR FAT-CONTROLLED DIETS *

Foods to Use	Foods to Avoid
Milk list	
Skim milk	Whole milk, homogenized milk, canned milk
Nonfat dry milk	Sweet cream, powdered cream
Buttermilk	Ice cream unless homemade with nonfat dry milk
	Sour cream
	Whole-milk buttermilk and yogurt
	Cheese made from whole milk

Vegetables
See List 2, Table A–2

Fruits
See List 3, Table A–2

Breads, cereals list

Foods to Use	Foods to Avoid
1 slice bread (white, whole-wheat, raisin, rye, pumpernickel, French, Italian, or Boston brown bread)	Commercial biscuits, muffins, corn breads, griddle cakes, waffles, cookies, crackers
1 roll (2 to 3 in. across)	Mixes for biscuits, muffins, and cakes (except angel food)
1 homemade biscuit or muffin (2 to 3 in. across)	Coffee cakes, cakes (except angel food), pies, sweet rolls, doughnuts, and pastries
1 square of homemade corn bread (1½ by 1½ in.)	

TABLE 24–2 FOOD LISTS FOR FAT-CONTROLLED DIETS—*Continued*

Foods to Use	Foods to Avoid

1 griddle cake (4 in. across) made with skim milk and with fat or oil from day's allowance

4 pieces Melba toast (3½ by 1½ by ⅛ in.)

1 piece matzo (5 by 5 in.)

¾ oz bread sticks, rye wafers, or pretzels

1½ cups popcorn (popped at home with fat or oil from day's allowance)

½ cup cooked cereal

¾ cup dry cereal

½ cup cooked rice, grits, hominy, barley, or buckwheat groats

½ cup cooked spaghetti, noodles or macaroni

¼ cup dry bread crumbs

3 tablespoons flour

2½ tablespoons corn meal

½ cup cooked dried peas, beans, lentils, or chickpeas

⅓ cup corn, kernels or cream style

1 ear corn on the cob (4 in. long)

1 small white potato

¼ cup sweet potato, cooked

Meat, fish, and poultry list

Selections from this group for 11 of the 14 main meals

Foods to Use	Foods to Avoid
Poultry without skin: chicken, turkey, Cornish hen, squab	Skin of chicken or turkey
Fish: any kind except shellfish	Duck or goose
Veal: any lean cut	Fish roe; caviar
Meat substitute: cottage cheese (preferably uncreamed), yogurt from partially skimmed milk, dried peas or beans, peanut butter, nuts (especially walnuts)	Fish canned in olive oil
	Shellfish (shrimp, crab, lobster, clams)
	Note: 2 oz may be used *in place of* 1 egg

Selections from this group for 3 of the 14 main meals

Foods to Use	Foods to Avoid
Beef:	Beef high in fat or marbled
Hamburger—ground round or chuck	Lamb high in fat
Roasts, pot roasts, stew meats—sirloin tip, round, rump, chuck, arm	Pork high in fat
Steaks—flank, sirloin, T-bone, porterhouse, tenderloin, round, cube	Bacon, salt pork, spareribs
Soup meats—shank or shin	Frankfurters, sausage, cold cuts
Other—dried chipped beef	Canned meats
Lamb:	Organ meats such as kidney, brain, sweetbreads, liver
Roast or steak—leg	Note: 2 oz liver, sweetbreads, or heart may be substituted for 1 egg
Chops, loin, rib, shoulder	Any visible fat on meat
Pork:	
Roast—loin, center cut ham	
Chops—loin	
Tenderloin	

TABLE 24–2   FOOD LISTS FOR FAT-CONTROLLED DIETS—*Continued*

Foods to Use	*Foods to Avoid*

Ham:
    Baked, center cut steaks, picnic, butt,
      Canadian bacon

Fat list

Corn oil	Butter
Cottonseed oil	Ordinary margarines
Safflower oil	Ordinary solid shortenings
Sesame seed oil	Lard
Soybean oil	Salt pork
Sunflower oil	Chicken fat
Mayonnaise (1 teaspoon mayonnaise equals 1 teaspoon oil)	Coconut oil
	Olive oil
French dressing made with allowed oil (1½ teaspoons dressing equals 1 teaspoon oil)	Chocolate

Sugars and sweets list

White, brown, or maple sugar
Corn syrup or maple syrup
Honey
Molasses
Jelly, jam, or marmalade

Dessert list

Each serving listed is equal to
    1 tablespoon sugar—about 50 calories.
    All except sugar cookies are fat-free

¼ cup tapioca or cornstarch pudding made with fruit and fruit juice or with skim milk from milk allowance	Puddings, custards, and ice creams unless homemade with skim milk or nonfat dry milk
¼ cup fruit whip (prune, apricot)	Whipped-cream desserts
⅓ cup gelatin dessert	Cookies unless homemade with allowed fat or oil
¼ cup sherbet (preferably water ice)	
⅓ cup canned or frozen fruit (sweetened fruit equals 1 portion fruit and 1 tablespoon sugar)	
1 small slice angel food cake	
2 sugar cookies made with oil from day's allowance	
3 cornflake or nut meringues	
¾ cup sweetened carbonated beverage	
⅔ cup cocoa (not chocolate) made with skim milk from milk allowance	
Candies: 3 medium or 14 small gum drops; 3 marshallows; 4 hard fruit drops; or 2 mint patties (not chocolate)	

Miscellaneous (use as desired)

Coffee, tea, coffee substitutes	Sauces and gravies unless made with allowed fat or oil or made from skimmed stock
Unsweetened carbonated beverages	
Lemons and lemon juice	

TABLE 24–2   FOOD LISTS FOR FAT-CONTROLLED DIETS—*Continued*

Foods to Use	Foods to Avoid
Egg white	Commercially fried foods such as potato
Unsweetened gelatin	chips, French fried potatoes, fried fish
Artificial sweeteners	Creamed soups and other creamed dishes
Fat-free consommé or bouillon	Frozen or packaged dinners
Pickles, relishes, catsup	Olives
Vinegar, mustard, seasonings	Macadamia nuts
	Avocado
	Chocolate
	Candies made with chocolate, butter, cream, or coconut
	Coconut
	Foods made with egg yolk unless counted as part of allowance
	Fudge, chocolate
	Commercial popcorn
	Substitutes for coffee cream

* Adapted from *Planning Fat-Controlled Meals for 1200 and 1800 Calories*, Revised. New York: American Heart Association, 1966.

TABLE 24–3   SAMPLE MENUS FOR TWO TYPES OF MODIFIED FAT DIETS

Very Low-Fat Diet (Calories Unrestricted)	Fat-Controlled Diet (1800 calories)
Breakfast	*Breakfast*
Stewed apricots	Honeydew melon—1 slice
Cooked cereal	Dry cereal—¾ cup
Sugar	Sugar—1 teaspoon
Toast	Whole-wheat toast—2 slices
Jelly	Special margarine—2 teaspoons
Skim milk	Jelly—2 teaspoons
Coffee, if desired	Skim milk—1 cup
Luncheon	*Luncheon*
Salad:	Sandwich:
Cottage cheese—½ cup	Rye bread—2 slices
Peach halves, canned	Sliced turkey—2 oz
Escarole	Mayonnaise—2 teaspoons
Rolls, soft	Cabbage–green pepper salad—½ cup
Jelly	Mayonnaise—1 tablespoon
Raspberry sherbet	Banana—1 small
Angel food cake	Skim milk—1 cup
Cocoa made with skim milk, sugar, cocoa	

256

Dinner
Grapefruit sections
Roast leg of veal—4 oz
Baked noodles and tomatoes
Asparagus tips
Dinner roll
Jelly
Apple tapioca pudding
Coffee or tea, if desired

Dinner
Broiled flounder—4 oz
  Oil—1 teaspoon
Parslied potato—1 small *with*
  Oil—1 teaspoon
Mixed diced carrots and celery—½ cup
Dinner roll—1
Special margarine—1 teaspoon
Tomato aspic on water cress *with*
  French dressing—1 tablespoon
Angel cake—1 small piece

The discussion on page 250 pertaining to food preparation for fat-restricted diets also applies to the preparation of foods for fat-controlled diets. Because oils are used in the latter diet, some guidance is usually needed for incorporating them into the diet. Some of the fat allowed may be combined with herbs and lemon juice, tomato juice, or vinegar or wine for a *marinade* for meat. The meat is brushed with the oil-herb-juice mixture and allowed to stand in the refrigerator for several hours, turning the meat often and brushing the sides again with the mixture. The liquid is drained off before the meat is broiled or roasted; the liquid is used to baste the meat from time to time.

Other uses for the vegetable oils are the following:

1. Pan-fry meat, chicken, fish, eggs, pancakes.

2. Substitute oil for solid fat in muffin, biscuit, pancake, and waffle recipes.

3. Mix with a pinch of herbs to flavor vegetables; or add to vegetables with a teaspoon or two of water before cooking, cover tightly, and cook until tender but still crisp.

4. Add to mashed potatoes with skim milk.

5. Use in mayonnaise, French dressing, and cooked salad dressings.

6. Use in place of solid fats for making white sauces with skim milk.

7. Use for pie crust and chiffon cakes.

REVIEW QUESTIONS AND PROBLEMS

1. What is the difference between a fat-restricted and a fat-controlled diet?

2. Prepare a list of foods that are high in cholesterol; in saturated fats; in polyunsaturated fatty acids.

3. What is the reason for using a low-fat diet for patients with gallbladder disease? What foods, other than fat, sometimes cause discomfort?

4. What is meant by atherosclerosis? What factors lead to it?

5. What is the effect of saturated fat on the blood cholesterol? Of polyunsaturated fat?

6. Write a menu for a patient restricted to about 25 gm fat and allowing about 1800 calories. What problems might arise in preparing this diet?

7. Why does a physician sometimes prescribe vitamin A for a patient on a very low-fat diet?

8. Keep a record of your own food intake for one day. Modify this food intake so that it would be high in polyunsaturated fatty acids. When is it desirable to change the pattern of diet?

9. In any cookbook look up the recipes for biscuits, buttered vegetables, creamed chicken, pie crust. How could you change these recipes so that they would be suitable for a patient who requires a diet high in polyunsaturated fatty acids?

REFERENCES

American Heart Association publications: Diet and Heart Disease, 1968. Planning Fat-Controlled Meals for 1200 and 1800 Calories, Revised, 1966. Planning Fat-Controlled Meals for 2000 to 2600 Calories, Revised, 1967. Recipes for Fat-Controlled, Low Cholesterol Meals, 1968. Reduce Your Risk of Heart Attack, 1966. The Way to a Man's Heart, 1968.

Brown, H. B., et al. "Design of Practical Fat Controlled Diets. Foods, Fat Composition, and Cholesterol Content," J. Amer. Med. Ass., 196:205, 1966.

Brown, H. B., and Farrand, M. E. "Pitfalls in Constructing a Fat-Controlled Diet," J. Amer. Diet. Ass., 49:303, 1966.

Hashim, S. A. "The Relation of Diet to Atherosclerosis and Infarction," Amer. J. Nurs., 60:348, 1960.

Mason, M. A. Basic Medical-Surgical Nursing, 2nd ed. New York: The Macmillan Company, 1967, Chaps. 9 and 16.

Robinson, C. H. Proudfit-Robinson's Normal and Therapeutic Nutrition, 13th ed. New York: The Macmillan Company, 1967, Chap. 41.

Stamler, J., et al. "Coronary Proneness and Approaches to Preventing Heart Attacks," Amer. J. Nurs., 66:1788, 1966.

Stare, F. J. "Nutritional Suggestions for the Primary Prevention of Coronary Heart Disease," J. Amer. Diet. Ass., 48:88, 1966.

DIETS RESTRICTED IN SODIUM OR POTASSIUM

Sodium-Restricted Diets

NOMENCLATURE

Normally the daily sodium intake is 3 to 7 gm (3000 to 7000 mg). A sodium-restricted diet is limited to a specified amount of sodium, and may range from a mild to severe restriction. Terms such as "salt free," "salt poor," and "low salt" should not be used. Such terms are so indefinite that the patient might well receive a diet with much more sodium than he should have or, perhaps, one with less than he could have.

The levels of sodium restriction described in booklets published by the American Heart Association are:

250 mg sodium, Very Low-Sodium Diet. Used primarily for hospital patients.
500 mg sodium, Strict Low-Sodium Diet. Used primarily for hospital patients.
1000 mg sodium, Moderate Sodium-Restricted Diet. Often used as a maintenance diet for patients at home.
Mild Sodium Restriction. Sodium content of this diet may vary from about 2400 to 4500 mg. This is essentially a normal diet that omits salty foods and the use of salt at the table. This is frequently prescribed as a maintenance diet for patients at home.

259

INDICATIONS

A sodium-restricted diet is used primarily for the prevention, control, or elimination of edema. As pointed out in Chapter 9, sodium occurs chiefly in the extracellular fluid and is important for maintaining water balance. Normal persons promptly excrete excess sodium, no matter how high their dietary intake. In certain conditions sodium cannot be eliminated. Additional water will then be held in the body to keep the sodium concentration of the fluid at a constant level. As a result, swelling of the tissues occurs, and is readily noticeable in the ankles and other body locations.

A level of sodium restriction that prevents or controls edema in some patients will be too high for others. The physician orders the level appropriate for each patient, and may adjust it upward or downward according to the patient's progress. Typical examples are given below, but these are by no means arbitrary rules.

Congestive heart failure. When the heart is unable to maintain adequate circulation to the tissues, *decompensation* is said to have taken place. With the decompensation, the reduced level of circulation allows sodium to accumulate in the tissues. To hold the sodium in solution, fluid also accumulates in the chest cavity and thus interferes with further heart action. In such a condition the physician may prescribe diuretics and a sodium restriction at 500 and occasionally 250 mg. When the edema has been eliminated, a 1000-mg or mild sodium-restricted diet may be used to prevent further fluid accumulation.

Several associated factors must be considered in planning the diet for the patient with congestive failure. Shortness of breath, fatigue, distention of the abdomen, and poor appetite are frequent problems for patients with heart disease. Rest is the chief consideration during the first stages of acute illness. Diet is ordered as the patient improves and is adjusted from day to day, according to individual tolerance.

In order to reduce the work of the heart as much as possible a low-calorie diet (1000 calories or less) is usually ordered. If the patient is obese, the low-calorie diet is continued until a satisfactory weight level is reached. The 1800-calorie diet is a good basis for the patient who returns to activity and who is not overweight.

Acutely ill patients may need to be fed, using soft or even puréed foods that require a minimum of chewing (see 500-mg-sodium, 1000-calorie soft diet, Table 25–2). Five to six small feedings may be given daily to avoid excessive heart action for the digestive process. Legumes, melons, and strongly flavored vegetables, such as onions and cabbage, cause discomfort for many, and are best avoided during the acute stages of illness. (See Fig. 25–1.)

The *Karell diet* sometimes ordered for cardiac patients originated almost a century ago. It consists of four feedings of 7 oz of milk given at

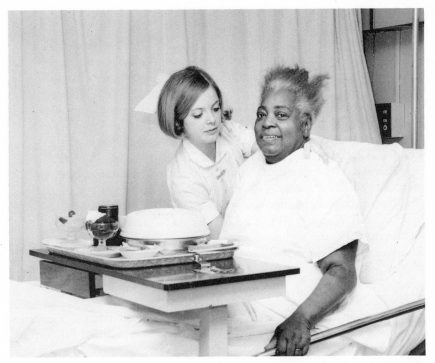

FIGURE 25–1 By adjusting the patient's position, the nurse helps to reduce the energy the patient must exert in eating her meal. (*Courtesy Thomas Jefferson University Hospital.*)

four-hourly intervals. This simple regimen furnishes 680 calories and 480 mg sodium. As the patient improves, toast, eggs, fruit, and cream soups may be added.

Hypertension. Many physicians recommend some restriction of sodium for patients with hypertension. Some years ago the 250-mg-sodium diet was used frequently. However, the severe restriction required very careful adherence to a diet that is difficult for some patients to understand, and is, moreover, quite unpalatable. Effective medications for hypertension have made such severe restrictions unnecessary for most patients. A mild restriction of sodium, and occasionally a 1000-mg-sodium diet may be ordered.

Hypertensive patients may be overweight and thus any restriction in sodium might be incorporated into a 1000-to-1200-calorie diet. The role of fat in the diet has been discussed in Chapter 24.

Renal diseases. When edema is present in nephritis or nephrosis, a sodium restriction at 1000 mg is usually satisfactory. Once the edema fluid has disappeared, many patients can be maintained with a mild sodium restriction.

In renal failure a careful balance must be maintained between the sodium, potassium, and protein intake and the body's ability to eliminate the wastes. See Potassium-Restricted Diets in the section following.

Diseases of the liver. In severe cirrhosis of the liver a serious complication may be ascites (fluid in the abdomen). Diets restricted to 250 mg sodium may be prescribed in an effort to control the edema.

Patients with cirrhosis of the liver are often depleted of protein. A protein intake of 100 gm at a sodium level of 250 mg is possible when low-sodium milk is substituted for regular milk in the 500-mg-sodium, 1800-calorie diet plan (see Table 25–1). In this plan 8 oz of meat and 4 cups low-sodium milk would be included.

Toxemias of pregnancy. Some pregnant women retain sodium and water as shown by swelling of the ankles. A 1000-mg-sodium diet will usually control this condition.

Hormone therapy. When ACTH or cortisone is used for conditions such as arthritis, the additional hormones may lead to sodium and water retention. A 1000-mg or mild sodium-restricted diet is usually satisfactory.

SOURCES OF SODIUM

The principal source of sodium in the diet is salt used (1) in numerous ways in food processing; for example, bacon, sauerkraut, dried fish, canned vegetables and meats, and many others; (2) in baking or cooking of foods; and (3) at the table. Salt is about 40 per cent sodium. Thus a teaspoon of salt that weighs about 6 gm would provide 2400 mg sodium. If a recipe requires one teaspoon salt and serves six people, you can see that one serving of that food alone would give 400 mg sodium from the addition of the salt.

All living things, plants as well as animals, require some sodium. Hence one would expect to find some sodium in foods as they naturally occur before they are processed by the manufacturer or cooked in the home. Animal foods are relatively high in sodium, and plant foods, with few exceptions, are low. You will note that 2 cups of milk alone provide almost half the sodium in the calculation of the 500-mg-sodium, 1800-calorie diet (see Table 25–1). Meat, fish, and poultry are naturally high in sodium, and their amounts must be controlled on all levels except the mild sodium restriction. Shellfish are higher than meat and poultry and are therefore avoided. Eggs are also high in sodium, one egg containing about 65 mg. Most of the sodium is in the white, so it is possible to omit the white in some preparations and to use only the yolk.

Most vegetables are low in sodium, but several, such as beets and spinach, are "salt-loving" in their growth, and therefore contain too much sodium except for diets permitting 1000 mg or more per day.

Fruits, unsalted cereals, unsalted bread, unsalted butter, and sugar contain small amounts of sodium or none at all, and may be used without restriction as far as sodium is concerned.

Numerous compounds containing sodium are used by the manufacturer or in home preparation to improve the flavor or texture of foods. Among the more common ones are:

Baking powder   Sodium benzoate
Baking soda   Sodium citrate
Monosodium glutamate   Sodium propionate
Sodium acetate   Sodium sulfite
Sodium alginate

It is not important that you know why each of these compounds is added to foods. But it is essential that you form the habit of looking for the words *sodium*, *salt*, and *soda* on any label (see Fig. 25–2). However,

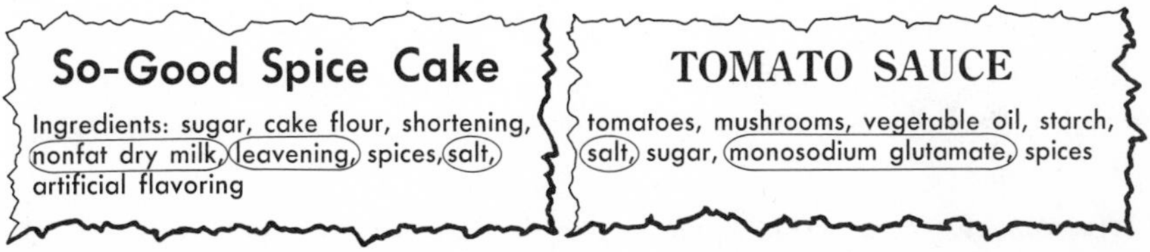

So-Good Spice Cake

Ingredients: sugar, cake flour, shortening, nonfat dry milk, leavening, spices, salt, artificial flavoring

TOMATO SAUCE

tomatoes, mushrooms, vegetable oil, starch, salt, sugar, monosodium glutamate, spices

FIGURE 25–2 Watch for the words "salt" and "sodium" when selecting foods for sodium-restricted diets. Leavenings and nonfat dry milk also contribute much sodium.

the label provides no information for such foods as mayonnaise and catsup, which are standardized according to the regulations of the Food and Drug Administration.

Some drinking waters are high in sodium, especially if water softeners are used. Many drugs contain sodium. The patient needs to be warned against self-medication with baking soda or various antacids.

FOOD SELECTION

The Food Exchange Lists (see Table A–2 in the Appendix) have been adapted by the American Heart Association in its booklets for the sodium-restricted diet. All foods used for these diets must be processed and prepared without salt or other sodium compounds. Canned foods, for example, must be eliminated if they contain salt; canned fruits would be the only exception. Many low-sodium dietetic canned foods are suitable if the labeling indicates that they are no higher in sodium than the fresh product.

The table of exchange lists in the Appendix may be used for calculating diets, provided that the following foods within each list are avoided.

List 1, Milk and related products: avoid buttermilk, soda fountain beverages, ice cream, ice milk, sherbet

List 2, Vegetables: avoid beet greens, beets, carrots, celery, chard, dandelion greens, kale, mustard greens, sauerkraut, spinach, white turnips; any canned vegetables unless canned without salt; frozen peas, if salted

List 3, Fruits: avoid dried fruit if treated with sodium sulfite; maraschino cherries; glazed fruit

List 4, Breads and cereals: avoid any products containing salt, baking powder, or baking soda; regular yeast breads, muffins, rolls; all dry breakfast cereals except puffed wheat, puffed rice, and shredded wheat; quick breads, muffins, pancakes, waffles; quick bread, biscuit, muffin, pancake, waffle mixes; self-rising flour; pretzels; popcorn; potato chips; canned baked beans, corn, or Lima beans; frozen Lima beans

List 5, Meat: avoid fresh or canned shellfish, including clams, crabs, lobsters, oysters, scallops, shrimp; all kinds of cheese; canned, dried, or smoked meat, such as bologna, chipped or corned beef, frankfurters, ham, kosher meat, luncheon meat, sausage, smoked tongue; frozen fish fillets; canned, salted, or smoked fish, including anchovies, caviar, salted and dried cod, herring, sardines; canned salmon, tuna; and peanut butter, except low-sodium

List 6, Fats: avoid salted butter or margarine; bacon and bacon fat; salt pork; olives; commercial French dressing, mayonnaise, or salad dressing; salted nuts

Miscellaneous foods: avoid bouillon cubes, commercial candies, catsup, celery salt, chili sauce, garlic salt, sweetened gelatin mixes, meat and steak sauces, prepared horseradish, prepared mustard, monosodium glutamate, onion salt, pickles, pudding mixes, relishes, soy sauce

DIETARY PLANS

The selection of foods for three calorie levels of a 500-mg-sodium diet is shown below. The calculations for sodium in the 1800-calorie diet are based on average values assigned to each food list.

TABLE 25–1   500-MG-SODIUM DIET AT THREE CALORIE LEVELS

Food List	1000 Calories Exchanges	1200 Calories Exchanges	1800 Calories Exchanges	Sodium (mg)
1. Milk	2 skim	2 skim	2 whole	240
2. Vegetables, A group	1–2	1–2	1–2	18
B group	1	1	1	9
3. Fruit	3	3	3	6
4. Bread	4	4	6	30
5. Meat (only 1 egg daily)	6	6	7	175
6. Fat	0	4	6	—
Sugars and sweets	0	0	7 teaspoons	
				478

250 mg sodium: substitute low-sodium milk for regular milk.

1000 mg sodium: measure ¼ teaspoon salt into shaker and use on food during the day; *or* use 2 slices regular bread and 2 teaspoons regular butter in place of 2 slices unsalted bread and 2 teaspoons unsalted butter.

Mild sodium restriction: food may be lightly salted in cooking. Use regular bread and butter. Omit salt at the table. Omit salty foods, such as potato chips, pretzels, pickles, relishes, meat sauces, salty meats, fish and so on.

Unrestricted calories: provide additional calories from fruits, unsalted breads and cereals, unsalted fats, sugars and sweets.

TABLE 25–2 TWO SAMPLE MENUS FOR THE 500-MG-SODIUM DIET

1000-Calories Soft Diet *(No salt used in cooking)*	*1800-Calorie Regular Diet* *(No salt used in cooking)*
Breakfast	*Breakfast*
Orange sections	Orange sections
Puffed rice	Shredded wheat
Skim milk—½ cup	Milk, whole—1 cup
No sugar	Sugar—2 teaspoons
Poached egg—1 *on*	Soft cooked egg—1
Toast, unsalted—1 slice	Toast, unsalted—1 slice
No butter	Butter, unsalted—1 teaspoon
Luncheon	*Luncheon*
Sliced tender chicken (ground, if necessary)—2 oz	Salad bowl:
Asparagus tips with lemon wedge	Lettuce, endive, escarole, raw cauliflower, green pepper, tomato wedges
Roll, unsalted, soft—1	Sliced chicken strips—2 oz
No butter	French dressing, unsalted—1 tablespoon
Peaches, unsweetened, canned—2 halves	Roll, unsalted—1
Milk, skim—1 cup	Butter, unsalted—1 teaspoon
	Marmalade—2 teaspoons
	Milk, whole—1 cup
	Peaches, fresh, sliced
Dinner	*Dinner*
Tender roast beef (ground, if necessary)—3 oz	Roast beef—4 oz
	with currant jelly—1 tablespoon
Baked potato without skin—1 small	Potato, baked—1 medium
Peas, canned, unsalted	with chive butter—2 teaspoons
Milk, skim—½ cup	Fresh peas with mushrooms
Banana—½	Roll, unsalted—1
	Butter, unsalted—1 teaspoon
	Tokay grapes
NOTE: Fruit and milk may be given between meals if desired.	

PREPARATION OF FOOD

Patients who have always used much salt at the table are likely to complain bitterly about the flat taste of the food. Others, who prefer foods only lightly salted, find the diet to be more tolerable. In time most patients find that they can adjust to the restriction of sodium by learning to substitute other flavorings. Salt substitutes are useful to some. Because these compounds may be harmful to patients with damaged kidneys, they should be used only with a physician's prescription.

Many flavoring extracts, spices, and herbs may be used to lend interest to the diet. Usually a dash of spices or a small pinch of herbs is sufficient for most family-size recipes. The flavor should be delicate and subtle rather than strong and overpowering. Meats may be marinated in wine, vinegar, low-sodium French dressing, or sprinkled with lemon juice before cooking. A few suggestions for flavor combinations are provided below.*

MEAT, POULTRY, FISH, EGGS

Beef: bay leaf, lemon juice, marjoram, dry mustard, mushrooms, nutmeg, onion, green pepper, pepper, sage, thyme; currant or grape jelly

Chicken or turkey: basil, bay leaf, lemon juice, marjoram, onion, pepper, rosemary, sage, sesame seeds, thyme; cranberry sauce

Lamb: curry, garlic, mint, onion, oregano, parsley, rosemary, thyme; mint jelly, broiled pineapple

Pork: garlic, lemon juice, marjoram, sage; applesauce, spiced apples, cranberries

Veal: bay leaf, curry, dill seed, ginger, marjoram, oregano, summer savory; currant jelly; broiled apricots or peaches

Fish: bay leaf, curry, dill, garlic, lemon juice, mushrooms, mustard, onion, paprika, pepper

Eggs: basil, chives, curry, mustard, parsley, green pepper, rosemary, diced tomato

VEGETABLES

Add a dash of sugar while cooking vegetables to bring out flavor.

Asparagus: lemon juice, caraway; unsalted chopped nuts

Green beans: dill, lemon, marjoram, nutmeg, onion, rosemary; slivered almonds

Broccoli: lemon juice, oregano, tarragon

Corn: chives, parsley, green pepper, pimento, tomato

Peas: mint, mushroom, onion, parsley, green pepper

Potatoes: chives, mace, onion, parsley, green pepper

Squash: basil, ginger, mace, onion, oregano

Sweet potatoes: cinnamon, nutmeg; brown sugar

Tomatoes: basil, marjoram, oregano, parsley, sage

* Robinson, C. H., *Proudfit-Robinson's Normal and Therapeutic Nutrition*, 13th ed. The Macmillan Company, New York, 1967, pp. 759, 760.

Homemade quick breads, biscuits, and muffins may be made by using low-sodium baking powder instead of regular baking power. For each teaspoon of regular baking powder, it is necessary to use 1½ teaspoons low-sodium baking powder. The salt specified in the recipe should be omitted.

Homemade bread, waffles, and rolls may be made by using yeast and omitting the salt from the recipe. The yeast dough may be rolled out, spread with unsalted butter, and sprinkled with sugar and cinnamon for delicious cinnamon rolls.

The booklets prepared by the American Heart Association contain menu suggestions and helpful hints in the preparation of food, as well as guides for eating out.

Potassium-Restricted Diets

INDICATIONS

In severe renal damage potassium, nitrogenous wastes and sometimes sodium cannot be excreted satisfactorily. The use of very low-protein diets has been described in Chapter 23; these may be used for short periods of time. However, for patients who are maintained for longer periods of time, it is essential to regulate the potassium, protein, and sodium intakes at levels that prevent accumulation in the body. This regulation is also required for patients who are being maintained with an artificial kidney.

The breakdown of body tissues must be avoided because the potassium released by tissue catabolism would be just as harmful as an excess in the diet. If the calorie intake is adequate, a protein intake of approximately 40 gm will usually maintain nitrogen balance. Such a diet would supply about 1500 mg potassium daily; lower levels of potassium would be difficult to maintain without also lowering the protein. The sodium level may be adjusted as necessary, with 500-mg and 1000-mg restrictions being common.

DIETARY PLANNING

Sources of potassium. The normal intake of potassium varies from about 3000 to 8000 mg, being at the higher levels when protein and calorie intakes are also high. Potassium is widely distributed in all protein-rich foods, in vegetables, in whole-grain cereals and breads, and in fruits.

Potassium salts are quite soluble in water. Therefore, when a potassium-restricted diet is required, vegetables, fruits, and meats should be cooked in a relatively large volume of water to extract the potassium. The cooking liquid would not be used. Likewise, the liquid from canned foods would be discarded.

The food choices for a 1500-mg-potassium diet are listed in Table 25–3.

TABLE 25–3 FOOD SELECTION FOR POTASSIUM-RESTRICTED DIET

Foods to Include	Foods to Avoid (high in potassium and/or sodium)
Beverages—carbonated water, ginger ale, Koolade, Pepsi Cola, Royal Crown Cola, root beer, Seven-Up; tea, ⅔ cup daily	*Beverages*—coffee
Breads—low-sodium breads and rolls, white	*Breads*—all salted; cracked wheat, whole-wheat, Ry Krisp; dark rye; whole-wheat crackers
Cereals—cornmeal, farina, hominy grits; Puffed Wheat, Puffed Rice; macaroni, noodles, rice, spaghetti	*Cereals*—bran, bran flakes, Maltex, oatmeal, Ralston, shredded wheat, Wheatena, or other whole-grain cereal
Cheese—cream, low-sodium cottage	*Cheese*—all regular types
Eggs—prepared any way	
Fats—unsalted butter, margarine, cooking fats, oils	*Fats*—any salted
Fruits—canned applesauce, blackberries, blueberries, cherries, fruit cocktail, grapefruit, peaches, pears, pineapple. *Do not use liquid* Fresh apple, blueberries, pear	*Fruits*—all fresh except apple, blueberries, pear. Especially avoid: avocado, apricots, banana, cantaloupe, grapes, orange, plums; all dried fruits
Fruit juices—apple, cranberry, pear, peach, pineapple	*Fruit juices*—grapefruit, orange, prune, tangerine, tomato
Meat—beef, lamb, pork, veal; chicken, turkey; fish	*Meat*—products high in sodium; see page 264
Milk—whole milk, skim milk, nonfat dry milk, sour cream, cream	*Milk*—low-sodium (ion-exchange)
Sweets—plain candy, honey, jam, jelly, sugar	*Sweets*—candy with chocolate or nuts
Vegetables—canned asparagus, beets, green and wax beans, carrots, mushrooms, peas, tomatoes. *Do not use liquid* Fresh cooked cabbage, onions, squash Raw endive, lettuce, tomato	*Vegetables*—all raw except endive, lettuce, and tomato Cooked: Lima beans, beet greens, broccoli, Brussels sprouts, collards, kale, spinach, sweet potatoes, white potatoes; dried beans or peas
Miscellaneous—cornstarch, flour, tapico, vinegar, herbs, spices, flavoring extracts	*Miscellaneous*—broth, bouillon, chocolate, cocoa, molasses

When sodium restriction is also required, as is usually the case, only unsalted foods would be used. See also preceding discussion on sodium-restricted diets.

Daily food allowances. From the preceding discussion it should be apparent that the diet will have the following characteristics: (1) carefully measured quantities of all foods; (2) reduced amounts of milk, meat, poultry, fish, eggs, and cheese; (3) cooked foods rather than raw; (4) low sodium; and (5) restricted fluid content. A number of plans have been developed on the principle of Food Exchange Lists. (See references at the end of this chapter.)

The following food allowances would supply 1800 calories, 60 gm protein, 500 mg sodium, and 1500 mg potassium. A sample menu based upon these food allowances follows.

½ cup milk
½ cup light cream
1 oz cottage cheese, low-sodium
1 egg
3 oz meat, poultry, fish
2 servings vegetables
2 servings fruit and fruit juices
8 servings refined cereals and white breads
2 tablespoons or more fats
2 tablespoons or more sweets
1 cup carbonated beverages
⅔ cup weak tea, if desired

Sample Menu for 1500-mg-Potassium Diet
(all foods prepared without added salt)

Breakfast
Peaches, canned—2 halves
Puffed Rice—1 cup
Cream—½ cup
Poached egg—1
White toast—2 slices
Butter
Blackberry jelly
Tea—5 oz

Luncheon
Casserole:
 Macaroni—½ cup
 Beef, ground—1 oz
 Tomato, canned—⅓ cup
 Butter, unsalted

Green beans, canned—⅓ cup
White roll
Butter
Jelly
Pineapple, canned—2 slices
Cola beverages—8 oz

Dinner
Roast lamb—2 oz
Mint jelly
Noodles—½ cup
Peas, canned—⅓ cup
Lettuce with cottage cheese—1 oz
French dressing
Low-sodium cinnamon roll—1
Butter
Milk—½ cup

REVIEW QUESTIONS AND PROBLEMS

1. In which diseases is edema frequently seen? Why is sodium restriction often prescribed?

2. What is the chief source of sodium in the diet?

3. How do sodium-restricted diets compare with the normal diet in the amounts of sodium contained in them?

4. Classify the following foods as (1) low in sodium; (2) naturally high in sodium; or (3) containing much added salt: oranges, shredded wheat, corn-flakes, peaches, catsup, American cheese, skim milk, sardines, peanut butter, potato chips, sugar, fresh peas, canned apricots, canned tuna fish, roast beef, pickles.

5. For a patient with cardiac failure and edema, what factors would be important in dietary care in addition to sodium restriction?

6. How would you change a 500-mg-sodium diet to 250-mg-sodium? To 1000-mg-sodium?

7. List the foods that often cause discomfort and distention for cardiac patients.

8. How could you make each of the following foods more palatable for a sodium-restricted diet: sweet potatoes, frozen green beans, roast pork, unsalted bread?

9. A patient asks if he may use a salt substitute. What would you tell him?

10. Change the 1800-calorie, 500-mg-sodium diet on page 265 so that it will provide about 1000 mg sodium and sufficient protein and calcium for a pregnant woman.

11. When is a potassium-restricted diet prescribed?

12. What other nutrients are also restricted for low-potassium diets?

13. Why is the liquid from cooked and canned foods usually discarded in the potassium-restricted diet?

14. Write a menu for one day, using the food allowances for the 1500-mg-potassium diet. Check your food choices against the regulations for sodium restriction at 500 mg.

REFERENCES

Bagg, E. W. "Without a Grain of Salt," *Today's Health*, **42**:32, May 1964.
Bailey, G. L., and Sullivan, N. R. "Selected-Protein Diet in Terminal Uremia," *J. Amer. Diet. Ass.*, **52**:125, 1968.
Bakke, J., et al. "Sodium-Restricted Diets for Dialysis Patients," *Hospitals*, **40**:76, March 1, 1966.
de St. Jeor, S. T., et al. "Planning Low-Protein Diets for Use in Chronic Renal Failure," *J. Amer. Diet. Ass.*, **54**:34, 1969.
Jordan, W. L., et al. "Basic Pattern for Controlled Protein, Sodium, and Potassium Diet," *J. Amer. Diet. Ass.*, **50**:137, 1967.

Keller, M., and Segner, E. F. "When Heart and Hands Are Overburdened," *Amer. J. Nurs.*, **62**:92, June 1962.

Mason, M. A. *Basic Medical-Surgical Nursing*, 2nd ed. New York: The Macmillan Company, 1967, Chaps. 9 and 10.

Mitchell, M. C., and Smith, E. J. "Dietary Care of the Patient with Chronic Oliguria," *Amer. J. Clin. Nutr.*, **19**:163, 1966.

Robinson, C. H. *Proudfit-Robinson's Normal and Therapeutic Nutrition*, 13th ed. New York: The Macmillan Company, 1967, Chaps. 42 and 43.

Searight, M. W. "A Low-Sodium Potluck Luncheon," *Nurs. Outlook*, **16**:30, August 1968.

Your 500 Milligram Sodium Diet; Your 1000 Milligram Sodium Diet; Your Mild Sodium-Restricted Diet. New York: American Heart Association, 1958.

APPENDIXES

Appendix A

TABLE A–1 NUTRITIVE VALUES OF THE EDIBLE PART OF FOODS *

	Food, approximate measure, and weight (in grams)			Water	Food energy	Protein	Fat (total lipid)
	MILK, CREAM, CHEESE; RELATED PRODUCTS						
	Milk, cow's:		Grams	Per Cent	Calories	Grams	Grams
1	Fluid, whole (3.5% fat)	1 cup	244	87	160	9	9
2	Fluid, nonfat (skim)	1 cup	246	90	90	9	Trace
3	Buttermilk, cultured, from skim milk	1 cup	246	90	90	9	Trace
4	Evaporated, un- sweetened, undiluted	1 cup	252	74	345	18	20
5	Condensed, sweetened, undiluted	1 cup	306	27	980	25	27
6	Dry, whole	1 cup	103	2	515	27	28
7	Dry, nonfat, instant	1 cup	70	3	250	25	Trace
	Milk, goats':						
8	Fluid, whole	1 cup	244	88	165	8	10
	Cream:						
9	Half-and-half (cream	1 cup	242	80	325	8	28
10	and milk)	1 tablespoon	15	80	20	Trace	2
11	Light, coffee or table	1 cup	240	72	505	7	49
12		1 tablespoon	15	72	30	Trace	3
	Whipping, unwhipped (volume about double when whipped):						
13	Light	1 cup	239	62	715	6	75
14		1 tablespoon	15	62	45	Trace	5
15	Heavy	1 cup	238	57	840	5	89
16		1 tablespoon	15	57	55	Trace	6
	Cheese:						
17	Blue or Roquefort type	1 ounce	28	40	105	6	9
	Cheddar or American:						
18	Ungrated	1 inch cube	17	37	70	4	5
19	Grated	1 cup	112	37	445	28	36
20		1 tablespoon	7	37	30	2	2
21	Cheddar, process	1 ounce	28	40	105	7	9
22	Cheese foods, Cheddar	1 ounce	28	43	90	6	7
	Cottage cheese, from skim milk:						
23	Creamed	1 cup	225	78	240	31	9
24		1 ounce	28	78	30	4	1
25	Uncreamed	1 cup	225	79	195	38	1
26	.	1 ounce	28	79	25	5	Trace
27	Cream cheese	1 ounce	28	51	105	2	11
28		1 tablespoon	15	51	55	1	6
29	Swiss (domestic)	1 ounce	28	39	105	8	8
	Milk beverages:						
30	Cocoa	1 cup	242	79	235	9	11
31	Chocolate-flavored milk drink (made with skim milk)	1 cup	250	83	190	8	6
32	Malted milk	1 cup	270	78	280	13	12

[1] *Nutritive Values of Foods*, Home and Garden Bulletin No. 72, revised (Washington, D.C.: US Department of Agriculture, 1964).

[Dashes show that no basis could be found for imputing a value although there was some reason to believe that a measurable amount of the constituent might be present]

Fatty acids			Carbo-hydrate	Calcium	Iron	Vitamin A value	Thia-mine	Ribo-flavin	Niacin	Ascorbic acid	
Satu-rated (total)	Unsaturated										
	Oleic	Linoleic									
Grams	Grams	Grams	Grams	Milli-grams	Milli-grams	Inter-national units	Milli-grams	Milli-grams	Milli-grams	Milli-grams	
5	3	Trace	12	288	0.1	350	0.08	0.42	0.1	2	1
—	—	—	13	298	.1	10	.10	.44	.2	2	2
—	—	—	13	298	.1	10	.09	.44	.2	2	3
11	7	1	24	635	.3	820	.10	.84	.5	3	4
15	9	1	166	802	.3	1090	.23	1.17	.5	3	5
16	9	1	39	936	.5	1160	.30	1.50	.7	6	6
—	—	—	36	905	.4	20	.24	1.25	.6	5	7
6	2	Trace	11	315	.2	390	.10	.27	.7	2	8
16	9	1	11	261	.1	1160	.08	.38	.1	2	9
1	1	Trace	1	16	Trace	70	Trace	.02	Trace	Trace	10
27	16	1	10	245	.1	2030	.07	.36	.1	2	11
2	1	Trace	1	15	Trace	130	Trace	.02	Trace	Trace	12
41	25	2	9	203	.1	3070	.06	.30	.1	2	13
3	2	Trace	1	13	Trace	190	Trace	.02	Trace	Trace	14
49	29	3	7	178	.1	3670	.05	.26	.1	2	15
3	2	Trace	Trace	11	Trace	230	Trace	.02	Trace	Trace	16
5	3	Trace	1	89	.1	350	.01	.17	.1	0	17
3	2	Trace	Trace	128	.2	220	Trace	.08	Trace	0	18
20	12	1	2	840	1.1	1470	.03	.51	.1	0	19
1	1	Trace	Trace	52	.1	90	Trace	.03	Trace	0	20
5	3	Trace	1	219	.3	350	Trace	.12	Trace	0	21
4	2	Trace	2	162	.2	280	.01	.16	Trace	0	22
5	3	Trace	7	212	.7	380	.07	.56	.2	0	23
1	Trace	Trace	1	27	.1	50	.01	.07	Trace	0	24
Trace	Trace	Trace	6	202	.9	20	.07	.63	.2	0	25
—	—	—	1	26	.1	Trace	.01	.08	Trace	0	26
6	4	Trace	1	18	.1	440	Trace	.07	Trace	0	27
3	2	Trace	Trace	9	Trace	230	Trace	.04	Trace	0	28
4	3	Trace	1	262	.3	320	Trace	.11	Trace	0	29
6	4	Trace	26	286	.9	390	.09	.45	.4	2	30
3	2	Trace	27	270	.4	210	.09	.41	.2	2	31
—	—	—	32	364	.8	670	.17	.56	.2	2	32

275

Food, approximate measure, and weight (in grams)			Water	Food energy	Protein	Fat (total lipid)

MILK, CREAM, CHEESE: RELATED PRODUCTS—*Continued*

	Milk desserts:		Grams	Per Cent	Calories	Grams	Grams
33	Cornstarch pudding, plain (blanc mange)	1 cup	248	76	275	9	10
34	Custard, baked	1 cup	248	77	285	13	14
	Ice cream, plain, factory packed:						
35	Slice or cut brick, ⅛ of quart brick	1 slice or cut brick	71	62	145	3	9
36	Container	3½ fluid ounces	62	62	130	2	8
37	Container	8 fluid ounces	142	62	295	6	18
38	Ice milk	1 cup	187	67	285	9	10
39	Yoghurt, from partially skimmed milk	1 cup	246	89	120	8	4

EGGS

	Eggs, large, 24 ounces per dozen: Raw:						
40	Whole, without shell	1 egg	50	74	80	6	6
41	White of egg	1 white	33	88	15	4	Trace
42	Yolk of egg	1 yolk	17	51	60	3	5
	Cooked:						
43	Boiled, shell removed	2 eggs	100	74	160	13	12
44	Scrambled, with milk and fat	1 egg	64	72	110	7	8

MEAT, POULTRY, FISH, SHELLFISH; RELATED PRODUCTS

45	Bacon, broiled or fried, crisp	2 slices	16	8	100	5	8
	Beef, trimmed to retail basis,[2] cooked: Cuts braised, simmered, or pot-roasted:						
46	Lean and fat	3 ounces	85	53	245	23	16
47	Lean only	2.5 ounces	72	62	140	22	5
	Hamburger (ground beef), broiled:						
48	Lean	3 ounces	85	60	185	23	10
49	Regular	3 ounces	85.	54	245	21	17
	Roast, oven-cooked, no liquid added: Relatively fat, such as rib:						
50	Lean and fat	3 ounces	85	40	375	17	34
51	Lean only	1.8 ounces	51	57	125	14	7
	Relatively lean, such as heel of round:						
52	Lean and fat	3 ounces	85	62	165	25	7
53	Lean only	2.7 ounces	78	65	125	24	3

[2] Outer layer of fat on the cut was removed to within approximately ½ inch of the lean. Deposits of fat within the cut were not removed.

[Dashes show that no basis could be found for imputing a value although there was some reason to believe that a measurable amount of the constituent might be present]

Fatty acids			Carbo-hydrate	Calcium	Iron	Vitamin A value	Thia-mine	Ribo-flavin	Niacin	Ascorbic acid	
Satu-rated (total)	Unsaturated										
	Oleic	Linoleic									
Grams	Grams	Grams	Grams	Milli-grams	Milli-grams	Inter-national units	Milli-grams	Milli-grams	Milli-grams	Milli-grams	
5	3	Trace	39	290	0.1	390	0.07	0.40	0.1	2	33
6	5	1	28	278	1.0	870	.10	.47	.2	1	34
5	3	Trace	15	87	.1	370	.03	.13	.1	1	35
4	3	Trace	13	76	.1	320	.03	.12	.1	1	36
10	6	1	29	175	.1	740	.06	.27	.1	1	37
6	3	Trace	42	292	.2	390	.09	.41	.2	2	38
2	1	Trace	13	295	.1	170	.09	.43	.2	2	39
2	3	Trace	Trace	27	1.1	590	.05	.15	Trace	0	40
—	—	—	Trace	3	Trace	0	Trace	.09	Trace	0	41
2	2	Trace	Trace	24	.9	580	.04	.07	Trace	0	42
4	5	1	1	54	2.3	1180	.09	.28	.1	0	43
3	3	Trace	1	51	1.1	690	.05	.18	Trace	0	44
3	4	1	1	2	.5	0	.08	.05	.8	——	45
8	7	Trace	0	10	2.9	30	.04	.18	3.5	——	46
2	2	Trace	0	10	2.7	10	.04	.16	3.3	——	47
5	4	Trace	0	10	3.0	20	.08	.20	5.1	——	48
8	8	Trace	0	9	2.7	30	.07	.18	4.6	——	49
16	15	1	0	8	2.2	70	.05	.13	3.1	——	50
3	3	Trace	0	6	1.8	10	.04	.11	2.6	——	51
3	3	Trace	0	11	3.2	10	.06	.19	4.5	——	52
1	1	Trace	0	10	3.0	Trace	.06	.18	4.3	——	53

Food, approximate measure, and weight (in grams)			Water	Food energy	Protein	Fat (total lipid)

MEAT, POULTRY, FISH, SHELLFISH; RELATED PRODUCTS—*Continued*

			Grams	*Per Cent*	*Calories*	*Grams*	*Grams*
	Steak, broiled:						
	Relatively fat, such as sirloin:						
54	Lean and fat	3 ounces	85	44	330	20	27
55	Lean only	2.0 ounces	56	59	115	18	4
	Relative lean, such as round:						
56	Lean and fat	3 ounces	85	55	220	24	13
57	Lean only	2.4 ounces	68	61	130	21	4
	Beef, canned:						
58	Corned beef	3 ounces	85	59	185	22	10
59	Corned beef hash	3 ounces	85	67	155	7	10
60	Beef, dried or chipped	2 ounces	57	48	115	19	4
61	Beef and vegetable stew	1 cup	235	82	210	15	10
62	Beef potpie, baked: Individual pie, 4¼-inch diameter, weight before baking about 8 ounces	1 pie	227	55	560	23	33
	Chicken, cooked:						
63	Flesh only, broiled	3 ounces	85	71	115	20	3
	Breast, fried, ½ breast:						
64	With bone	3.3 ounces	94	58	155	25	5
65	Flesh and skin only	2.7 ounces	76	58	155	25	5
	Drumstick, fried:						
66	With bone	2.1 ounces	59	55	90	12	4
67	Flesh and skin only	1.3 ounces	38	55	90	12	4
68	Chicken, canned, boneless	3 ounces	85	65	170	18	10
	Chicken potpie. (*See* Poultry potpie)						
	Chile con carne, canned:						
69	With beans	1 cup	250	72	335	19	15
70	Without beans	1 cup	255	67	510	26	38
71	Heart, beef, lean, braised	3 ounces	85	61	160	27	5
	Lamb, trimmed to retail basis,[2] cooked:						
72	Chop, thick, with bone, broiled.	1 chop, 4.8 ounces	137	47	400	25	33
73	Lean and fat	4.0 ounces	112	47	400	25	33
74	Lean only	2.6 ounces	74	62	140	21	6
	Leg, roasted:						
75	Lean and fat	3 ounces	85	54	235	22	16
76	Lean only	2.5 ounces	71	62	130	20	5
	Shoulder, roasted:						
77	Lean and fat	2 ounces	85	50	285	18	23
78	Lean only	2.3 ounces	64	61	130	17	6
79	Liver, beef, fried	2 ounces	57	57	130	15	6
	Pork, cured, cooked:						
80	Ham, light cure, lean and fat, roasted	3 ounces	85	54	245	18	19
	Luncheon meat:						
81	Boiled ham, sliced	2 ounces	57	59	135	11	10

[Dashes show that no basis could be found for imputing a value although there was some reason to believe that a measurable amount of the constituent might be present]

Fatty acids			Carbo-hydrate	Calcium	Iron	Vitamin A value	Thia-mine	Ribo-flavin	Niacin	Ascorbic acid	
Satu-rated (total)	Unsaturated										
	Oleic	Linoleic									
Grams	Grams	Grams	Grams	Milli-grams	Milli-grams	Inter-national units	Milli-grams	Milli-grams	Milli-grams	Milli-grams	
13	12	1	0	9	2.5	50	0.05	0.16	4.0	——	54
2	2	Trace	0	7	2.2	10	.05	.14	3.6	——	55
6	6	Trace	0	10	3.0	20	.07	.19	4.8	——	56
2	2	Trace	0	9	2.5	10	.06	.16	4.1	——	57
5	4	Trace	0	17	3.7	20	.01	.20	2.9	——	58
5	4	Trace	9	11	1.7	——	.01	.08	1.8	——	59
2	2	Trace	0	11	2.9	——	.04	.18	2.2	——	60
5	4	Trace	15	28	2.8	2310	.13	.17	4.4	15	61
9	20	2	43	32	4.1	1860	.25	.27	4.5	7	62
1	1	1	0	8	1.4	80	.05	.16	7.4	——	63
1	2	1	1	9	1.3	70	.04	.17	11.2	——	64
1	2	1	1	9	1.3	70	.04	.17	11.2	——	65
1	2	1	Trace	6	.9	50	.03	.15	2.7	——	66
1	2	1	Trace	6	.9	50	.03	.15	2.7	——	67
3	4	2	0	18	1.3	200	.03	.11	3.7	3	68
7	7	Trace	30	80	4.2	150	.08	.18	3.2	——	69
18	17	1	15	97	3.6	380	.05	.31	5.6	——	70
——	——	——	1	5	5.0	20	.21	1.04	6.5	1	71
18	12	1	0	10	1.5	——	.14	.25	5.6	——	72
18	12	1	0	10	1.5	——	.14	.25	5.6	——	73
3	2	Trace	0	9	1.5	——	.11	.20	4.5	——	74
9	6	Trace	0	9	1.4	——	.13	.23	4.7	——	75
3	2	Trace	0	9	1.4	——	.12	.21	4.4	——	76
13	8	1	0	9	1.0	——	.11	.20	4.0	——	77
3	2	Trace	0	8	1.0	——	.10	.18	3.7	——	78
——	——	——	3	6	5.0	30,280	.15	2.37	9.4	15	79
7	8	2	0	8	2.2	0	.40	.16	3.1	——	80
4	4	1	0	6	1.6	0	.25	.09	1.5	——	81

Food, approximate measure, and weight (in grams)			Water	Food energy	Protein	Fat (total lipid)
MEAT, POULTRY, FISH, SHELLFISH, RELATED PRODUCTS—*Continued*						
Luncheon meat—*Continued*		Grams	Per Cent	Calories	Grams	Grams
82	Canned, spiced or unspiced	2 ounces	57	55	165	8	14
Pork, fresh, trimmed to retail basis,[2] cooked:						
83	Chop, thick, with bone	1 chop, 3.5 ounces	98	42	260	16	21
84	Lean and fat	2.3 ounces	66	42	260	16	21
85	Lean only	1.7 ounces	48	53	130	15	7
Roast, oven-cooked, no liquid added:						
86	Lean and fat	3 ounces	85	46	310	21	24
87	Lean only	2.4 ounces	68	55	175	20	10
Cuts, simmered:						
88	Lean and fat	3 ounces	85	46	320	20	26
89	Lean only	2.2 ounces	63	60	135	18	6
90	Poultry potpie (based on chicken potpie). Individual pie, 4¼-inch diameter, weight before baking about 8 ounces	1 pie	227	57	535	23	31
Sausage:						
91	Bologna, slice, 4.1 by 0.1 inch	8 slices	227	56	690	27	62
92	Frankfurter, cooked	1 frankfurter	51	58	155	6	14
93	Pork, links or patty, cooked	4 ounces	113	35	540	21	50
94	Tongue, beef, braised	3 ounces	85	61	210	18	14
Turkey potpie. *See* Poultry potpie.						
Veal, cooked:						
95	Cutlet, without bone, broiled	3 ounces	85	60	185	23	9
96	Roast, medium fat, medium done; lean and fat	3 ounces	85	55	230	23	14
Fish and shellfish:						
97	Bluefish, baked or broiled	3 ounces	85	68	135	22	4
Clams:						
98	Raw, meat only	3 ounces	85	82	65	11	1
99	Canned, solids and liquid	3 ounces	85	86	45	7	1
100	Crabmeat, canned	3 ounces	85	77	85	15	2
101	Fish sticks, breaded, cooked, frozen; stick, 3.8 by 1.0 by 0.5 inch	10 sticks or 8-ounce package	227	66	400	38	20
102	Haddock, fried	3 ounces	85	66	140	17	5
Mackerel:						
103	Broiled, Atlantic	3 ounces	85	62	200	19	13

280

[Dashes show that no basis could be found for imputing a value although there was some reason to believe that a measurable amount of the constituent might be present]

	Fatty acids		Carbo-hydrate	Calcium	Iron	Vitamin A value	Thia-mine	Ribo-flavin	Niacin	Ascorbic acid	
Satu-rated (total)	Unsaturated										
	Oleic	Linoleic									
Grams	Grams	Grams	Grams	Milli-grams	Milli-grams	Inter-national units	Milli-grams	Milli-grams	Milli-grams	Milli-grams	
5	6	1	1	5	1.2	0	0.18	0.12	1.6	——	82
8	9	2	0	8	2.2	0	.63	.18	3.8	——	83
8	9	2	0	8	2.2	0	.63	.18	3.8	——	84
2	3	1	0	7	1.9	0	.54	.16	3.3	——	85
9	10	2	0	9	2.7	0	.78	.22	4.7	——	86
3	4	1	0	9	2.6	0	.73	.21	4.4	——	87
9	11	2	0	8	2.5	0	.46	.21	4.1	——	88
2	3	1	0	8	2.3	0	.42	.19	3.7	——	89
10	15	3	42	68	3.0	3020	.25	.26	4.1	5	90
——	——	——	2	16	4.1	——	.36	.49	6.0	——	91
——	——	——	1	3	.8	——	.08	.10	1.3	——	92
18	21	5	Trace	8	2.7	0	.89	.39	4.2	——	93
——	——	——	Trace	6	1.9	——	.04	.25	3.0	——	94
5	4	Trace	——	9	2.7	——	.06	.21	4.6	——	95
7	6	Trace	0	10	2.9	——	.11	.26	6.6	——	96
——	——	——	0	25	.6	40	.09	.08	1.6	——	97
——	——	——	2	59	5.2	90	.08	.15	1.1	8	98
——	——	——	2	47	3.5	——	.01	.09	.9	——	99
——	——	——	1	38	.7	——	.07	.07	1.6	——	100
5	4	10	15	25	.9	——	.09	.16	3.6	——	101
1	3	Trace	5	34	1.0	——	.03	.06	2.7	2	102
——	——	——	0	5	1.0	450	.13	.23	6.5	——	103

Food, approximate measure, and weight (in grams)			Water	Food energy	Protein	Fat (total lipid)

MEAT, POULTRY, FISH, SHELLFISH; RELATED PRODUCTS—*Continued*

	Fish and shellfish—*Continued*		*Grams*	*Per Cent*	*Calories*	*Grams*	*Grams*
104	Canned, Pacific, solids and liquid[3]	3 ounces	85	66	155	18	9
105	Ocean perch, breaded (egg and bread-crumbs), fried	3 ounces	85	59	195	16	11
106	Oysters, meat only: Raw, 13–19 medium selects	1 cup	240	85	160	20	4
107	Oyster stew, 1 part oysters to 3 parts milk by volume, 3–4 oysters	1 cup	230	84	200	11	12
108	Salmon, pink, canned	3 ounces	85	71	120	17	5
109	Sardines, Atlantic, canned in oil, drained solids	3 ounces	85	62	175	20	9
110	Shad, baked	3 ounces	85	64	170	20	10
111	Shrimp, canned, meat only	3 ounces	85	70	100	21	1
112	Swordfish, broiled with butter or margarine	3 ounces	85	65	150	24	5
113	Tuna, canned in oil, drained solids	3 ounces	85	61	170	24	7

MATURE DRY BEANS AND PEAS, NUTS, PEANUTS; RELATED PRODUCTS

114	Almonds, shelled	1 cup	142	5	850	26	77
	Beans, dry:						
	Common varieties, such as Great Northern, navy, and others, canned:						
115	Red	1 cup	256	76	230	15	1
	White, with tomato sauce:						
116	With pork	1 cup	261	71	320	16	7
117	Without pork	1 cup	261	68	310	16	1
118	Lima, cooked	1 cup	192	64	260	16	1
119	Brazil nuts	1 cup	140	5	915	20	94
120	Cashew nuts, roasted	1 cup	135	5	760	23	62
	Coconut:						
121	Fresh, shredded	1 cup	97	51	335	3	34
122	Dried, shredded, sweetened	1 cup	62	3	340	2	24
123	Cowpeas or blackeye peas, dry, cooked	1 cup	248	80	190	13	1
	Peanuts, roasted, salted:						
124	Halves	1 cup	144	2	840	37	72

[3] Vitamin values based on drained solids.

[Dashes show that no basis could be found for imputing a value although there was some reason to believe that a measurable amount of the constituent might be present]

Fatty acids			Carbo-hydrate	Calcium	Iron	Vitamin A value	Thia-mine	Ribo-flavin	Niacin	Ascorbic acid	
Satu-rated (total)	Unsaturated										
	Oleic	Linoleic									
Grams	Grams	Grams	Grams	Milli-grams	Milli-grams	Inter-national units	Milli-grams	Milli-grams	Milli-grams	Milli-grams	
——	——	——	0	221	1.9	20	0.02	0.28	7.4	——	104
——	——	——	6	28	1.1	——	.08	.09	1.5	——	105
——	——	——	8	226	13.2	740	.33	.43	6.0	——	106
——	——	——	11	269	3.3	640	.13	.41	1.6	——	107
1	1	Trace	0	167[4]	.7	60	.03	.16	6.8	——	108
——	——	——	0	372	2.5	190	.02	.17	4.6	——	109
——	——	——	0	20	.5	20	.11	.22	7.3	——	110
——	——	——	1	98	2.6	50	.01	.03	1.5	——	111
——	——	——	0	23	1.1	1750	.03	.04	9.3	——	112
——	——	——	0	7	1.6	70	.04	.10	10.1	——	113
6	52	15	28	332	6.7	0	.34	1.31	5.0	Trace	114
——	——	——	42	74	4.6	Trace	.13	.10	1.5	——	115
3	3	1	50	141	4.7	340	.20	.08	1.5	5	116
——	——	——	60	177	5.2	160	.18	.09	1.5	5	117
——	——	——	48	56	5.6	Trace	.26	.12	1.3	Trace	118
19	45	24	15	260	4.8	Trace	1.34	.17	2.2	——	119
10	43	4	40	51	5.1	140	.58	.33	2.4	——	120
29	2	Trace	9	13	1.6	0	.05	.02	.5	3	121
21	2	Trace	33	10	1.2	0	.02	.02	.2	0	122
——	——	——	34	42	3.2	20	.41	.11	1.1	Trace	123
16	31	21	27	107	3.0	——	.46	.19	24.7	0	124

[4] Based on total contents of can. If bones are discarded, value will be greatly reduced.

Food, approximate measure, and weight (in grams)			Water	Food energy	Protein	Fat (total lipid)
MATURE DRY BEANS AND PEAS, NUTS, PEANUTS; RELATED PRODUCTS— *Continued*						
Peanuts, roasted, salted—*Continued*		Grams	Per Cent	Calories	Grams	Grams
125	Chopped	1 tablespoon	9	2	55	2	4
126	Peanut butter	1 tablespoon	16	2	95	4	8
127	Peas, split, dry, cooked	1 cup	250	70	290	20	1
	Pecans:						
128	Halves	1 cup	108	3	740	10	77
129	Chopped	1 tablespoon	7.5	3	50	1	5
	Walnuts, shelled:						
130	Black or native, chopped	1 cup	126	3	790	26	75
	English or Persian:						
131	Halves	1 cup	100	4	650	15	64
132	Chopped	1 tablespoon	8	4	50	1	5
VEGETABLES AND VEGETABLE PRODUCTS						
	Asparagus:						
133	Cooked, cut spears	1 cup	175	94	35	4	Trace
	Canned spears, medium:						
134	Green	6 spears	96	92	20	2	Trace
135	Bleached	6 spears	96	92	20	2	Trace
	Beans:						
136	Lima, immature, cooked	1 cup	160	71	180	12	1
	Snap, green: Cooked:						
137	In small amount of water, short time	1 cup	125	92	30	2	Trace
138	In large amount of water, long time	1 cup	125	92	30	2	Trace
	Canned:						
139	Solids and liquid	1 cup	239	94	45	2	Trace
140	Strained or chopped (baby food)	1 ounce	28	92	5	Trace	Trace
	Bean sprouts. *See* Sprouts.						
141	Beets, cooked, diced	1 cup	165	91	50	2	Trace
142	Broccoli spears, cooked	1 cup	150	91	40	5	Trace
143	Brussels sprouts, cooked	1 cup	130	88	45	5	1
	Cabbage: Raw:						
144	Finely shredded	1 cup	100	92	25	1	Trace
145	Coleslaw	1 cup	120	83	120	1	9
	Cooked:						
146	In small amount of water, short time	1 cup	170	94	35	2	Trace
147	In large amount of water, long time	1 cup	170	94	30	2	Trace

[Dashes show that no basis could be found for imputing a value although there was some reason to believe that a measurable amount of the constituent might be present]

Fatty acids			Carbo-hydrate	Calcium	Iron	Vitamin A value	Thia-mine	Ribo-flavin	Niacin	Ascorbic acid	
Satu-rated (total)	Unsaturated										
	Oleic	Linoleic									
Grams	Grams	Grams	Grams	Milli-grams	Milli-grams	Inter-national units	Milli-grams	Milli-grams	Milli-grams	Milli-grams	
1	2	1	2	7	0.2	——	0.03	0.01	1.5	0	125
2	4	2	3	9	.3	——	.02	.02	2.4	0	126
——	——	——	52	28	4.2	100	.37	.22	2.2	——	127
5	48	15	16	79	2.6	140	.93	.14	1.0	2	128
Trace	3	1	1	5	.2	10	.06	.01	.1	Trace	129
4	26	36	19	Trace	7.6	380	.28	.14	.9	——	130
4	10	40	16	99	3.1	30	.33	.13	.9	3	131
Trace	1	3	1	8	.2	Trace	.03	.01	.1	Trace	132
——	——	——	6	37	1.0	1580	.27	.32	2.4	46	133
——	——	——	3	18	1.8	770	.06	.10	.8	14	134
——	——	——	4	15	1.0	80	.05	.06	.7	14	135
——	——	——	32	75	4.0	450	.29	.16	2.0	28	136
——	——	——	7.	62	.8	680	.08	.11	.6	16	137
——	——	——	7	62	.8	680	.07	.10	.4	13	138
——	——	——	10	81	2.9	690	.08	.10	.7	9	139
——	——	——	1	9	.3	110	.01	.02	.1	Trace	140
——	——	——	12	23	.8	40	.04	.07	.5	11	141
——	——	——	7	132	1.2	3750	.14	.29	1.2	135	142
——	——	——	8	42	1.4	680	.10	.18	1.1	113	143
——	——	——	5	49	.4	130	.05	.05	.3	47	144
2	2	5	9	52	.5	180	.06	.06	.3	35	145
——	——	——	7	75	.5	220	.07	.07	.5	56	146
——	——	——	7	71	.5	200	.04	.04	.2	40	147

	Food, approximate measure, and weight (in grams)			Water	Food energy	Protein	Fat (total lipid)
	VEGETABLES AND VEGETABLE PRODUCTS—*Continued*						
	Cabbage, celery or Chinese:		*Grams*	*Per Cent*	*Calories*	*Grams*	*Grams*
148	Raw, leaves and stalk, 1-inch pieces	1 cup	100	95	15	1	Trace
149	Cabbage, spoon (or pakchoy), cooked	1 cup	150	95	20	2	Trace
	Carrots:						
	Raw:						
150	Whole, 5½ by 1 inch, (25 thin strips)	1 carrot	50	88	20	1	Trace
151	Grated	1 cup	110	88	45	1	Trace
152	Cooked, diced	1 cup	145	91	45	1	Trace
153	Canned, strained or chopped (baby food)	1 ounce	28	92	10	Trace	Trace
154	Cauliflower, cooked, flowerbuds	1 cup	120	93	25	3	Trace
	Celery, raw:						
155	Stalk, large outer, 8 by about 1½ inches, at root end	1 stalk	40	94	5	Trace	Trace
156	Pieces, diced	1 cup	100	94	15	1	Trace
157	Collards, cooked	1 cup	190	91	55	5	1
	Corn, sweet:						
158	Cooked, ear 5 by 1¾ inches[5]	1 ear	140	74	70	3	1
159	Canned, solids and liquid	1 cup	256	81	170	5	2
160	Cowpeas, cooked, immature seeds	1 cup	160	72	175	13	1
	Cucumbers, 10-ounce; 7½ by about 2 inches:						
161	Raw, pared	1 cucumber	207	96	30	1	Trace
162	Raw, pared, center slice ⅛-inch thick	6 slices	50	96	5	Trace	Trace
163	Dandelion greens, cooked	1 cup	180	90	60	4	1
164	Endive, curly (including escarole)	2 ounces	57	93	10	1	Trace
165	Kale, leaves including stems, cooked	1 cup	110	91	30	4	1
	Lettuce, raw:						
166	Butterhead, as Boston types; head, 4-inch diameter	1 head	220	95	30	3	Trace
167	Crisphead, as Iceberg: head, 4¾-inch diameter	1 head	454	96	60	4	Trace
168	Looseleaf, or bunching varieties, leaves	2 large	50	94	10	1	Trace

[5] Measure and weight apply to entire vegetable or fruit including parts not usually eaten.

[Dashes show that no basis could be found for imputing a value although there was some reason to believe that a measurable amount of the constituent might be present]

Saturated (total)	Oleic	Linoleic	Carbohydrate	Calcium	Iron	Vitamin A value	Thiamine	Riboflavin	Niacin	Ascorbic acid	
Grams	Grams	Grams	Grams	Milligrams	Milligrams	International units	Milligrams	Milligrams	Milligrams	Milligrams	
——	——	——	3	43	0.6	150	0.05	0.04	0.6	25	148
——	——	——	4	222	.9	4650	.07	.12	1.1	23	149
——	——	——	5	18	.4	5500	.03	.03	.3	4	150
——	——	——	11	41	.8	12100	.06	.06	.7	9	151
——	——	——	10	48	.9	15220	.08	.07	.7	9	152
——	——	——	2	7	.1	3690	.01	.01	.1	1	153
——	——	——	5	25	.8	70	.11	.10	.7	66	154
——	——	——	2	16	.1	100	.01	.01	.1	4	155
——	——	——	4	39	.3	240	.03	.03	.3	9	156
——	——	——	9	289	1.1	10260	.27	.37	2.4	87	157
——	——	——	16	2	.5	310[6]	.09	.08	1.0	7	158
——	——	——	40	10	1.0	690[6]	.07	.12	2.3	13	159
——	——	——	29	38	3.4	560	.49	.18	2.3	28	160
——	——	——	7	35	.6	Trace	.07	.09	.4	23	161
——	——	——	2	8	.2	Trace	.02	.02	.1	6	162
——	——	——	12	252	3.2	21060	.24	.29	——	32	163
——	——	——	2	46	1.0	1870	.04	.08	.3	6	164
——	——	——	4	147	1.3	8140	——	——	——	68	165
——	——	——	6	77	4.4	2130	.14	.13	.6	18	166
——	——	——	13	91	2.3	1500	.29	.27	1.3	29	167
——	——	——	2	34	.7	950	.03	.04	.2	9	168

[6] Based on yellow varieties; white varieties contain only a trace of cryptoxanthin and carotenes, the pigments in corn that have biological activity.

Food, approximate measure, and weight (in grams)			Water	Food energy	Protein	Fat (total lipid)	
	VEGETABLES AND VEGETABLE PRODUCTS—*Continued*						
			Grams	*Per Cent*	*Calories*	*Grams*	*Grams*
169	Mushrooms, canned, solids and liquid	1 cup	244	93	40	5	Trace
170	Mustard greens, cooked	1 cup	140	93	35	3	1
171	Okra, cooked, pod 3 by ⅝ inch	8 pods	85	91	25	2	Trace
	Onions:						
	Mature:						
172	Raw, onion 2½-inch diameter	1 onion	110	89	40	2	Trace
173	Cooked	1 cup	210	92	60	3	Trace
174	Young green, small, without tops	6 onions	50	88	20	1	Trace
175	Parsley, raw, chopped	1 tablespoon	3.5	85	1	Trace	Trace
176	Parsnips, cooked	1 cup	155	82	100	2	1
	Peas, green:						
177	Cooked	1 cup	160	82	115	9	1
178	Canned, solids and liquid	1 cup	249	83	165	9	1
179	Canned, strained (baby food)	1 ounce	28	86	15	1	Trace
180	Peppers, hot, red, without seeds, dried (ground chili powder, added seasonings)	1 tablespoon	15	8	50	2	2
	Peppers, sweet:						
	Raw, medium, about 6 per pound:						
181	Green pod without stem and seeds	1 pod	62	93	15	1	Trace
182	Red pod without stem and seeds	1 pod	60	91	20	1	Trace
183	Canned, pimentos, medium	1 pod	38	92	10	Trace	Trace
	Potatoes, medium (about 3 per pound raw):						
184	Baked, peeled after baking	1 potato	99	75	90	3	Trace
	Boiled:						
185	Peeled after boiling	1 potato	136	80	105	3	Trace
186	Peeled before boiling	1 potato	122	83	80	2	Trace
	French-fried, piece 2 by ½ by ½ inch:						
187	Cooked in deep fat	10 pieces	57	45	155	2	7
188	Frozen, heated	10 pieces	57	53	125	2	5
	Mashed:						
189	Milk added	1 cup	195	83	125	4	1

288

[Dashes show that no basis could be found for imputing a value although there was some reason to believe that a measurable amount of the constituent might be present]

Fatty acids			Carbo-hydrate	Calcium	Iron	Vitamin A value	Thia-mine	Ribo-flavin	Niacin	Ascorbic acid	
Satu-rated (total)	Unsaturated										
	Oleic	Linoleic									
Grams	Grams	Grams	Grams	Milli-grams	Milli-grams	Inter-national units	Milli-grams	Milli-grams	Milli-grams	Milli-grams	
—	—	—	6	15	1.2	Trace	0.04	0.60	4.8	4	169
—	—	—	6	193	2.5	8120	.11	.19	.9	68	170
—	—	—	5	78	.4	420	.11	.15	.8	17	171
—	—	—	10	30	.6	40	.04	.04	.2	11	172
—	—	—	14	50	.8	80	.06	.06	.4	14	173
—	—	—	5	20	.3	Trace	.02	.02	.2	12	174
—	—	—	Trace	7	.2	300	Trace	.01	Trace	6	175
—	—	—	23	70	.9	50	.11	.13	.2	16	176
—	—	—	19	37	2.9	860	.44	.17	3.7	33	177
—	—	—	31	50	4.2	1120	.23	.13	2.2	22	178
—	—	—	3	3	.4	140	.02	.02	.4	3	179
—	—	—	8	40	2.3	9750	.03	.17	1.3	2	180
—	—	—	3	6	.4	260	.05	.05	.3	79	181
—	—	—	4	8	.4	2670	.05	.05	.3	122	182
—	—	—	2	3	.6	870	.01	.02	.1	36	183
—	—	—	21	9	.7	Trace	.10	.04	1.7	20	184
—	—	—	23	10	.8	Trace	.13	.05	2.0	22	185
—	—	—	18	7	.6	Trace	.11	.04	1.4	20	186
2	2	4	20	9	.7	Trace	.07	.04	1.8	12	187
1	1	1	19	5	1.0	Trace	.08	.01	1.5	12	188
—	—	—	25	47	.8	50	.16	.10	2.0	19	189

Food, approximate measure, and weight (in grams)			Water	Food energy	Protein	Fat (total lipid)	

VEGETABLES AND VEGETABLE PRODUCTS—*Continued*

Potatoes—*Continued*

				Grams	*Per Cent*	*Calories*	*Grams*	*Grams*
	Mashed:							
190	Milk and butter added	1 cup	195	80	185	4	8
191	Potato chips, medium, 2-inch diameter	10 chips	20	2	115	1	8
192	Pumpkin, canned	1 cup	228	90	75	2	1
193	Radish, raw, small, without tops	4 radishes	40	94	5	Trace	Trace
194	Sauerkraut, canned, solids and liquid	1 cup	235	93	45	2	Trace
	Spinach:						
195	Cooked	1 cup	180	92	40	5	1
196	Canned, drained solids	1 cup	180	91	45	5	1
197	Canned, strained or chopped (baby food)	1 ounce	28	88	10	1	Trace
	Sprouts, raw:						
198	Mung bean	1 cup	90	89	30	3	Trace
199	Soybean	1 cup	107	89	40	6	2
	Squash:						
	Cooked:						
200	Summer, diced	1 cup	210	96	30	2	Trace
201	Winter, baked, mashed	1 cup	205	81	130	4	1
202	Canned, winter, strained and chopped (baby food)	1 ounce	28	92	10	Trace	Trace
	Sweetpotatoes:						
	Cooked, medium, 5 by 2 inches, weight raw about 6 ounces:						
203	Baked, peeled after baking	1 sweetpotato	110	64	155	2	1
204	Boiled, peeled after boiling	1 sweetpotato	147	71	170	2	1
205	Candied, 3½ by 2¼ inches	1 sweetpotato	175	60	295	2	6
206	Canned, vacuum or solid pack	1 cup	218	72	235	4	Trace
	Tomatoes:						
207	Raw, medium, 2 by 2½ inches, about 3 per pound	1 tomato	150	94	35	2	Trace
208	Canned	1 cup	242	94	50	2	Trace
209	Tomato juice, canned	1 cup	242	94	45	2	Trace
210	Tomato catsup	1 tablespoon	17	69	15	Trace	Trace

[Dashes show that no basis could be found for imputing a value although there was some reason to believe that a measurable amount of the constituent might be present]

Fatty acids			Carbo-hydrate	Calcium	Iron	Vitamin A value	Thia-mine	Ribo-flavin	Niacin	Ascorbic acid	
Satu-rated (total)	Unsaturated										
	Oleic	Linoleic									
Grams	Grams	Grams	Grams	Milli-grams	Milli-grams	Inter-national units	Milli-grams	Milli-grams	Milli-grams	Milli-grams	
4	3	Trace	24	47	0.8	330	0.16	0.10	1.9	18	190
2	2	4	10	8	.4	Trace	.04	.01	1.0	3	191
——	——	——	18	57	.9	14590	.07	.12	1.3	12	192
——	——	——	1	12	.4	Trace	.01	.01	.1	10	193
——	——	——	9	85	1.2	120	.07	.09	.4	33	194
——	——	——	6	167	4.0	14580	.13	.25	1.0	50	195
——	——	——	6	212	4.7	14400	.03	.21	.6	24	196
——	——	——	2	18	.2	1420	.01	.04	.1	2	197
——	——	——	6	17	1.2	20	.12	.12	.7	17	198
——	——	——	4	46	.7	90	.17	.16	.8	4	199
——	——	——	7	52	.8	820	.10	.16	1.6	21	200
——	——	——	32	57	1.6	8610	.10	.27	1.4	27	201
——	——	——	2	7	.1	510	.01	.01	.1	1	202
——	——	——	36	44	1.0	8910	.10	.07	.7	24	203
——	——	——	39	47	1.0	11610	.13	.09	.9	25	204
2	3	1	60	65	1.6	11030	.10	.08	.8	17	205
——	——	——	54	54	1.7	17000	.10	.10	1.4	30	206
——	——	——	7	20	.8	1350	.10	.06	1.0	34[7]	207
——	——	——	10	15	1.2	2180	.13	.07	1.7	40	208
——	——	——	10	17	2.2	1940	.13	.07	1.8	39	209
——	——	——	4	4	.1	240	.02	.01	.3	3	210

[7] Year-round average. Samples marketed from November through May average around 15 milligrams per 150-gram tomato; from June through October, around 39 milligrams.

Food, approximate measure, and weight (in grams)			Water	Food energy	Protein	Fat (total lipid)

VEGETABLES AND VEGETABLE PRODUCTS—*Continued*

			Grams	Per Cent	Calories	Grams	Grams
211	Turnips, cooked, diced	1 cup	155	94	35	1	Trace
	Turnip greens:						
	Cooked:						
212	In small amount of water, short time	1 cup	145	93	30	3	Trace
213	In large amount of water, long time	1 cup	145	94	25	3	Trace
214	Canned, solids and liquid	1 cup	232	94	40	3	1

FRUITS AND FRUIT PRODUCTS

215	Apples, raw, medium, 2½-inch diameter, about 3 per pound[5]	1 apple	150	85	70	Trace	Trace
216	Apple brown betty	1 cup	230	64	345	4	8
217	Apple juice, bottled or canned	1 cup	249	88	120	Trace	Trace
	Applesauce, canned:						
218	Sweetened	1 cup	254	76	230	1	Trace
219	Unsweetened or artificially sweetened	1 cup	239	88	100	Trace	Trace
220	Applesauce and apricots, canned, strained or junior (baby food)	1 ounce	28	77	25	Trace	Trace
	Apricots						
221	Raw, about 12 per pound[5]	3 apricots	114	85	55	1	Trace
	Canned in heavy sirup:						
222	Halves and sirup	1 cup	259	77	220	2	Trace
223	Halves (medium) and sirup	4 halves; 2 tablespoons sirup	122	77	105	1	Trace
	Dried:						
224	Uncooked, 40 halves, small	1 cup	150	25	390	8	1
225	Cooked, unsweetened, fruit and liquid	1 cup	285	76	240	5	1
226	Apricot nectar, canned	1 cup	250	85	140	1	Trace
	Avocados, raw:						
	California varieties, mainly Fuerte:						
227	10-ounce avocado, about 3⅓ by 4¼ inches, peeled, pitted	½ avocado	108	74	185	2	18
228	½-inch cubes	1 cup	152	74	260	3	26
	Florida varieties:						
229	13-ounce avocado, about 4 by 3 inches, peeled, pitted	½ avocado	123	78	160	2	14

[Dashes show that no basis could be found for imputing a value although there was some reason to believe that a measurable amount of the constituent might be present]

Fatty acids			Carbo-hydrate	Calcium	Iron	Vitamin A value	Thia-mine	Ribo-flavin	Niacin	Ascorbic acid	
Satu-rated (total)	Unsaturated										
	Oleic	Linoleic									
Grams	Grams	Grams	Grams	Milli-grams	Milli-grams	Inter-national units	Milli-grams	Milli-grams	Milli-grams	Milli-grams	
—	—	—	8	54	0.6	Trace	0.06	0.08	0.5	33	211
—	—	—	5	267	1.6	9140	.21	.36	.8	100	212
—	—	—	5	252	1.4	8260	.14	.33	.8	68	213
—	—	—	7	232	3.7	10900	.04	.21	1.4	44	214
—	—	—	18	8	.4	50	.04	.02	.1	3	215
4	3	Trace	68	41	1.4	230	.13	.10	.9	3	216
—	—	—	30	15	1.5	—	.01	.04	.2	2	217
—	—	—	60	10	1.3	100	.05	.03	.1	3	218
—	—	—	26	10	1.2	100	.04	.02	.1	2	219
—	—	—	6	1	.1	170	Trace	Trace	Trace	1	220
—	—	—	14	18	.5	2890	.03	.04	.7	10	221
—	—	—	57	28	.8	4510	.05	.06	.9	10	222
—	—	—	27	13	.4	2120	.02	.03	.4	5	223
—	—	—	100	100	8.2	16350	.02	.23	4.9	19	224
—	—	—	62	63	5.1	8550	.01	.13	2.8	8	225
—	—	—	36	22	.5	2380	.02	.02	.5	7	226
4	8	2	6	11	.6	310	.12	.21	1.7	15	227
5	12	3	9	15	.9	440	.16	.30	2.4	21	228
3	6	2	11	12	.7	360	.13	.24	2.0	17	229

	Food, approximate measure, and weight (in grams)			Water	Food energy	Protein	Fat (total lipid)
	FRUITS AND FRUIT PRODUCTS— *Continued*						
	Avocados—*Continued*		Grams	Per Cent	Calories	Grams	Grams
230	½-inch cubes	1 cup	152	78	195	2	17
231	Bananas, raw, 6 by 1½ inches, about 3 per pound[5]	1 banana	150	76	85	1	Trace
232	Blackberries, raw	1 cup	144	84	85	2	1
233	Blueberries, raw	1 cup	140	83	85	1	1
234	Cantaloups, raw; medium, 5-inch diameter, about 1⅔ pounds	½ melon	385	91	60	1	Trace
	Cherries:						
235	Raw, sweet, with stems[5]	1 cup	130	80	80	2	Trace
236	Canned, red, sour, pitted, heavy sirup	1 cup	260	76	230	2	1
237	Cranberry juice cocktail, canned	1 cup	250	83	160	Trace	Trace
238	Cranberry sauce, sweetened, canned, strained	1 cup	277	62	405	Trace	1
239	Dates, domestic, natural and dry, pitted, cut	1 cup	178	22	490	4	1
	Figs:						
240	Raw, small, 1½-inch diameter, about 12 per pound	3 figs	114	78	90	1	Trace
241	Dried, large, 2 by 1 inch	1 fig	21	23	60	1	Trace
242	Fruit cocktail, canned in heavy sirup, solids and liquid	1 cup	256	80	195	1	1
	Grapefruit:						
	Raw, medium, 4¼-inch diameter, size 64:						
243	White[5]	½ grapefruit	285	89	55	1	Trace
244	Pink or red[5]	½ grapefruit	285	89	60	1	Trace
245	Raw sections, white	1 cup	194	89	75	1	Trace
	Canned, white:						
246	Sirup pack, solids and liquid	1 cup	249	81	175	1	Trace
247	Water pack, solids and liquid	1 cup	240	91	70	1	Trace
	Grapefruit juice:						
248	Fresh	1 cup	246	90	95	1	Trace
	Canned, white:						
249	Unsweetened	1 cup	247	89	100	1	Trace
250	Sweetened	1 cup	250	86	130	1	Trace

[Dashes show that no basis could be found for imputing a value although there was some reason to believe that a measurable amount of the constituent might be present]

Fatty acids			Carbo-hydrate	Calcium	Iron	Vitamin A value	Thia-mine	Ribo-flavin	Niacin	Ascorbic acid	
Satu-rated (total)	Unsaturated										
	Oleic	Linoleic									
Grams	Grams	Grams	Grams	Milli-grams	Milli-grams	Inter-national units	Milli-grams	Milli-grams	Milli-grams	Milli-grams	
3	8	2	13	15	0.9	440	0.16	0.30	2.4	21	230
—	—	—	23	8	.7	190	.05	.06	.7	10	231
—	—	—	19	46	1.3	290	.05	.06	.5	30	232
—	—	—	21	21	1.4	140	.04	.08	.6	20	233
—	—	—	14	27	.8	6540[8]	.08	.06	1.2	63	234
—	—	—	20	26	.5	130	.06	.07	.5	12	235
—	—	—	59	36	.8	1680	.07	.06	.4	13	236
—	—	—	41	12	.8	Trace	.02	.02	.1	(9)	237
—	—	—	104	17	.6	40	.03	.03	.1	5	238
—	—	—	130	105	5.3	90	.16	.17	3.9	0	239
—	—	—	23	40	.7	90	.07	.06	.5	2	240
—	—	—	15	26	.6	20	.02	.02	.1	0	241
—	—	—	50	23	1.0	360	.04	.03	1.1	5	242
—	—	—	14	22	.6	10	.05	.02	.2	52	243
—	—	—	15	23	.6	640	.05	.02	.3	52	244
—	—	—	20	31	.8	20	.07	.03	.3	72	245
—	—	—	44	32	.7	20	.07	.04	.5	75	246
—	—	—	18	31	.7	20	.07	.04	.5	72	247
—	—	—	23	22	.5	(10)	.09	.04	.4	92	248
—	—	—	24	20	1.0	20	.07	.04	.4	84	249
—	—	—	32	20	1.0	20	.07	.04	.4	78	250

[8] Value based on varieties with orange-colored flesh, for green-fleshed varieties value is about 540 I.U. per ½ melon.

[9] About 5 milligrams per 8 fluid ounces is from cranberries. Ascorbic acid is usually added to approximately 100 milligrams per 8 fluid ounces.

[10] For white-fleshed varieties value is about 20 I.U. per cup; for red-fleshed varieties, 1080 I.U. per cup.

Food, approximate measure, and weight (in grams)			Water	Food energy	Protein	Fat (total lipid)
FRUITS AND FRUIT PRODUCTS— *Continued*						
Grapefruit juice—*Continued*						
Frozen, concentrate, unsweetened:		*Grams*	*Per Cent*	*Calories*	*Grams*	*Grams*
251	Undiluted, can, 6 fluid ounces	1 can	207	62	300	4	1
252	Diluted with 3 parts water, by volume	1 cup	247	89	100	1	Trace
Frozen, concentrate, sweetened:						
253	Undiluted, can, 6 fluid ounces	1 can	211	57	350	3	1
254	Diluted with 3 parts water, by volume	1 cup	249	88	115	1	Trace
Dehydrated:						
255	Crystals, can, net weight 4 ounces	1 can	114	1	430	5	1
256	Prepared with water (1 pound yields about 1 gallon)	1 cup	247	90	100	1	Trace
Grapes, raw:						
257	American type (slip skin), such as Concord, Delaware, Niagara, Catawba, and Scuppernong	1 cup	153	82	65	1	1
258	European type (adherent skin), such as Malaga, Muscat, Thompson Seedless, Emperor, and Flame Tokay[5]	1 cup	160	81	95	1	Trace
259	Grape juice, bottled or canned	1 cup	254	83	165	1	Trace
260	Lemons, raw, medium, 2⅕-inch diameter, size 150[5]	1 lemon	106	90	20	1	Trace
Lemon juice:						
261	Fresh	1 cup	246	91	60	1	Trace
262		1 tablespoon	15	91	5	Trace	Trace
263	Canned, unsweetened	1 cup	245	92	55	1	Trace
Lemonade concentrate, frozen, sweetened:						
264	Undiluted, can, 6 fluid ounces	1 can	220	48	430	Trace	Trace
265	Diluted with 4⅓ parts water, by volume	1 cup	248	88	110	Trace	Trace
Lime juice:						
266	Fresh,	1 cup	246	90	65	1	Trace
267	Canned	1 cup	246	90	65	1	Trace
Limeade concentrate, frozen, sweetened:						
268	Undiluted, can, 6 fluid ounces	1 can	218	50	410	Trace	Trace

[Dashes show that no basis could be found for imputing a value although there was some reason to believe that a measurable amount of the constituent might be present]

Fatty acids			Carbo-hydrate	Calcium	Iron	Vitamin A value	Thia-mine	Ribo-flavin	Niacin	Ascorbic acid	
Satu-rated (total)	Unsaturated										
	Oleic	Linoleic									
Grams	Grams	Grams	Grams	Milli-grams	Milli-grams	Inter-national units	Milli-grams	Milli-grams	Milli-grams	Milli-grams	
—	—	—	72	70	0.8	60	0.29	0.12	1.4	286	251
—	—	—	24	25	.2	20	.10	.04	.5	96	252
—	—	—	85	59	.6	50	.24	.11	1.2	245	253
—	—	—	28	20	.2	20	.08	.03	.4	82	254
—	—	—	103	99	1.1	90	.41	.18	2.0	399	255
—	—	—	24	22	.2	20	.10	.05	.5	92	256
—	—	—	15	15	.4	100	.05	.03	.2	3	257
—	—	—	25	17	.6	140	.07	.04	.4	6	258
—	—	—	42	28	.8	——	.10	.05	.6	Trace	259
—	—	—	6	18	.4	10	.03	.01	.1	38	260
—	—	—	20	17	.5	40	.08	.03	.2	113	261
—	—	—	1	1	Trace	Trace	Trace	Trace	Trace	7	262
—	—	—	19	17	.5	40	.07	.03	.2	102	263
—	—	—	112	9	.4	40	.05	.06	.7	66	264
—	—	—	28	2	.1	10	.01	.01	.2	17	265
—	—	—	22	22	.5	30	.05	.03	.3	80	266
—	—	—	22	22	.5	30	.05	.03	.3	52	267
—	—	—	108	11	.2	Trace	.02	.02	.2	26	268

Food, approximate measure, and weight (in grams)			Water	Food energy	Protein	Fat (total lipid)

FRUITS AND FRUIT PRODUCTS— *Continued*

	Food, approximate measure, and weight (in grams)			Water	Food energy	Protein	Fat (total lipid)
	Limeade concentrate, frozen, sweetened—*Continued*		Grams	Per Cent	Calories	Grams	Grams
269	Diluted with 4⅓ parts water, by volume	1 cup	248	90	105	Trace	Trace
	Oranges, raw:						
270	California, Navel (winter), 2⅘-inch diameter, size 88[5]	1 orange	180	85	60	2	Trace
271	Florida, all varieties, 3-inch diameter[5]	1 orange	210	86	75	1	Trace
	Orange juice:						
	Fresh:						
272	California, Valencia (summer)	1 cup	249	88	115	2	1
	Florida varieties:						
273	Early and mid-season	1 cup	247	90	100	1	Trace
274	Late, season Valencia	1 cup	248	88	110	1	Trace
275	Canned, unsweetened	1 cup	249	87	120	2	Trace
	Frozen concentrate:						
276	Undiluted, can, 6 fluid ounces	1 can	210	58	330	5	Trace
277	Diluted with 3 parts water, by volume	1 cup	248	88	110	2	Trace
	Dehydrated:						
278	Crystals, can, net weight 4 ounces	1 can	113	1	430	6	2
279	Prepared with water, 1 pound yields about 1 gallon	1 cup	248	88	115	1	Trace
	Orange and grapefruit juice:						
	Frozen concentrate:						
280	Undiluted, can, 6 fluid ounces	1 can	209	59	325	4	1
281	Diluted with 3 parts water, by volume	1 cup	248	88	110	1	Trace
282	Papayas, raw, ½-inch cubes	1 cup	182	89	70	1	Trace
	Peaches:						
	Raw:						
283	Whole, medium, 2-inch diameter, about 4 per pound[5]	1 peach	114	89	35	1	Trace

[Dashes show that no basis could be found for imputing a value although there was some reason to believe that a measurable amount of the constituent might be present]

Fatty acids			Carbo-hydrate	Calcium	Iron	Vitamin A value	Thia-mine	Ribo-flavin	Niacin	Ascorbic acid	
Satu-rated (total)	Unsaturated										
	Oleic	Linoleic									
Grams	Grams	Grams	Grams	Milli-grams	Milli-grams	Inter-national units	Milli-grams	Milli-grams	Milli-grams	Milli-grams	
———	———	———	27	2	Trace	Trace	Trace	Trace	Trace	6	269
———	———	———	16	49	.5	240	.12	.05	.5	75	270
———	———	———	19	67	.3	310	.16	.06	.6	70	271
———	———	———	26	27	.7	500	.22	.06	.9	122	272
———	———	———	23	25	.5	490	.22	.06	.9	127	273
———	———	———	26	25	.5	500	.22	.06	.9	92	274
———	———	———	28	25	1.0	500	.17	.05	.6	100	275
———	———	———	80	69	.8	1490	.63	.10	2.4	332	276
———	———	———	27	22	.2	500	.21	.03	.8	112	277
———	———	———	100	95	1.9	1900	.76	.24	3.3	406	278
———	———	———	27	25	.5	500	.20	.06	.9	108	279
———	———	———	78	61	.8	790	.47	.06	2.3	301	280
———	———	———	26	20	.2	270	.16	.02	.8	102	281
———	———	———	18	36	.5	3190	.07	.08	.5	102	282
———	———	———	10	9	.5	1320[11]	.02	.05	1.0	7	283

[11] Based on yellow-fleshed varieties; for white-fleshed varieties value is about 50 I.U. per 114-gram peach and 80 I.U. per cup of sliced peaches.

Food, approximate measure, and weight (in grams)			Water	Food energy	Protein	Fat (total lipid)

FRUITS AND FRUIT PRODUCTS— *Continued*

	Peaches—*Continued*		*Grams*	*Per Cent*	*Calories*	*Grams*	*Grams*
284	Sliced	1 cup	168	89	65	1	Trace
	Canned, yellow-fleshed, solids and liquid:						
	Sirup pack, heavy:						
285	Halves or slices	1 cup	257	79	200	1	Trace
286	Halves (medium) and sirup	2 halves and 2 table-spoons sirup	117	79	90	Trace	Trace
287	Water pack	1 cup	245	91	75	1	Trace
288	Strained or chopped (baby food)	1 ounce	28	78	25	Trace	Trace
	Dried:						
289	Uncooked	1 cup	160	25	420	5	1
290	Cooked, unsweet-ened, 10–12 halves and 6 tablespoons liquid	1 cup	270	77	220	3	1
	Frozen:						
291	Carton, 12 ounces, not thawed	1 carton	340	76	300	1	Trace
292	Can, 16 ounces, not thawed	1 can	454	76	400	2	Trace
293	Peach nectar, canned	1 cup	250	87	120	Trace	Trace
	Pears:						
294	Raw, 3 by 2½-inch diameter[5]	1 pear	182	83	100	1	1
	Canned, solids and liquid:						
	Sirup pack, heavy:						
295	Halves or slices	1 cup	255	80	195	1	1
296	Halves (medium) and sirup	2 halves and 2 table-spoons sirup	117	80	90	Trace	Trace
297	Water pack	1 cup	243	91	80	Trace	Trace
298	Strained or chopped (baby food)	1 ounce	28	82	20	Trace	Trace
299	Pear nectar, canned	1 cup	250	86	130	1	Trace
300	Persimmons, Japanese or kaki, raw, seedless, 2½-inch diameter[5]	1 persimmon	125	79	75	1	Trace
	Pineapple:						
301	Raw, diced	1 cup	140	85	75	1	Trace
	Canned, heavy sirup pack, solids and liquid:						
302	Crushed	1 cup	260	80	195	1	Trace

Table A–1—Continued

[Dashes show that no basis could be found for imputing a value although there was some reason to believe that a measurable amount of the constituent might be present]

Fatty acids			Carbo-hydrate	Calcium	Iron	Vitamin A value	Thia-mine	Ribo-flavin	Niacin	Ascorbic acid	
Satu-rated (total)	Unsaturated										
	Oleic	Linoleic									
Grams	Grams	Grams	Grams	Milli-grams	Milli-grams	Inter-national units	Milli-grams	Milli-grams	Milli-grams	Milli-grams	
———	———	———	16	15	0.8	2230[11]	0.03	0.08	1.6	12	284
———	———	———	52	10	.8	1100	.02	.06	1.4	7	285
———	———	———	24	5	.4	500	.01	.03	.7	3	286
———	———	———	20	10	.7	1100	.02	.06	1.4	7	287
———	———	———	6	2	.1	140	Trace	.01	.2	1	288
———	———	———	109	77	9.6	6240	.02	.31	8.5	28	289
———	———	———	58	41	5.1	3290	.01	.15	4.2	6	290
———	———	———	77	14	1.7	2210	.03	.14	2.4	135[12]	291
———	———	———	103	18	2.3	2950	.05	.18	3.2	181[12]	292
———	———	———	31	10	.5	1080	.02	.05	1.0	1	293
———	———	———	25	13	.5	30	.04	.07	.2	7	294
———	———	———	50	13	.5	Trace	.03	.05	.3	4	295
———	———	———	23	6	.2	Trace	.01	.02	.2	2	296
———	———	———	20	12	.5	Trace	.02	.05	.3	4	297
———	———	———	5	2	.1	10	Trace	.01	.1	1	298
———	———	———	33	8	.2	Trace	.01	.05	Trace	1	299
———	———	———	20	6	.4	2740	.03	.02	.1	11	300
———	———	———	19	24	.7	100	.12	.04	.3	24	301
———	———	———	50	29	.8	120	.20	.06	.5	17	302

[12] Average weighted in accordance with commercial freezing practices. For products without added ascorbic acid, value is about 37 milligrams per 12-ounce carton and 50 milligrams per 16-ounce can; for those with added ascorbic acid, 139 milligrams per 12 ounces and 186 milligrams per 16 ounces.

301

	Food, approximate measure, and weight (in grams)			Water	Food energy	Protein	Fat (total lipid)
	FRUITS AND FRUIT PRODUCTS— *Continued*						
	Pineapple—*Continued*		*Grams*	*Per Cent*	*Calories*	*Grams*	*Grams*
303	Sliced, slices and juice	2 small or 1 large and 2 tablespoons juice	122	80	90	Trace	Trace
304	Pineapple juice, canned	1 cup	249	86	135	1	Trace
	Plums, all except prunes:						
305	Raw, 2-inch diameter, about 2 ounces[5]	1 plum	60	87	25	Trace	Trace
	Canned, sirup pack (Italian prunes):						
306	Plums (with pits) and juice[5]	1 cup	256	77	205	1	Trace
307	Plums (without pits) and juice	3 plums and 2 tablespoons juice	122	77	100	Trace	Trace
	Prunes, dried, "softenized," medium:						
308	Uncooked	4 prunes	32	28	70	1	Trace
309	Cooked, unsweetened, 17–18 prunes and ⅓ cup liquid[5]	1 cup	270	66	295	2	1
310	Prunes with tapioca, canned, strained or junior (baby food)	1 ounce	28	77	25	Trace	Trace
311	Prune juice, canned	1 cup	256	80	200	1	Trace
312	Raisins, dried	1 cup	160	18	460	4	Trace
	Raspberries, red:						
313	Raw	1 cup	123	84	70	1	1
314	Frozen, 10-ounce carton, not thawed	1 carton	284	74	275	2	1
315	Rhubarb, cooked, sugar added	1 cup	272	63	385	1	Trace
	Strawberries:						
316	Raw, capped	1 cup	149	90	55	1	1
317	Frozen, 10-ounce carton, not thawed	1 carton	284	71	310	1	1
318	Frozen 16-ounce can, not thawed	1 can	454	71	495	2	1
319	Tangerines, raw, medium, 2½-inch diameter, about 4 per pound[5]	1 tangerine	114	87	40	1	Trace
	Tangerine juice:						
320	Canned, unsweetened	1 cup	248	89	105	1	Trace
	Frozen concentrate:						
321	Undiluted, can, 6 fluid ounces	1 can	210	58	340	4	1
322	Diluted with 3 parts water, by volume	1 cup	248	88	115	1	Trace

[Dashes show that no basis could be found for imputing a value although there was some reason to believe that a measurable amount of the constituent might be present]

Fatty acids			Carbo-hydrate	Calcium	Iron	Vitamin A value	Thia-mine	Ribo-flavin	Niacin	Ascorbic acid	
Satu-rated (total)	Unsaturated										
	Oleic	Linoleic									
Grams	Grams	Grams	Grams	Milli-grams	Milli-grams	Inter-national units	Milli-grams	Milli-grams	Milli-grams	Milli-grams	
—	—	—	24	13	0.4	50	0.09	0.03	0.2	8	303
—	—	—	34	37	.7	120	.12	.04	.5	22	304
—	—	—	7	7	.3	140	.02	.02	.3	3	305
—	—	—	53	22	2.2	2970	.05	.05	.9	4	306
—	—	—	26	11	1.1	1470	.03	.02	.5	2	307
—	—	—	18	14	1.1	440	.02	.04	.4	1	308
—	—	—	78	60	4.5	1860	.08	.18	1.7	2	309
—	—	—	6	2	.3	110	.01	.02	.1	1	310
—	—	—	49	36	10.5	—	.02	.03	1.1	4	311
—	—	—	124	99	5.6	30	.18	.13	.9	2	312
—	—	—	17	27	1.1	160	.04	.11	1.1	31	313
—	—	—	70	37	1.7	200	.06	.17	1.7	59	314
—	—	—	98	212	1.6	220	.06	.15	.7	17	315
—	—	—	13	31	1.5	90	.04	.10	1.0	88	316
—	—	—	79	40	2.0	90	.06	.17	1.5	150	317
—	—	—	126	64	3.2	150	.09	.27	2.4	240	318
—	—	—	10	34	.3	350	.05	.02	.1	26	319
—	—	—	25	45	.5	1040	.14	.04	.3	56	320
—	—	—	80	130	1.5	3070	.43	.12	.9	202	321
—	—	—	27	45	.5	1020	.14	.04	.3	67	322

Food, approximate measure, and weight (in grams)			Water	Food energy	Protein	Fat (total lipid)	
	FRUITS AND FRUIT PRODUCTS— *Continued*						
			Grams	*Per Cent*	*Calories*	*Grams*	*Grams*
323	Watermelon, raw, wedge, 4 by 8 inches ($^1/_{16}$ of 10 by 16-inch melon, about 2 pounds with rind)[5]	1 wedge	925	93	115	2	1
	GRAIN PRODUCTS						
324	Barley, pearled, light, uncooked	1 cup	203	11	710	17	2
325	Biscuits, baking powder with enriched flour, 2½-inch diameter	1 biscuit	38	27	140	3	6
326	Bran flakes (40 percent bran) added thiamine	1 ounce	28	3	85	3	1
	Breads:						
327	Boston brown bread, slice, 3 by ¾ inch	1 slice	48	45	100	3	1
	Cracked-wheat bread:						
328	Loaf, 1-pound, 20 slices	1 loaf	454	35	1190	39	10
329	Slice	1 slice	23	35	60	2	1
	French or vienna bread:						
330	Enriched, 1-pound loaf	1 loaf	454	31	1315	41	14
331	Unenriched, 1-pound loaf	1 loaf	454	31	1315	41	14
	Italian bread:						
332	Enriched, 1-pound loaf	1 loaf	454	32	1250	41	4
333	Unenriched, 1-pound loaf	1 loaf	454	32	1250	41	4
	Raisin bread:						
334	Loaf, 1-pound, 20 slices	1 loaf	454	35	1190	30	13
335	Slice	1 slice	23	35	60	2	1
	Rye bread:						
	American, light (⅓ rye, ⅔ wheat):						
336	Loaf, 1-pound, 20 slices	1 loaf	454	36	1100	41	5
337	Slice	1 slice	23	36	55	2	Trace
338	Pumpernickel, loaf, 1 pound	1 loaf	454	34	1115	41	5
	White bread, enriched:						
	1 to 2 per cent nonfat dry milk:						
339	Loaf, 1-pound, 20 slices	1 loaf	454	36	1225	39	15

Table A–1—*Continued*

[Dashes show that no basis could be found for imputing a value although there was some reason to believe that a measurable amount of the constituent might be present]

Fatty acids			Carbo-hydrate	Calcium	Iron	Vitamin A value	Thia-mine	Ribo-flavin	Niacin	Ascorbic acid	
Satu-rated (total)	Unsaturated										
	Oleic	Linoleic									
Grams	Grams	Grams	Grams	Milli-grams	Milli-grams	Inter-national units	Milli-grams	Milli-grams	Milli-grams	Milli-grams	
—	—	—	27	30	2.1	2510	0.13	0.13	0.7	30	323
Trace	1	1	160	32	4.1	0	.25	.17	6.3	0	324
2	3	1	17	46	.6	Trace	.08	.08	.7	Trace	325
—	—	—	23	20	1.2	0	.11	.05	1.7	0	326
—	—	—	22	43	.9	0	.05	.03	.6	0	327
2	5	2	236	399	5.0	Trace	.53	.42	5.8	Trace	328
—	—	—	12	20	.3	Trace	.03	.02	.3	Trace	329
3	8	2	251	195	10.0	Trace	1.26	.98	11.3	Trace	330
3	8	2	251	195	3.2	Trace	.39	.39	3.6	Trace	331
Trace	1	2	256	77	10.0	0	1.31	.93	11.7	0	332
Trace	1	2	256	77	3.2	0	.39	.27	3.6	0	333
3	8	2	243	322	5.9	Trace	.24	.42	3.0	Trace	334
—	—	—	12	16	.3	Trace	.01	.02	.2	Trace	335
—	—	—	236	340	7.3	0	.81	.33	6.4	0	336
—	—	—	12	17	.4	0	.04	.02	.3	0	337
—	—	—	241	381	10.9	0	1.05	.63	5.4	0	338
3	8	2	229	318	10.9	Trace	1.13	.77	10.4	Trace	339

Food, approximate measure, and weight (in grams)			Water	Food energy	Protein	Fat (total lipid)

GRAIN PRODUCTS—*Continued*

Breads—*Continued*

			Grams	*Per Cent*	*Calories*	*Grams*	*Grams*
	White bread, enriched—*Continued*						
340	Slice	1 slice	23	36	60	2	1
	3 to 4 per cent nonfat dry milk:[13]						
341	Loaf, 1-pound	1 loaf	454	36	1225	39	15
342	Slice, 20 per loaf	1 slice	23	36	60	2	1
343	Slice, toasted	1 slice	20	25	60	2	1
344	Slice, 26 per loaf	1 slice	17	36	45	1	1
	5 to 6 per cent nonfat dry milk:						
345	Loaf, 1-pound, 20 slices	1 loaf	454	35	1245	41	17
346	Slice	1 slice	23	35	65	2	1
	White bread, unenriched:						
	1 to 2 per cent nonfat dry milk:						
347	Loaf, 1-pound, 20 slices	1 loaf	454	36	1225	39	15
348	Slice	1 slice	23	36	60	2	1
	3 to 4 per cent nonfat dry milk:[13]						
349	Loaf, 1-pound	1 loaf	454	36	1225	39	15
350	Slice, 20 per loaf	1 slice	23	36	60	2	1
351	Slice, toasted	1 slice	20	25	60	2	1
352	Slice, 26 per loaf	1 slice	17	36	45	1	1
	5 to 6 per cent nonfat dry milk:						
353	Loaf, 1 pound, 20 slices	1 loaf	454	35	1245	41	17
354	Slice	1 slice	23	35	65	2	1
	Whole-wheat bread, made with 2 per cent nonfat dry milk:						
355	Loaf, 1-pound, 20 slices	1 loaf	454	36	1105	48	14
356	Slice	1 slice	23	36	55	2	1
357	Slice, toasted	1 slice	19	24	55	2	1
358	Breadcrumbs, dry, grated	1 cup	88	6	345	11	4
	Cakes:[14]						
359	Angelfood cake; sector, 2-inch ($1/12$ of 8-inch-diameter cake)	1 sector	40	32	110	3	Trace
360	Chocolate cake, chocolate icing; sector, 2-inch ($1/16$ of 10-inch-diameter layer cake)	1 sector	120	22	445	5	20
361	Fruitcake, dark (made with enriched flour); piece, 2 by 2 by $1/2$ inch	1 piece	30	18	115	1	5

[13] When the amount of nonfat dry milk in commercial white bread is unknown, values for bread with 3 to 4 per cent nonfat dry milk are suggested.

[14] Unenriched cake flour and vegetable cooking fat used unless otherwise specified.

TABLE A–1—*Continued*

[Dashes show that no basis could be found for imputing a value although there was some reason to believe that a measurable amount of the constituent might be present]

Fatty acids			Carbo-hydrate	Calcium	Iron	Vitamin A value	Thia-mine	Ribo-flavin	Niacin	Ascorbic acid	
Satu-rated (total)	Unsaturated										
	Oleic	Linoleic									
Grams	Grams	Grams	Grams	Milli-grams	Milli-grams	Inter-national units	Milli-grams	Milli-grams	Milli-grams	Milli-grams	
Trace	Trace	Trace	12	16	0.6	Trace	0.06	0.04	0.5	Trace	340
3	8	2	229	381	11.3	Trace	1.13	.95	10.8	Trace	341
Trace	Trace	Trace	12	19	.6	Trace	.06	.05	.6	Trace	342
Trace	Trace	Trace	12	19	.6	Trace	.05	.05	.6	Trace	343
Trace	Trace	Trace	9	14	.4	Trace	.04	.04	.4	Trace	344
4	10	2	228	435	11.3	Trace	1.22	.91	11.0	Trace	345
Trace	Trace	Trace	12	22	.6	Trace	.06	.05	.6	Trace	346
3	8	2	229	318	3.2	Trace	.40	.36	5.6	Trace	347
Trace	Trace	Trace	12	16	.2	Trace	.02	.02	.3	Trace	348
3	8	2	229	381	3.2	Trace	.31	.39	5.0	Trace	349
Trace	Trace	Trace	12	19	.2	Trace	.02	.02	.3	Trace	350
Trace	Trace	Trace	12	19	.2	Trace	.01	.02	.3	Trace	351
Trace	Trace	Trace	9	14	.1	Trace	.01	.01	.2	Trace	352
4	10	2	228	435	3.2	Trace	.32	.59	4.1	Trace	353
Trace	Trace	Trace	12	22	.2	Trace	.02	.03	.2	Trace	354
3	6	3	216	449	10.4	Trace	1.17	.56	12.9	Trace	355
Trace	Trace	Trace	11	23	.5	Trace	.06	.03	.7	Trace	356
Trace	Trace	Trace	11	22	.5	Trace	.05	.03	.6	Trace	357
1	2	1	65	107	3.2	Trace	.19	.26	3.1	Trace	358
——	——	——	24	4	.1	0	Trace	.06	.1	0	359
8	10	1	67	84	1.2	190[15]	.03	.12	.3	Trace	360
1	3	1	18	22	.8	40[15]	.04	.04	.2	Trace	361

[15] If the fat used in the recipe is butter or fortified margarine, the vitamin A value for chocolate cake with chocolate icing will be 490 I.U. per 2-inch sector, item 360; 100 I.U. for fruitcake, item 361; for plain cake without icing, 300 I.U. per piece, item 363; 220 I.U. per cupcake, item 364; for plain cake with icing, 440 I.U. per 2-inch sector, item 365; 220 I.U. per cupcake, item 366; and 300 I.U. for poundcake, item 367.

Food, approximate measure, and weight (in grams)			Water	Food energy	Protein	Fat (total lipid)

GRAIN PRODUCTS—*Continued*

	Cakes[14]—*Continued*		Grams	Per Cent	Calories	Grams	Grams
362	Gingerbread (made with enriched flour); piece, 2 by 2 by 2 inches	1 piece	55	31	175	2	6
	Plain cake and cupcakes, without icing:						
363	Piece, 3 by 2 by 1½ inches	1 piece	55	24	200	2	8
364	Cupcake, 2¾-inch diameter	1 cupcake	40	24	145	2	6
	Plain cake and cupcakes, with chocolate icing:						
365	Sector, 2-inch (1/16 of 10-inch-layer cake)	1 sector	100	21	370	4	14
366	Cupcake, 2¾-inch diameter	1 cupcake	50	21	185	2	7
367	Poundcake, old-fashioned (equal weights flour, sugar, fat, eggs); slice, 2¾ by 3 by ⅝ inch	1 slice	30	17	140	2	9
368	Sponge cake; sector, 2-inch (1/12 of 8-inch-diameter cake)	1 sector	40	32	120	3	2
	Cookies:						
369	Plain and assorted, 3-inch diameter	1 cooky	25	3	120	1	5
370	Fig bars, small	1 fig bar	16	14	55	1	1
371	Corn, rice and wheat flakes, mixed, added nutrients	1 ounce	28	3	110	2	Trace
	Corn flakes, added nutrients:						
372	Plain	1 ounce	28	4	110	2	Trace
373	Sugar-covered	1 ounce	28	2	110	1	Trace
	Corn grits, degermed, cooked:						
374	Enriched	1 cup	242	87	120	3	Trace
375	Unenriched	1 cup	242	87	120	3	Trace
	Cornmeal, white or yellow, dry:						
376	Whole ground, unbolted	1 cup	118	12	420	11	5
377	Degermed, enriched	1 cup	145	12	525	11	2
378	Corn muffins, made with enriched degermed cornmeal and enriched flour; muffin, 2¾-inch diameter	1 muffin	48	33	150	3	5
379	Corn, puffed, pre-sweetened, added nutrients	1 ounce	28	5	110	1	Trace

Table A-1—*Continued*

[Dashes show that no basis could be found for imputing a value although there was some reason to believe that a measurable amount of the constituent might be present]

Fatty acids			Carbo-hydrate	Calcium	Iron	Vitamin A value	Thia-mine	Ribo-flavin	Niacin	Ascorbic acid	
Satu-rated (total)	Unsaturated										
	Oleic	Linoleic									
Grams	Grams	Grams	Grams	Milli-grams	Milli-grams	Inter-national units	Milli-grams	Milli-grams	Milli-grams	Milli-grams	
1	4	Trace	29	37	1.3	50	0.06	0.06	0.5	0	362
2	5	1	31	35	.2	90[15]	.01	.05	.1	Trace	363
1	3	Trace	22	26	.2	70[15]	.01	.03	.1	Trace	364
5	7	1	59	63	.6	180[15]	.02	.09	.2	Trace	365
2	4	Trace	30	32	.3	90[15]	.01	.04	.1	Trace	366
2	5	1	14	6	.2	80[15]	.01	.03	.1	0	367
1	1	Trace	22	12	.5	180	.02	.06	.1	Trace	368
—	—	—	18	9	.2	20	.01	.01	.1	Trace	369
—	—	—	12	12	.2	20	.01	.01	.1	Trace	370
—	—	—	24	11	.5	0	.11	—	.9	0	371
—	—	—	24	5	.4	0	.12	.02	.6	0	372
—	—	—	26	3	.3	0	.12	.01	.5	0	373
—	—	—	27	2	.7[16]	150[17]	.10[16]	.07[16]	1.0[16]	0	374
—	—	—	27	2	.2	150[17]	.05	.02	.5	0	375
1	2	2	87	24	2.8	600[17]	.45	.13	2.4	0	376
Trace	1	1	114	9	4.2[16]	640[17]	.64[16]	.38[16]	5.1[16]	0	377
2	2	Trace	23	50	.8	80[18]	.09	.11	.8	Trace	378
—	—	—	26	3	.5	0	.12	.05	.6	0	379

[16] Iron, thiamine, riboflavin, and niacin are based on the minimum levels of enrichment specified in standards of identity promulgated under the Federal Food, Drug, and Cosmetic Act.
[17] Vitamin A value based on yellow product. White product contains only a trace.
[18] Based on recipe using white cornmeal; if yellow cornmeal is used, the vitamin A value is 140 I.U. per muffin.

	Food, approximate measure, and weight (in grams)			Water	Food energy	Protein	Fat (total lipid)
	GRAIN PRODUCTS—*Continued*						
			Grams	*Per Cent*	*Calories*	*Grams*	*Grams*
380	Corn, shredded, added nutrients	1 ounce	28	3	110	2	Trace
	Crackers:						
381	Graham, plain	4 small or 2 medium	14	6	55	1	1
382	Saltines, 2 inches square	2 crackers	8	4	35	1	1
	Soda:						
383	Cracker, 2½ inches square	2 crackers	11	4	50	1	1
384	Oyster crackers	10 crackers	10	4	45	1	1
385	Cracker meal	1 tablespoon	10	6	45	1	1
386	Doughnuts, cake type	1 doughnut	32	24	125	1	6
387	Farina, regular, enriched, cooked	1 cup	238	90	100	3	Trace
	Macaroni, cooked:						
	Enriched:						
388	Cooked, firm stage (8 to 10 minutes; undergoes additional cooking in a food mixture)	1 cup	130	64	190	6	1
389	Cooked until tender	1 cup	140	72	155	5	1
	Unenriched:						
390	Cooked, firm stage (8 to 10 minutes; undergoes additional cooking in a food mixture)	1 cup	130	64	190	6	1
391	Cooked until tender	1 cup	140	72	155	5	1
392	Macaroni (enriched) and cheese, baked	1 cup	220	58	470	18	24
393	Muffins, with enriched white flour: muffin, 2¾-inch diameter	1 muffin	48	38	140	4	5
	Noodles (egg noodles), cooked:						
394	Enriched	1 cup	160	70	200	7	2
395	Unenriched	1 cup	160	70	200	7	2
396	Oats (with or without corn) puffed, added nutrients	1 ounce	28	3	115	3	2
397	Oatmeal or rolled oats, regular or quick-cooking, cooked	1 cup	236	86	130	5	2
	Pancakes (griddlecakes), 4-inch diameter:						
398	Wheat, enriched flour (home recipe)	1 cake	27	50	60	2	2

[Dashes show that no basis could be found for imputing a value although there was some reason to believe that a measurable amount of the constituent might be present]

Fatty acids			Carbohydrate	Calcium	Iron	Vitamin A value	Thiamine	Riboflavin	Niacin	Ascorbic acid	
Saturated (total)	Unsaturated										
	Oleic	Linoleic									
Grams	Grams	Grams	Grams	Milligrams	Milligrams	International units	Milligrams	Milligrams	Milligrams	Milligrams	
——	——	——	25	1	0.7	0	0.12	0.05	0.6	0	380
——	——	——	10	6	.2	0	.01	.03	.2	0	381
——	——	——	6	2	.1	0	Trace	Trace	.1	0	382
Trace	1	Trace	8	2	.2	0	Trace	Trace	.1	0	383
Trace	1	Trace	7	2	.2	0	Trace	Trace	.1	0	384
Trace	1	Trace	7	2	.1	0	.01	Trace	.1	0	385
1	4	Trace	16	13	.4[19]	30	.05[19]	.05[19]	.4[19]	Trace	386
——	——	——	21	10	.7[16]	0	.11[16]	.07[16]	1.0[16]	0	387
——	——	——	39	14	1.4[16]	0	.23[16]	.14[16]	1.9[16]	0	388
——	——	——	32	11	1.3[16]	0	.19[16]	.11[16]	1.5[16]	0	389
——	——	——	39	14	.6	0	.02	.02	.5	0	390
——	——	——	32	11	.6	0	.02	.02	.4	0	391
11	10	1	44	398	2.0	950	.22	.44	2.0	Trace	392
1	3	Trace	20	50	.8	50	.08	.11	.7	Trace	393
1	1	Trace	37	16	1.4[16]	110	.23[16]	.14[16]	1.8[16]	0	394
1	1	Trace	37	16	1.0	110	.04	.03	.7	0	395
Trace	1	1	21	50	1.3	0	.28	.05	.5	0	396
Trace	1	1	23	21	1.4	0	.19	.05	.3	0	397
Trace	1	Trace	9	27	.4	30	.05	.06	.3	Trace	398

[19] Based on product made with enriched flour. With unenriched flour, approximate values per doughnut are: Iron, 0.2 milligram; thiamine, 0.01 milligram; riboflavin, 0.03 milligram; niacin, 0.2 milligram.

Food, approximate measure, and weight (in grams)			Water	Food energy	Protein	Fat (total lipid)	

GRAIN PRODUCTS—*Continued*

	Pancakes—*Continued*		Grams	Per Cent	Calories	Grams	Grams	
399	Buckwheat (buckwheat pancake mix, made with egg and milk)	1 cake	27	58	55	2	2	
	Piecrust, plain, baked: Enriched flour:							
400	Lower crust, 9-inch shell	1 crust	135	15	675	8	45	
401	Double crust, 9-inch pie	1 double crust	270	15	1350	16	90	
	Unenriched flour:							
402	Lower crust, 9-inch shell	1 crust	135	15	675	8	45	
403	Double crust, 9-inch pie	1 double crust	270	15	1350	16	90	
	Pies (piecrust made with unenriched flour); sector, 4-inch, $1/7$ of 9-inch-diameter pie:							
404	Apple	1 sector	135	48	345	3	15	
405	Cherry	1 sector	135	47	355	4	15	
406	Custard	1 sector	130	58	280	8	14	
407	Lemon meringue	1 sector	120	47	305	4	12	
408	Mince	1 sector	135	43	365	3	16	
409	Pumpkin	1 sector	130	59	275	5	15	
410	Pizza (cheese); 5½-inch sector; ⅛ of 14-inch-diameter pie	1 sector	75	45	185	7	6	
411	Popcorn, popped, with added oil and salt	1 cup	14	3	65	1	3	
412	Pretzels, small stick	5 sticks	5	8	20	Trace	Trace	
	Rice, white (fully milled or polished), enriched, cooked:							
413	Common commercial varieties, all types	1 cup	168	73	185	3	Trace	
414	Long grain, parboiled	1 cup	176	73	185	4	Trace	
415	Rice, puffed, added nutrients (without salt)	1 cup	14	4	55	1	Trace	
416	Rice flakes, added nutrients	1 cup	30	3	115	2	Trace	
	Rolls:							
	Plain, pan; 12 per 16 ounces:							
417	Enriched	1 roll	38	31	115	3	2	
418	Unenriched	1 roll	38	31	115	3	2	
419	Hard, round; 12 per 22 ounces	1 roll	52	25	160	5	2	
420	Sweet, pan; 12 per 18 ounces	1 roll	43	32	135	4	4	

[Dashes show that no basis could be found for imputing a value although there was some reason to believe that a measurable amount of the constituent might be present]

| Saturated (total) | Unsaturated | | Carbo-hydrate | Calcium | Iron | Vitamin A value | Thiamine | Riboflavin | Niacin | Ascorbic acid | |
	Oleic	Linoleic									
Grams	Grams	Grams	Grams	Milligrams	Milligrams	International units	Milligrams	Milligrams	Milligrams	Milligrams	
1	1	Trace	6	59	0.4	60	0.03	0.04	0.2	Trace	399
10	29	3	59	19	2.3	0	.27	.19	2.4	0	400
21	58	7	118	38	4.6	0	.55	.39	4.9	0	401
10	29	3	59	19	.7	0	.04	.04	.6	0	402
21	58	7	118	38	1.4	0	.08	.07	1.3	0	403
4	9	1	51	11	.4	40	.03	.02	.5	1	404
4	10	1	52	19	.4	590	.03	.03	.6	1	405
5	8	1	30	125	.8	300	.07	.21	.4	0	406
4	7	1	45	17	.6	200	.04	.10	.2	4	407
4	10	1	56	38	1.4	Trace	.09	.05	.5	1	408
5	7	1	32	66	.6	3210	.04	.13	.6	Trace	409
2	3	Trace	27	107	.7	290	.04	.12	.7	4	410
2	Trace	Trace	8	1	.3	——	——	.01	.2	0	411
——	——	——	4	1	0	0	Trace	Trace	Trace	0	412
——	——	——	41	17	1.5[20]	0	.19[20]	.01[20]	1.6[20]	0	413
——	——	——	41	33	1.4[20]	0	.19[20]	.02[20]	2.0[20]	0	414
——	——	——	13	3	.3	0	.06	.01	.6	0	415
——	——	——	26	9	.5	0	.10	.02	1.6	0	416
Trace	1	Trace	20	28	.7	Trace	.11	.07	.8	Trace	417
Trace	1	Trace	20	28	.3	Trace	.02	.03	.3	Trace	418
Trace	1	Trace	31	24	.4	Trace	.03	.05	.4	Trace	419
1	2	Trace	21	37	.3	30	.03	.06	.4	Trace	420

[20] Iron, thiamine, and niacin are based on the minimum levels of enrichment specified in standards of identity promulgated under the Federal Food, Drug, and Cosmetic Act. Riboflavin is based on unenriched rice. When the minimum level of enrichment for riboflavin specified in the standards of identity becomes effective the value will be 0.12 milligram per cup of parboiled rice and of white rice.

	Food, approximate measure, and weight (in grams)			Water	Food energy	Protein	Fat total (lipid)
	GRAIN PRODUCTS—*Continued*						
			Grams	*Per Cent*	*Calories*	*Grams*	*Grams*
421	Rye wafers, whole-grain, 1⅞ by 3½ inches	2 wafers	13	6	45	2	Trace
	Spaghetti:						
	Cooked, tender stage (14 to 20 minutes):						
422	Enriched	1 cup	140	72	155	5	1
423	Unenriched	1 cup	140	72	155	5	1
424	Spaghetti with meat balls in tomato sauce (home recipe)	1 cup	250	70	335	19	12
425	Spaghetti in tomato sauce with cheese (home recipe)	1 cup	250	77	260	9	9
426	Waffles, with enriched flour, ½ by 4½ by 5½ inches	1 waffle	75	41	210	7	7
	Wheat, puffed						
427	With added nutrients (without salt)	1 ounce	28	3	105	4	Trace
428	With added nutrients, with sugar and honey	1 ounce	28	3	105	2	1
429	Wheat, rolled; cooked	1 cup	236	80	175	5	1
430	Wheat, shredded, plain (long, round, or bite-size)	1 ounce	28	7	100	3	1
431	Wheat and malted barley flakes, with added nutrients	1 ounce	28	3	110	2	Trace
432	Wheat flakes, with added nutrients	1 ounce	28	4	100	3	Trace
	Wheat flours:						
433	Whole-wheat, from hard wheats, stirred	1 cup	120	12	400	16	2
	All-purpose or family flour:						
434	Enriched, sifted	1 cup	110	12	400	12	1
435	Unenriched, sifted	1 cup	110	12	400	12	1
436	Self-rising, enriched	1 cup	110	11	385	10	1
437	Cake or pastry flour, sifted	1 cup	100	12	365	8	1
438	Wheat germ, crude, commercially milled	1 cup	68	11	245	18	7
	FATS, OILS						
	Butter, 4 sticks per pound:						
439	Sticks, 2	1 cup	227	16	1625	1	184
440	Stick, ⅛	1 tablespoon	14	16	100	Trace	11

[Dashes show that no basis could be found for imputing a value although there was some reason to believe that a measurable amount of the constituent might be present]

Fatty acids			Carbo-hydrate	Calcium	Iron	Vitamin A value	Thia-mine	Ribo-flavin	Niacin	Ascorbic acid	
Satu-rated (total)	Unsaturated										
	Oleic	Linoleic									
Grams	Grams	Grams	Grams	Milli-grams	Milli-grams	Inter-national units	Milli-grams	Milli-grams	Milli-grams	Milli-grams	
——	——	——	10	7	0.5	0	0.04	0.03	0.2	0	421
——	——	——	32	11	1.3[16]	0	.19[16]	.11[16]	1.5[16]	0	422
——	——	——	32	11	.6	0	.02	.02	.4	0	423
4	6	1	39	125	3.8	1600	.26	.30	4.0	22	424
2	5	1	37	80	2.2	1080	.24	.18	2.4	14	425
2	4	1	28	85	1.3	250	.13	.19	1.0	Trace	426
——	——	——	22	8	1.2	0	.15	.07	2.2	0	427
——	——	——	25	7	.9	0	.14	.05	1.8	0	428
——	——	——	40	19	1.7	0	.17	.06	2.1	0	429
——	——	——	23	12	1.0	0	.06	.03	1.2	0	430
——	——	——	24	14	.7	0	.13	.03	1.1	0	431
——	——	——	23	12	1.2	0	.18	.04	1.4	0	432
Trace	1	1	85	49	4.0	0	.66	.14	5.2	0	433
Trace	Trace	Trace	84	18	3.2[16]	0	.48[16]	.29[16]	3.8[16]	0	434
Trace	Trace	Trace	84	18	.9	0	.07	.05	1.0	0	435
Trace	Trace	Trace	82	292	3.2[16]	0	.49[16]	.29[16]	3.9[16]	0	436
Trace	Trace	Trace	79	17	.5	0	.03	.03	.7	0	437
1	2	4	32	49	6.4	0	1.36	.46	2.9	0	438
101	61	6	1	45	0	7500[21]	——	——	——	0	439
6	4	Trace	Trace	3	0	460[21]	——	——	——	0	440

[21] Year-round average.

	Food, approximate measure, and weight (in grams)			Water	Food energy	Protein	Fat (total lipid)
	FATS, OILS—*Continued*						
	Butter—*Continued*		Grams	Per Cent	Calories	Grams	Grams
441	Pat or square (64 per pound)	1 pat	7	16	50	Trace	6
	Fats, cooking:						
442	Lard	1 cup	220	0	1985	0	220
443	Lard	1 tablespoon	14	0	125	0	14
444	Vegetable fats	1 cup	200	0	1770	0	200
445	Vegetable fats	1 tablespoon	12.5	0	110	0	12
	Margarine, 4 sticks per pound:						
446	Sticks, 2	1 cup	227	16	1635	1	184
447	Stick, ⅛	1 tablespoon	14	16	100	Trace	11
448	Pat or square (64 per pound)	1 pat	7	16	50	Trace	6
	Oils, salad or cooking:						
449	Corn	1 tablespoon	14	0	125	0	14
450	Cottonseed	1 tablespoon	14	0	125	0	14
451	Olive	1 tablespoon	14	0	125	0	14
452	Soybean	1 tablespoon	14	0	125	0	14
	Salad dressings:						
453	Blue cheese	1 tablespoon	16	32	80	1	8
454	Commercial, mayonnaise type	1 tablespoon	15	41	65	Trace	6
455	French	1 tablespoon	15	39	60	Trace	6
456	Home cooked, boiled	1 tablespoon	17	68	30	1	2
457	Mayonnaise	1 tablespoon	15	15	110	Trace	12
458	Thousand island	1 tablespoon	15	32	75	Trace	8
	SUGARS, SWEETS						
	Candy:						
459	Caramels	1 ounce	28	8	115	1	3
460	Chocolate, milk, plain	1 ounce	28	1	150	2	9
461	Fudge, plain	1 ounce	28	8	115	1	3
462	Hard candy	1 ounce	28	1	110	0	Trace
463	Marshmallows	1 ounce	28	17	90	1	Trace
464	Chocolate sirup, thin type	1 tablespoon	20	32	50	Trace	Trace
465	Honey, strained or extracted	1 tablespoon	21	17	65	Trace	0
466	Jams and preserves	1 tablespoon	20	29	55	Trace	Trace
467	Jellies	1 tablespoon	20	29	55	Trace	Trace
	Molasses, cane:						
468	Light (first extraction)	1 tablespoon	20	24	50	——	——
469	Blackstrap (third extraction)	1 tablespoon	20	24	45	——	——
470	Sirup, table blends (chiefly corn, light and dark)	1 tablespoon	20	24	60	0	0

[Dashes show that no basis could be found for imputing a value although there was some reason to believe that a measurable amount of the constituent might be present]

Fatty acids			Carbo-hydrate	Calcium	Iron	Vitamin A value	Thia-mine	Ribo-flavin	Niacin	Ascorbic acid	
Satu-rated (total)	Unsaturated										
	Oleic	Linoleic									
Grams	Grams	Grams	Grams	Milli-grams	Milli-grams	Inter-national units	Milli-grams	Milli-grams	Milli-grams	Milli-grams	
3	2	Trace	Trace	1	0	230[21]	——	——	——	0	441
84	101	22	0	0	0	0	0	0	0	0	442
5	6	1	0	0	0	0	0	0	0	0	443
46	130	14	0	0	0	——	0	0	0	0	444
3	8	1	0	0	0	——	0	0	0	0	445
37	105	33	1	45	0	7500[22]	——	——	——	0	446
2	6	2	Trace	3	0	460[22]	——	——	——	0	447
1	3	1	Trace	1	0	230[22]	——	——	——	0	448
1	4	7	0	0	0	——	0	0	0	0	449
4	3	7	0	0	0	——	0	0	0	0	450
2	11	1	0	0	0	——	0	0	0	0	451
2	3	7	0	0	0	——	0	0	0	0	452
2	2	4	1	13	Trace	30	Trace	0.02	Trace	Trace	453
1	1	3	2	2	Trace	30	Trace	Trace	Trace	——	454
1	1	3	3	2	.1	——	——	——	——	——	455
1	1	Trace	3	15	.1	80	.01	.03	Trace	Trace	456
2	3	6	Trace	3	.1	40	Trace	.01	Trace	——	457
1	2	4	2	2	.1	50	Trace	Trace	Trace	Trace	458
2	1	Trace	22	42	.4	Trace	.01	.05	Trace	Trace	459
5	3	Trace	16	65	.3	80	.02	.09	.1	Trace	460
2	1	Trace	21	22	.3	Trace	.01	.03	.1	Trace	461
——	——	——	28	6	.5	0	0	0	0	0	462
——	——	——	23	5	.5	0	0	Trace	Trace	0	463
Trace	Trace	Trace	13	3	.3	——	Trace	.01	.1	0	464
——	——	——	17	1	.1	0	Trace	.01	.1	Trace	465
——	——	——	14	4	.2	Trace	Trace	.01	Trace	Trace	466
——	——	——	14	4	.3	Trace	Trace	.01	Trace	1	467
——	——	——	13	33	.9	——	.01	.01	Trace	——	468
——	——	——	11	137	3.2	——	.02	.04	.4	——	469
——	——	——	15	9	.8	0	0	0	0	0	470

[22] Based on the average vitamin A content of fortified margarine. Federal specifications for fortified margarine require a minimum of 15,000 I.U. of vitamin A per pound.

317

	Food, approximate measure, and weight (in grams)			Water	Food energy	Protein	Fat (total lipid)
			Grams	Per Cent	Calories	Grams	Grams
	SUGARS, SWEETS—*Continued*						
	Sugars (cane or beet):						
471	Granulated	1 cup	200	Trace	770	0	0
472		1 tablespoon	12	Trace	45	0	0
473	Lump, 1⅛ by ¾ by ⅜	1 lump	6	Trace	25	0	0
474	Powdered, stirred be-	1 cup	128	Trace	495	0	0
475	fore measuring	1 tablespoon	8	Trace	30	0	0
476	Brown, firm-packed	1 cup	220	2	820	0	0
477		1 tablespoon	14	2	50	0	0
	MISCELLANEOUS ITEMS						
478	Beer (average 3.6 per cent alcohol by weight)	1 cup	240	92	100	1	0
	Beverages, carbonated:						
479	Cola type	1 cup	240	90	95	0	0
480	Ginger ale	1 cup	230	92	70	0	0
481	Bouillon cube, ⅝ inch	1 cube	4	4	5	1	Trace
	Chili powder. *See* Vegetables, peppers						
482	Chili sauce (mainly tomatoes)	1 tablespoon	17	68	20	Trace	Trace
	Chocolate:						
483	Bitter or baking	1 ounce	28	2	145	3	15
484	Sweet	1 ounce	28	1	150	1	10
	Cider. *See* Fruits, apple juice						
	Gelatin, dry:						
485	Plain	1 tablespoon	10	13	35	9	Trace
486	Dessert powder, 3-ounce package	½ cup	85	2	315	8	0
	Gelatin dessert, ready-to-eat						
487	Plain	1 cup	239	84	140	4	0
488	With fruit	1 cup	241	82	160	3	Trace
	Olives, pickled:						
489	Green	4 medium or 3 extra large or 2 giant	16	78	15	Trace	2
490	Ripe: Mission	3 small or 2 large	10	73	15	Trace	2
	Pickles, cucumber:						
491	Dill, large, 4 by 1¾ inches	1 pickle	135	93	15	1	Trace
492	Sweet, 2¾ by ¾ inches	1 pickle	20	61	30	Trace	Trace
	Popcorn. *See* Grain products						
493	Sherbet, orange	1 cup	193	67	260	2	2
	Soups, canned; ready-to-serve (prepared with equal volume of water):						
494	Bean with pork	1 cup	250	84	170	8	6

[Dashes show that no basis could be found for imputing a value although there was some reason to believe that a measurable amount of the constituent might be present]

Fatty acids			Carbo-hydrate	Calcium	Iron	Vitamin A value	Thia-mine	Ribo-flavin	Niacin	Ascorbic acid	
Satu-rated (total)	Unsaturated										
	Oleic	Linoleic									
Grams	Grams	Grams	Grams	Milli-grams	Milli-grams	Inter-national units	Milli-grams	Milli-grams	Milli-grams	Milli-grams	
----	----	----	199	0	0.2	0	0	0	0	0	471
----	----	----	12	0	Trace	0	0	0	0	0	472
----	----	----	6	0	Trace	0	0	0	0	0	473
----	----	----	127	0	.1	0	0	0	0	0	474
----	----	----	8	0	Trace	0	0	0	0	0	475
----	----	----	212	187	7.5	0	.02	.07	.4	0	476
----	----	----	13	12	.5	0	Trace	Trace	Trace	0	477
----	----	----	9	12	Trace	----	.01	.07	1.6	----	478
----	----	----	24	----	----	0	0	0	0	0	479
----	----	----	18	----	----	0	0	0	0	0	480
----	----	----	Trace	----	----	----	----	----	----	----	481
----	----	----	4	3	.1	240	.02	.01	.3	3	482
8	6	Trace	8	22	1.9	20	.01	.07	.4	0	483
6	4	Trace	16	27	.4	Trace	.01	.04	.1	Trace	484
----	----	----	----	----	----	----	----	----	----	----	485
----	----	----	75	----	----	----	----	----	----	----	486
----	----	----	34	----	----	----	----	----	----	----	487
----	----	----	40	----	----	----	----	----	----	----	488
Trace	2	Trace	Trace	8	.2	40	----	----	----	----	489
Trace	2	Trace	Trace	9	.1	10	Trace	Trace	----	----	490
----	----	----	3	35	1.4	140	Trace	.03	Trace	8	491
----	----	----	7	2	.2	20	Trace	Trace	Trace	1	492
----	----	----	59	31	Trace	110	.02	.06	Trace	4	493
1	2	2	22	62	2.2	650	.14	.07	1.0	2	494

	Food, approximate measure, and weight (in grams)			Water	Food energy	Protein	Fat (total lipid)

MISCELLANEOUS ITEMS—*Continued*

Soups, canned: ready-to-serve—*Continued*

			Grams	Per Cent	Calories	Grams	Grams
495	Beef noodle	1 cup	250	93	70	4	3
496	Beef bouillon, broth, consomme	1 cup	240	96	30	5	0
497	Chicken noodle	1 cup	250	93	65	4	2
498	Clam chowder	1 cup	255	92	85	2	3
499	Cream soup (mushroom)	1 cup	240	90	135	2	10
500	Minestrone	1 cup	245	90	105	5	3
501	Pea, green	1 cup	245	86	130	6	2
502	Tomato	1 cup	245	90	90	2	2
503	Vegetable with beef broth	1 cup	250	92	80	3	2
504	Starch (cornstarch)	1 cup	128	12	465	Trace	Trace
505		1 tablespoon	8	12	30	Trace	Trace
506	Tapioca, quick-cooking	1 cup	152	13	535	1	Trace
507	granulated, dry, stirred before measuring	1 tablespoon	10	13	35	Trace	Trace
508	Vinegar	1 tablespoon	15	——	2	0	——
509	White sauce, medium	1 cup	265	73	430	10	33
	Yeast:						
	Baker's:						
510	Compressed	1 ounce	28	71	25	3	Trace
511	Dry active	1 ounce	28	5	80	10	Trace
512	Brewer's dry, debittered	1 tablespoon	8	5	25	3	Trace
	Yoghurt. *See* Milk, cream, cheese; related products						

[Dashes show that no basis could be found for imputing a value although there was some reason to believe that a measurable amount of the constituent might be present]

Fatty acids			Carbo-hydrate	Calcium	Iron	Vitamin A value	Thia-mine	Ribo-flavin	Niacin	Ascorbic acid	
Satu-rated (total)	Unsaturated										
	Oleic	Linoleic									
Grams	Grams	Grams	Grams	Milli-grams	Milli-grams	Inter-national units	Milli-grams	Milli-grams	Milli-grams	Milli-grams	
1	1	1	7	8	1.0	50	0.05	0.06	1.1	Trace	495
0	0	0	3	Trace	.5	Trace	Trace	.02	1.2	—	496
Trace	1	1	8	10	0.5	50	.02	.02	.8	Trace	497
—	—	—	13	36	1.0	920	.03	.03	1.0	—	498
1	3	5	10	41	.5	70	.02	.12	.7	Trace	499
—	—	—	14	37	1.0	2350	.07	.05	1.0	—	500
1	1	Trace	23	44	1.0	340	.05	.05	1.0	7	501
Trace	1	1	16	15	.7	1000	.06	.05	1.1	12	502
—	—	—	14	20	.8	3250	.05	.02	1.2	—	503
—	—	—	112	0	0	0	0	0	0	0	504
—	—	—	7	0	0	0	0	0	0	0	505
—	—	—	131	15	.6	0	0	0	0	0	506
—	—	—	9	1	Trace	0	0	0	0	0	507
—	—	—	1	1	.1	—	—	—	—	—	508
18	11	1	23	305	.5	1220	.12	.44	.6	Trace	509
—	—	—	3	4	1.4	Trace	.20	.47	3.2	Trace	510
—	—	—	11	12	4.6	Trace	.66	1.53	10.4	Trace	511
—	—	—	3	17	1.4	Trace	1.25	.34	3.0	Trace	512

TABLE A–2 FOOD EXCHANGE LISTS FOR CALCULATING DIETS *
Foods are divided into six groups, according to their composition.

| Food Exchange | Quantity for One Exchange | | | | | |
	Measure	Weight (gm)	Carbo-hydrate (gm)	Protein (gm)	Fat (gm)	Calories
Milk	8 oz	240	12	8	10	170
Vegetables—A	As desired	—	—	—	—	—
Vegetables—B	½ cup	100	7	2	—	36
Fruit	Varies	—	10	—	—	40
Bread	Varies	—	15	2	—	68
Meat	1 oz	30	—	7	5	73
Fat	1 teaspoon	5	—	—	—	45

* Caso, E. K. "Calculation of Diabetic Diets," *J. Amer. Diet. Ass.*, 26:575, 1950.

LIST 1—MILK EXCHANGES

PER EXCHANGE: CARBOHYDRATE, 12 GM; PROTEIN, 8 GM; FAT, 10 GM.

	Measure
Milk, whole (plain or homogenized)	1 cup (8 ounces)
Milk, skim, liquid *	1 cup
Milk, evaporated	½ cup
Milk, powdered whole	3–5 tablespoons †
Milk, nonfat dry *	3–5 tablespoons †
Buttermilk (from whole milk)	1 cup
Buttermilk (from skim milk) *	1 cup

* Because these forms of milk contain no fat, two fat exchanges may be added to the diet when they are used; or one exchange of these forms of milk may be calculated as carbohydrate 12; protein, 8; and fat, 0.

† The amount of milk powder to use depends upon the brand used; read package direction for the equivalent for 1 cup liquid milk.

LIST 2—VEGETABLE EXCHANGES

GROUP A VEGETABLES—NEGLIGIBLE CARBOHYDRATE, PROTEIN, AND FAT IF 1 CUP (200 GM) OR LESS IS USED. COUNT EACH ADDITIONAL CUP AS ONE EXCHANGE OF GROUP B VEGETABLE.

Asparagus
Beans, string, young
Broccoli *
Brussels sprouts
Cabbage
Cauliflower
Celery
Chicory *
Cucumbers
Escarole *

Eggplant
Greens *
　beet greens
　chard, Swiss
　collard
　dandelion
　kale
　mustard
　spinach
　turnip greens

Lettuce
Mushrooms
Okra
Pepper *
Radish
Sauerkraut
Squash, summer
Tomatoes *
Watercress *

GROUP B VEGETABLES—PER EXCHANGE: CARBOHYDRATE, 7 GM; PROTEIN, 2 GM; FAT, NEGLIGIBLE. ONE EXCHANGE = ½ CUP = 100 GM.

Beets	Peas, green	Squash, winter *
Carrots *	Pumpkin *	Turnip
Onion	Rutabaga	

* These vegetables have high vitamin A value. At least one serving should be included in the diet each day.

LIST 3—FRUIT EXCHANGES

PER EXCHANGE: CARBOHYDRATE, 10 GM; PROTEIN, AND FAT, NEGLIGIBLE. FRUITS MAY BE USED FRESH, COOKED, CANNED, OR FROZEN, UNSWEETENED.

	Measure
Apple	1 small, 2-in. diameter
Applesauce	½ cup
Apricots, dried	4 halves
Apricots, fresh	2 medium
Banana	½ small
Blackberries	1 cup
Blueberries	⅔ cup
Cantaloupe *	¼, 6-in. diameter
Cherries	10 large
Dates	2
Figs, dried	1 small
Figs, fresh	2 large
Grapefruit *	½ small
Grapefruit juice *	½ cup
Grape juice	¼ cup
Grapes	12
Honeydew melon *	⅛, 7-in. diameter
Mango	½ small
Nectarines	1 medium
Orange *	1 small
Orange juice *	½ cup
Papaya	⅓ medium
Peach	1 medium
Pear	1 small
Pineapple	½ cup cubed
Pineapple juice	⅓ cup
Plums	2 medium
Prunes, dried	2 medium
Raisins	2 tablespoons
Raspberries	1 cup
Strawberries *	1 cup
Tangerine	1 large
Watermelon	1 cup diced

* These fruits are rich sources of ascorbic acid. At least one exchange should be included in the diet each day.

List 4—Bread Exchanges

Per Exchange: carbohydrate, 15 gm; protein, 2 gm; fat, negligible.

	Measure
Bread	1 slice
biscuit, roll (2-in. diameter)	1
muffin	1 medium
cornbread	1½-inch cube
Cereal, cooked	½ cup
Cereal, dry	¾ cup
Crackers, graham	2
oyster	20 (½ cup)
saltines (2-in. square)	5
soda (2½-in. square)	3
round, thin (1½-in. diameter)	6–8
Flour	2½ tablespoons
Grits	½ cup cooked
Ice cream, vanilla (omit two fat exchanges)	⅛ quart
Macaroni	½ cup cooked
Matzoth	½ (6½-in. square)
Noodles	½ cup cooked
Rice	½ cup cooked
Spaghetti	½ cup cooked
Sponge cake, no icing	1½-inch cube
Vegetables	
beans, baked; no pork	¼ cup
beans and peas, dried (includes kidney, Lima, navy beans, black-eyed, split, and cowpeas, etc.)	½ cup cooked
beans, Lima, fresh	½ cup
corn, popped	1 cup
corn, fresh	⅓ cup or ½ small ear
parsnips	⅔ cup
potatoes, white	1 small (2-in. diameter)
potatoes, white, mashed	½ cup
potatoes, sweet or yam	¼ cup

List 5—Meat Exchanges

Per Exchange: carbohydrate, negligible; protein, 7 gm; fat, 5 gm. Measures and weights are for cooked meat.

	Measure
Meat, fish, and poultry (medium fat) (beef, lamb, pork, veal, liver, chicken, turkey, etc.)	1 oz
cold cuts (bologna, liver sausage, luncheon loaf, boiled ham, salami, etc.)	1 slice, ⅛-in. thick

frankfurt	1
cod, haddock, halibut, herring, etc.	1 oz
crab, lobster, salmon, tuna	¼ cup
clams, oysters, shrimp	5 small
sardines	3 medium
Cheese, Cheddar	1 oz
cottage	¼ cup
Egg	1
Peanut butter *	2 tablespoons

* Limit to one exchange daily, or adjust for carbohydrate. Deduct 5 gm carbohydrate for each additional exchange.

List 6—Fat Exchanges

Per Exchange: fat, 5 gm; protein and carbohydrate, negligible.

	Measure
Butter or margarine	1 teaspoon
Bacon, crisp	1 slice
Cream, light, 20 per cent	2 tablespoons
Cream, heavy, 35–40 per cent	1 tablespoon
Cream cheese	1 tablespoon
French dressing	1 tablespoon
Mayonnaise	1 teaspoon
Nuts	6 small
Oil or cooking fat	1 teaspoon
Olives	5 small
Avocado	⅛, 4-in. diameter

Foods Allowed As Desired

Protein, Fat, and Carbohydrate Negligible.

Coffee	Gelatin, unsweetened	Vinegar
Tea	Rennet tablets	Cranberries, unsweetened
Clear broth	Cyclamate, sodium or	Lemon
Bouillon	calcium	Mustard, dry
(fat-free)	Saccharin	Pickle, dill, unsweetened
Herbs	Spices	Rhubarb, unsweetened

TABLE A-3   SUGGESTED WEIGHTS FOR HEIGHTS FOR MEN AND WOMEN *

Height in Inches (without shoes)	Weights for Men (without clothing)			Weights for Women (without clothing)		
	Low	Median	High	Low	Median	High
	Pounds	Pounds	Pounds	Pounds	Pounds	Pounds
60				100	109	118
61				104	112	121
62				107	115	125
63	(118)	(129)	(141)	110	118	128
64	(122)	(133)	(145)	113	122	132
65	126	137	149	116	125	135
66	130	142	155	120	129	139
67	134	147	161	123	132	142
68	139	151	166	126	136	146
69	143	155	170	130	140	151
70	147	159	174	133	144	156
71	150	163	178	(137)	(148)	(161)
72	154	167	183	(141)	(152)	(166)
73	158	171	188			
74	162	175	192			
75	165	178	195			

* Hathaway, M. L., and Foard, E. D., *Heights and Weights of Adults in The United States*. Home Economics Research Report No. 10. Washington, D.C.: U.S. Government Printing Office, Table 80, p. 111, 1960.

Appendix B

A LIST OF REFERENCE MATERIALS

BOOKS

Eppright, E., Pattison, M., and Barbour, H. *Teaching Nutrition*, 2nd ed. Ames, Iowa: Iowa State University Press, 1963.

Gerard, R. W. *Food for Life*. Chicago: University of Chicago Press, 1965.

Hasler, D., and Hasler, N. B. *Personal, Home, and Community Health*. New York: The Macmillan Company, 1967.

Howe, P. S. *Nutrition for Practical Nurses*, 4th ed. Philadelphia: W. B. Saunders Company, 1967.

Krause, M. V. *Nutrition and Diet Therapy*, 4th ed. Philadelphia: W. B. Saunders Company, 1966.

Leverton, R. M. *Food Becomes You*, 3rd ed. Ames, Iowa: Iowa State University Press, 1965.

Lowenberg, M., et al. *Food and Man*. New York: John Wiley & Sons, 1968.

Martin, E. A. *Nutrition in Action*, 2nd ed. New York: Holt, Rinehart and Winston, 1965.

Mason, M. A. *Basic Medical-Surgical Nursing*, 2nd ed. New York: The Macmillan Company, 1967.

Mickelson, O. *Nutrition Science and You*. Englewood Cliffs, N.J.: Scholastic Books, 1964.

Mitchell, H. S., Rynbergen, H. J., Anderson, L., and Dibble, M. V. *Cooper's Nutrition in Health and Disease*, 15th ed. Philadelphia: J. B. Lippincott Company, 1968.

Peyton, A. B. *Practical Nutrition*. Philadelphia: J. B. Lippincott Company, 1962.

Rasmussen, S. *Foundations of Practical and Vocational Nursing*. New York: The Macmillan Company, 1967.

Robinson, C. H. *Proudfit-Robinson's Normal and Therapeutic Nutrition*, 13th ed. New York: The Macmillan Company, 1967.

Shackelton, A. D. *Practical Nurse Nutrition Education*, 2nd ed. Philadelphia: W. B. Saunders Company, 1966.

Stare, F. J. *Eating for Good Health*. Garden City, N.Y.: Doubleday, 1964.

Stefferud, A. (ed.). *Food, the Yearbook of Agriculture 1959*. Washington, D.C.: Government Printing Office, 1959.

White, P. L. *Let's Talk About Food*. Chicago: American Medical Association, 1967.

JOURNALS

American Journal of Nursing
American Journal of Public Health
Geriatrics
Journal of the American Dietetic Association
Journal of the American Medical Association
Nursing Outlook
Nutrition Reviews
Nutrition Today
Today's Health

SOURCES OF NUTRITION EDUCATION MATERIALS

American Can Company. 730 Park Avenue, New York, N.Y. 10017.

American Diabetes Association. 18 East 48th Street, New York, N.Y. 10017.

American Dietetic Association. 620 North Michigan Avenue, Chicago, Ill. 60611.

American Heart Association. 44 East 23rd Street, New York, N.Y. 10010.

American Home Economics Association. 1600 Twentieth Street, N.W., Washington, D.C. 20009.

American Institute of Baking. Consumer Service Department, 400 East Ontario Street, Chicago, Ill. 60611.

American Public Health Association. 1790 Broadway, New York, N.Y. 10019.

American School Food Service Association. P.O. Box 10095, Denver, Colo. 80210.

The Borden Company. 350 Madison Avenue, New York, N.Y. 10017.

Home Economics Department, The Campbell Soup Company. 385 Memorial Avenue, Camden, N.J.

Cereal Institute, Inc., Educational Director. 135 South LaSalle Street, Chicago, Ill. 60603.

Chicago Dietetic Supply House, Inc. 405 E. Shawnut Ave., P.O. Box 529, La Grange, Ill. 60525.

Children's Bureau. Department of Health, Education, and Welfare. Washington, D.C.

Council on Foods and Nutrition. American Medical Association. 535 North Dearborn Street, Chicago, Ill. 60610.

Evaporated Milk Association. 228 North LaSalle Street, Chicago, Ill. 60601.

Food and Drug Administration. Department of Health, Education, and Welfare. Washington, D.C.

Food and Nutrition Board, National Research Council. 2101 Constitution Avenue, Washington, D.C.

General Foods Corporation. 250 North Street, White Plains, N.Y.

Public Relations Department. General Mills, Inc. 9200 Wayzata Boulevard, Minneapolis, Minn. 55426.

Gerber Products. Department of Nutrition. Fremont, Mich.

John Hancock Life Insurance Company. 200 Berkeley Street, Boston, Mass. 02117.

Department of Home Economics Services. Kellogg Company. 215 Porter Street, Battle Creek, Mich.

Metropolitan Life Insurance Company. Health and Welfare Division. One Madison Avenue, New York, N.Y. 10010.

National Dairy Council. 111 North Canal Street, Chicago, Ill. 60606.

National Live Stock and Meat Board, Home Economics Department. 36 South Wabash Avenue, Chicago, Ill. 60603.

The Nutrition Foundation, Inc. 99 Park Avenue, New York, N.Y. 10016.

Poultry and Egg National Board. 250 West 57th Street, New York, N.Y. 10019.

School Lunch Branch, Food Distribution Division, Agricultural Marketing Service, U.S. Department of Agriculture, Washington, D.C. 20250.

Superintendent of Documents, U.S. Government Printing Office, Washington, D.C. 20402.

Office of Information, U.S. Department of Agriculture, Washington, D.C. 20250.

Appendix C

GLOSSARY

FOREWORD TO THE STUDENT

The first step in the study of any subject is gaining an understanding of the vocabulary. Every student should have a standard dictionary and should form the habit of using it whenever he comes across a word he does not know.

This glossary includes words frequently used in medicine and nutrition and that are not, for the most part, defined fully in the text. Many terms directly related to nutrition are defined in the text, and the student should refer to the chapters in which these terms are discussed. Consult the index for page references to such terms.

absorption. In physiology, the uptake of nutrients by the walls of the small intestine for transfer to the circulation.

acetone bodies. Intermediate products in the oxidation of fatty acids; acetone, acetoacetic acid, and beta-hydroxy-butyric acid.

acidosis. Abnormal accumulation of acids in the body, or loss of base.

ACTH (adrenocorticotropic hormone). A hormone produced by the pituitary gland that controls the action of the adrenal cortex; sodium metabolism, for example.

acute. Sudden, severe symptoms of short duration.

adipose. Fatty tissue; body stores of fat.

adrenal. Organ near the kidney that secretes several hormones.

331

amylase (amylopsin). An enzyme in saliva or pancreatic juice that digests starch.

anemia. A decrease in the number of red blood cells or hemoglobin or both.

anorexia. Loss of appetite.

antibiotic. A substance that checks the growth of microorganisms.

antibody. A protein substance produced within the body that destroys bacteria.

antioxidant. A substance that prevents oxidation; often added to foods to prevent rancidity.

ascites. Accumulation of fluid in the abdominal cavity.

avitaminosis. Deficiency or lack of vitamins in the diet, or failure to absorb them; specific symptoms result from each vitamin deficiency.

bile. Secretion of the liver that aids in fat digestion and absorption.

blanch. To preheat in boiling water or steam; used to inactivate enzymes before freezing food, or to remove the skins of fruits.

bland. Mild in flavor.

braise. To cook food in a tightly covered pan with a small amount of liquid.

buffer. A substance that lessens the change in pH that otherwise would occur with the addition of acids or alkalies.

calcification. Hardening of tissue by deposits of calcium salts; bone, for example.

caliper. An instrument for measuring the thickness of an object; used in medicine to measure thickness of fat layers.

calorimeter. An instrument for measuring heat change. A bomb calorimeter measures calories in food; a respiration calorimeter measures oxygen and carbon dioxide exchange of an individual.

candling. Holding an egg against a controlled source of light in order to view the interior quality of the egg.

carboxylase. An enzyme necessary for the metabolism of glucose; thiamine is a component.

catalyst. A substance that speeds up a chemical reaction.

cecum. The large blind pouch in which the large intestine begins.

cellular. Pertaining to the function of cells that make up the tissues.

chlorophyll. The green coloring matter in plants that is responsible for the process of photosynthesis.

cholecystokinin. A hormone secreted in the wall of the duodenum when fat is present; causes contraction of the gallbladder and flow of bile.

chronic. Of long duration; opposed to acute.

chyme. The liquid food mass that has been digested in the stomach and is ready for passage through the duodenum.

coagulation. Change from a fluid to a semisolid or solid state; curd; clot.

coenzyme. A substance such as a vitamin that is a part of an enzyme.

colitis. Inflammation of the colon.

colon. The large intestine, beginning at the cecum.

coma. Unconsciousness; may result from accumulation of acids as in diabetes mellitus.

congenital. Present at birth.

consistency. Refers to the texture of a diet; liquid, soft, low-fiber, etc.

convulsion. Involuntary contraction of the muscles; may occur in eclampsia, uremic poisoning, and many other conditions.

cortisone. A hormone of the adrenal gland.

cretin. An individual who has inadequate physical and mental development because of insufficient thyroid secretion.

cultural. In study of food habits, refers to social, religious, national habits of a group of people.

decompensation, heart. Failure of the heart to adequately pump blood through the circulation.

dehydration. Abnormal loss of water from the body. Also, removal of water from food.

delirium. Mental disturbance characterized by physical restlessness, excitement, confusion, and delusions.

denaturation. The change of the physical state of a substance; for example, the coagulation of a protein.

dentine. The major calcified portion of the tooth; covered by enamel over the crown, and by cementum on the root portion of the tooth.

dermatitis. Inflammation of the skin.

dextrose. A single sugar; also called glucose.

dietetic food. A food prepared for specific uses in modified diets; for example, low-sodium, or packed without sugar.

distention. The state of stretching or enlarging; often refers to the accumulation of gases in the intestinal tract and the resultant feeling of fullness.

diuretic. Any substance that increases the volume of urine.

duodenum. The first part of the small intestine beginning at the pylorus.

dysentery. An inflammation of the colon; often caused by bacterial or parasitic infection.

edema. Accumulation of fluid in the body.

embryo. Early stage of development of the fetus.

emulsification. The breaking up of large particles into much smaller particles and suspending them in another liquid; for example, bile breaks up fat into minute droplets for digestion.

endemic. Refers to a disease being prevalent in a particular area.

endocrine. Any of the ductless glands such as the thyroid, adrenal, pituitary that secrete hormones into the blood circulation.

endosperm. The starchy portion of the cereal grain.

enzyme. A substance formed by living cells that speeds up chemical reactions; a living catalyst.

epithelium. Outer layer of the skin; includes the linings of the hollow organs, the respiratory, gastrointestinal, and genitourinary tracts.

erepsin. A group of protein-splitting enzymes secreted by the small intestine.

esophageal varices. Varicose veins of the esophagus.

extracellular. Around the cells.

extractive, meat. Nonprotein, nitrogen-containing, water-soluble substances in meat.

fallout. The radioactive dust that settles following explosion of a nuclear bomb.

feces. Excretion from the bowels.

fetus. Unborn young, especially in the later stages of development.

fibrinogen. A protein in blood necessary for clotting.

fortify. To add nutrients to food so that it contains more than was originally present; fortified margarine and milk, for example.

gastrectomy. Operation for removal of part or all of the stomach.

gastritis. Inflammation of the stomach.

genitourinary. Pertaining to the organs of reproduction and the urinary tract.

geriatrics. Branch of medicine concerned with diseases of older people.

glycerol. The organic compound to which fatty acids are attached to form a fat.

gristle. The tough connective-tissue fibers of meat.

hemicellulose. A complex, indigestible carbohydrate found in cell walls of plants.

hemoglobin. Red pigment in blood cells that carries oxygen.

hemorrhage. Loss of blood.

hepatic. Refers to the liver.

herbs. Group of plants having odors and flavors useful in the seasoning of foods; for example, sage, marjoram, thyme, and many others.

homogenized. Broken up into minute particles to maintain uniform texture or quality; for example, cream does not rise in homogenized milk.

hormone. Chemical substance produced by a gland of the body and transported by the blood for activity in other tissues; thyroxine, insulin, and others.

hydrolysis. The splitting of a substance into simpler compounds by the addition of water.

hyper-. A prefix meaning increased, or greater than normal.

hyperglycemia. Increased level of glucose in the blood.

hypertension. High blood pressure.

hypervitaminosis. Excess of vitamin storage in the body; for example, an overdosage of vitamin A or D.

hypo-. A prefix meaning below normal.

hypochromic. Less color than normal; for example, hypochromic anemia.

hypothyroidism. Inadequate secretion of thyroid gland.

ileum. Lower part of the small intestine.

insulin. Hormone secreted by the islands of Langerhans in the pancreas; changes blood glucose to glycogen, increases uptake of glucose by the cell, and facilitates the formation of fat.

intracellular. Within the cell.

intravenous. Within the veins.

irradiation.   Exposure to rays such as ultraviolet rays, x-rays.

jejunum.   Middle part of the small intestine, beginning at the duodenum and extending to the ileum.

ketosis.   Condition resulting from the accumulation of ketones (acetone bodies) as a result of incomplete oxidation of fatty acids.

labile.   Easily destroyed.
lacteal.   A small lymphatic vessel that takes up fatty substances from the intestinal wall.
lactase.   Enzyme produced by the small intestine; splits lactose to glucose and galactose.
legumes.   Class of plant foods including beans, lentils, peas, peanuts.
lignin.   Indigestible carbohydrate found in the cell wall of plants.
lipase.   Enzyme produced by the pancreas that digests fats.

macrocyte.   Giant red blood cell.
malabsorption.   Failure to absorb the various nutrients from the intestinal tract; occurs in celiac disease, sprue, dysentery, diarrhea.
maltase.   Enzyme that splits maltose to two molecules of glucose.
marbled.   Referring to meat, fine streaks of fat appearing throughout the lean portion of meat.
marinate.   To soak meat, fish, or salad ingredients in a seasoned mixture such as wine, vinegar, French dressing.
median.   The middle point; half of the values in a series of measurements will be above and half below this point.
micro-.   Prefix meaning small; for example, *microcyte* is a very small cell; *microorganisms* include bacteria, yeasts, molds.
myo-.   Refers to muscle; *myocardium* is the heart muscle; *myoglobin* is the iron-containing pigment in muscle.

nausea.   Sick at the stomach with tendency to vomit.
nephritis.   Inflammation of the kidney.
nyctalopia.   Night blindness.

osmosis.   Passage of fluid through membranes from weaker to stronger solution.
ossification.   Hardening of the bone.
oxidase.   A class of enzymes that brings about oxidation of products in metabolism.
oxidation.   Combination of a substance with oxygen; an increase in the positive valence of an atom through the loss of electrons.

parathyroid.   Gland located near the thyroid that secretes hormone for control of calcium metabolism.
parenteral.   Outside the gastrointestinal tract; for example, injection into vein, under the skin.

pasta. Spaghetti, macaroni, noodles, and the like made from durum wheat flour.

pathogenic. Disease-producing.

pectin. A complex, indigestible carbohydrate that has the capacity to hold water; found in many fruits such as apples.

pepsin. Enzyme secreted by the stomach for digestion of proteins.

peptidases. Class of enzymes that split peptides to amino acids.

peptones. Intermediate products in protein digestion.

peristalsis. Waves of contraction of muscle fibers in the intestinal tract that cause food to move through the tract.

photosynthesis. The process by which plants synthesize carbohydrates from carbon dioxide and water in the presence of light.

placenta. Organ attached to the wall of the uterus through which the fetus receives nourishment.

plasma. Fluid portion of the blood.

poly-. Prefix meaning much or many.

polydipsia. Excessive thirst.

polyneuritis. Inflammation of the nerves as in thiamine deficiency.

polypeptide. Groups of amino acids; intermediate stage in protein digestion.

polyphagia. Excessive appetite.

polyuria. Excessive amount of urine.

protease. Group of enzymes that digest proteins.

ptyalin. Starch-splitting enzyme in the saliva; also known as amylase.

purée. The pulp obtained by pressing food through a sieve to remove the fiber.

purines. Nitrogen-containing substances of a nonprotein nature occurring especially in meats; metabolized to uric acid.

pylorus. Circular opening of the stomach into the duodenum.

rancid. Having a disagreeable flavor or odor; usually affects foods high in fat content.

rectum. The lower part of the large intestine extending to the anal canal.

regimen. Dietary program.

rehabilitation. Restoration of health and efficiency as much as possible by physical, dietary, or other therapy.

renal. Referring to the kidney.

rennin. Enzyme secreted by the stomach that brings about coagulation of milk.

retina. The layer of the eye that receives the image and is connected to the brain by the optic nerve.

sauté. To cook in a small amount of fat.

secretin. Hormone produced by the duodenum; stimulates pancreatic activity.

sedentary. Occupied in quiet activities; sitting, for example.

serum. Clear liquid that separates from clotted blood.

simmer. To cook in liquid just below the boiling point.

sphincter. A muscle surrounding and closing an opening; for example, pyloric sphincter.

spore. Reproductive part of a microrganism; very resistant to heat.

stabilizer. A substance added to food to help maintain quality over a period of time.

steapsin. Enzyme in the small intestine that digests fat; also called lipase.

steatorrhea. Excessive amount of fat in the feces.

subcutaneous. Beneath the skin.

sucrase. Enzyme produced by the small intestine that splits sucrose to glucose and fructose.

supplementary. Additional.

syndrome. A number of symptoms occurring together that are typical of a certain disease; for example, malabsorption syndrome.

synthesis. Formation of complex substances from simpler substances.

tenderizer. An enzyme preparation that partially breaks down meat fibers, thereby making the meat more tender.

toxemia. Condition in which the blood contains poisonous substances; for example, excess of nitrogenous wastes.

toxin. Poisonous product produced by cells; for example, botulin.

trypsin. Protein-splitting enzyme produced by the pancreas.

ultraviolet rays. Light rays of shorter wave length than visible rays.

urea. The chief nitrogenous waste product in the urine.

uric acid. Nitrogenous product resulting from the breakdown of purines.

uterus. The womb.

vascular. Refers to the blood and lymph vessels in the body.

villus. Tiny fingerlike projection on the mucous lining of the small intestine; supplied with blood and lymph vessels.

viosterol. Activated ergosterol; vitamin D.

visual purple. Organic compound in retina of the eye that is changed to yellow by light; vitamin A is required for its synthesis.

INDEX

Illustrations are indicated by numbers in boldface type.